OBESITY INTERVENTIONS IN UNDERSERVED COMMUNITIES

OBESITY Interventions in UNDERSERVED Communities

Evidence and Directions

EDITED BY
VIRGINIA M. BRENNAN
Journal of Health Care for the Poor and Underserved
Meharry Medical College
Nashville, Tennessee

SHIRIKI K. KUMANYIKA
Department of Biostatistics and Epidemiology and
Department of Pediatrics
University of Pennsylvania, Perelman School of Medicine
Philadelphia, Pennsylvania

RUTH ENID ZAMBRANA
Department of Women's Studies and Consortium
on Race, Gender, and Ethnicity
University of Maryland, College Park
College Park, Maryland

JOHNS HOPKINS UNIVERSITY PRESS
BALTIMORE

© 2014 Johns Hopkins University Press
All rights reserved. Published 2014
Printed in the United States of America on acid-free paper
9 8 7 6 5 4 3 2 1

Johns Hopkins University Press
2715 North Charles Street
Baltimore, Maryland 21218-4363
www.press.jhu.edu

Library of Congress Cataloging-in-Publication Data

Obesity interventions in underserved communities : evidence and directions /
edited by Virginia M. Brennan, Shiriki K. Kumanyika, and Ruth Enid Zambrana.
     p. ; cm.
   Includes bibliographical references and index.
   ISBN 978-1-4214-1544-4 (hardcover : alk. paper) — ISBN 1-4214-1544-5
(hardcover : alk. paper) — ISBN 978-1-4214-1545-1 (pbk. : alk. paper) —
ISBN 1-4214-1545-3 (pbk. : alk. paper) — ISBN 978-1-4214-1546-8 (electronic) —
ISBN 1-4214-1546-1 (electronic)
   I. Brennan, Virginia M., editor.   II. Kumanyika, Shiriki Kinika, 1945–, editor.
III. Zambrana, Ruth E., editor.
   [DNLM: 1. Obesity—prevention & control—United States.   2. Health
Promotion—methods—United States.   3. Minority Groups—United States.
4. Vulnerable Populations—United States. WD 210]
   RA645.O23
   362.1963'98—dc23   2014008683

A catalog record for this book is available from the British Library.

*Special discounts are available for bulk purchases of this book. For more information,
please contact Special Sales at 410-516-6936 or specialsales@press.jhu.edu.*

Johns Hopkins University Press uses environmentally friendly book materials,
including recycled text paper that is composed of at least 30 percent
post-consumer waste, whenever possible.

CONTENTS

FOREWORD

Gillian Regina Barclay, DDS, MPH, DrPH, Vice President, Aetna Foundation

Howell Wechsler, EdD, MPH, Chief Executive Officer, Alliance for a Healthier Generation

This book highlights the contributions that research can make to the national and local movements to address the burden of obesity and overweight for underserved and vulnerable communities in the United States. It features literature reviews and commentaries from leading national experts, along with 21 brief reports on innovative interventions from the field. The authors translate complex information and present it in a simplified and user-friendly format with a major emphasis on identifying lessons learned that can guide future work in this area. The focus of the work presented in this book is where it needs to be: on people and where they live, eat, learn, play, and socialize. At the same time, however, the authors do not lose sight of the historical legacy of inequity that has shaped the less-than-favorable conditions of local environments that constrain the choices available to underserved communities. It is now clearly understood that obesity is not simply a consequence of individual lifestyle choices, but rather a symptom of formidable underlying root causes that are historical, economic, social, and cultural in nature.

The research findings, intervention descriptions, and commentaries in this book address an exceptionally wide range of intervention settings, populations served, and geographical regions covered. The book describes interventions that have been developed and implemented in settings such as schools, faith-based communities, health care institutions, correctional facilities, and the military, and with diverse actors and stakeholders differentiated by race/ethnicity, culture, and intellectual and developmental disabilities. The work highlighted has been done in diverse geographic locations such as rural communities in Appalachia and Idaho, urban communities in Los Angeles and Milwaukee, and American Indian, Native Hawaiian, and Pacific Islander communities.

The editors of this book have carefully chosen examples that highlight how adverse health and social outcomes may be mitigated by intervention strategies that are catalytic, cross-sectoral, and collaborative, with a strong focus on policy change and community involvement. These examples show how engaging people and communities may lead to societal benefit through opportunities for healthier school meals, safe neighborhoods, community nutrition education at mobile markets, local food systems that provide fresh, affordable, and accessible food, and health promotion through faith-based organizations.

The work highlighted in this book demonstrates the emergence of a social movement focused on reducing historically intractable racial and ethnic disparities in health outcomes such as obesity. By pulling together in one volume the most up-to-date scientific information on efforts to address obesity in underserved and vulnerable communities, this book can play a critical role in guiding future advances of this social movement. Let us indeed hope that the insights gleaned from this book will contribute to the needed social change and, thereby, increase the likelihood that future generations will be healthier generations.

OBESITY INTERVENTIONS IN UNDERSERVED COMMUNITIES

Advancing a New Conversation about Obesity in the Underserved

Virginia Brennan, PhD, MA, Shiriki K. Kumanyika, PhD, MPH, and Ruth Enid Zambrana, PhD

The obesity epidemic in the United States has a disproportionate impact on children and adults in populations that are affected by social and economic disadvantages and are underserved from the perspective of health equity.[1–7] Although most people affected by obesity in the United States are non-Hispanic Whites and have incomes above the poverty line, data from national surveys clearly indicate that in one or both of the sexes, obesity prevalence is higher among Hispanics/Latinos,* Blacks / African Americans, American Indians, Native Hawaiians, Pacific Islanders, and populations with low socioeconomic status (SES) than among their White or higher-SES counterparts.[2,8–10] Asian Americans are the exception in that obesity rates are significantly lower than those for non-Hispanic Whites and other minority populations. However, standard definitions of obesity may underestimate obesity-related health risks in populations of Asian descent.[11] Relationships between obesity and SES are complex, change over time, and differ for different populations and by gender.[7,12,13] Furthermore, although low SES is more common among racial/ethnic minority populations, low SES does not account for the excess obesity-related risks in these populations. Other high-risk, underserved populations with respect to obesity include those living in rural compared with urban or suburban areas.[14] In addition, physical and mental disabilities may confer excess obesity-related risks.[2,7]

The chapters in this book provide perspectives on obesity in these high-risk and underserved populations. The coverage is not encyclopedic but rather is intended to explore the many facets of these disparities and their potential solutions in ways that

---

* For the purpose of this book, and consistent with federal standards for racial and ethnic data, the terms *Hispanic* and *Latino* are used interchangeably or jointly. These words differ in important ways when examined closely but are used in free variation in contemporary American English. (For more on this subject, see Zambrana RE. Latinos in American society: families and communities in transition. Ithaca, NY: Cornell University Press, 2011.) See also the discussion of related issues in chapter 4 of this book.

will generate interest in and stimulate thinking about new directions in efforts to eliminate such disparities.

A striking lack of data hinders efforts to lower obesity prevalence in high-risk populations and eliminate disparities. For some high-risk populations, the data necessary to characterize the problem and monitor trends in the impact of interventions are lacking, even when such interventions exist.[15,16] The bigger problem, though, is a lack of evidence about interventions with demonstrated effectiveness within physical, economic, social, and cultural contexts that are relevant to socially disadvantaged and underserved populations. Although much remains to be learned, there is guidance about several types of interventions that, alone or in combination, will be critical for success in combating the obesity epidemic in the U.S. population as a whole.[2,15,17–20] How to address disparities in obesity is another and far more challenging question. It is more challenging because doing so will require implementing targeted interventions that will work *better* than average in populations and settings where the difficulty of effecting change of any sort is *greater*. The difficulty is greater due to a combination of variables in the relevant sociocultural, economic, and physical contexts that may work against achieving the desired intervention effects—including many of the same structural factors that predispose to higher obesity prevalence in the first place and, more generally, to poorer health in racial/ethnic minority and low-SES populations.[21–23]

An evident need for new ways to talk about and think about obesity interventions for underserved, high-risk communities motivated this book. While people concerned with public health have been talking about obesity for some time and are aware of the sociodemographic disparities, actual solutions have been slow to emerge. Some recent data suggest a modicum of success in stabilizing or even reversing the trajectory of increasing obesity.[24,25] Rates remain high, however, especially in socially disadvantaged populations. Furthermore, some data show that while overall trends may be improving, sociodemographic disparities have persisted or even increased.[24,26–28]

To elicit new perspectives, we extended a broad invitation to researchers and professionals around the United States to offer reviews and commentaries that could shed light on the status of current research, identify research gaps related to obesity in high-risk and underserved populations, and identify novel ways of looking at relevant conceptual or methodological issues. In addition, we invited reports from the field to highlight promising intervention approaches that have not yet reached the evidence base but provide potentially useful lessons for others seeking to address obesity and overweight in their own communities. The remainder of this introduction provides background and context for the central themes covered in the book.

An Overview of Obesity in High-Risk and Underserved Populations

Some facts are cited repeatedly throughout this volume because they have motivated a wealth of research and because they cry out for interventions. In the opening paragraphs of this introduction we pointed to the broadest generalizations about inequities among populations in the United States in the distribution of obesity and overweight. Here we provide a brief history of the problem and establish its importance in terms of disease burden and variability over the life course.

International and U.S. health agencies define obesity and overweight in terms of body mass index (BMI),[29,30] a weight-to-height ratio.* Weight and height are relatively easy to measure. Body mass index can be used to set public health targets for population weight levels, for first-level clinical screening, and for tracking change over time. Uncertainty and criticism are sometimes voiced regarding the value of BMI because it is not a "perfect" measure of obesity-related health risk. Whereas obesity refers to excess body fat, BMI does not reflect differences in body composition associated with fat versus muscle. Body mass index is defined in the same way for adults of both sexes and, using a different but standard approach, for male and female children and adolescents. This facilitates comparisons by sex and across race/ethnicity, although it does not work equally well for all racial and ethnic groups or for all individuals as a predictor of weight-related health problems. A given BMI level or category might overestimate or underestimate health risks for a given population group or individual. Additionally, a BMI in the normal weight range does not always reflect healthy eating or physical activity lifestyles in all respects. In general, however, BMI and body fat are highly correlated, and high BMI values are associated with increased risks of obesity-related diseases.[30†]

In the summer of 2013, the American Medical Association began classifying obesity as a disease, noting that it contributes to 112,000 preventable deaths and costs in the neighborhood of $150 billion in the United States per year,[31,32] Higher body weights are associated with a higher incidence of type 2 diabetes,[33–36] cardiovascular disease,[33,36] non-alcoholic fatty liver disease,[33] gallbladder disease,[33] osteoarthritis,[33] certain cancers,[37,38] asthma,[39–44] and increased risk of disability.[33,45,46] Additionally, higher body weights are associated with stigmatization[47–49] and mental illness and their sequelae,[50–52] among other conditions. These disease consequences are seen in the high-risk and underserved populations that are the focus of this book. For example,

---

* Body mass index (BMI) is a weight-to-height ratio: divide a person's weight in kilograms by the square of his or her height in meters. Direct interpretation of BMI using inches and pounds requires dividing weight in pounds by the square of height in inches and then multiplying by 703 to convert the result to the metric scale. BMIs of $> 25\,kg/m^2$ and $> 30\,kg/m^2$ are the standard cutoffs used as public health or clinical action levels for defining adult overweight and obesity, respectively.[29] Some additional or alternative cutoffs vary by country or by population within a country, as is the case for some Asians.[11] For children and adolescents (whose weight, height, and body fatness change during development), BMI is interpreted relative to growth curves that are age- and sex-specific, with > 85th and > 95th percentiles of the reference distributions used to designate overweight and obesity, respectively. Different reference distributions exist. Generally, in the United States, the CDC growth charts are used. The cut points on the growth charts have stayed the same over time. The terminology, however, has changed. See http://cdc.gov/nchs/data/nhsr /nhsr025.pdf. Furthermore, the World Health Organization and U.S. growth curves used for this purpose differ.[24] BMI levels used to characterize obesity and the terminology to describe them in the United States have varied over time. Trend data are adjusted to recalculate older data to the current standard.

† Because an excess of body fat in the abdominal area is related to health risk somewhat independently of body weight, waist measurements are sometimes used in addition to BMI to identify health risks.

the prevalence of type 2 diabetes and associated years of life lost for Blacks and Latinos are disproportionately high relative to those for non-Hispanic Whites.[31,34,35,53] The prevalence of type 2 diabetes is higher at lower levels of income and educational attainment.[54] The Diabetes Prevention Program clearly demonstrated that modest weight loss can prevent the onset of type 2 diabetes in high-risk adults, including in Blacks, Hispanics, and American Indians,[55] under the ideal conditions of a tightly controlled research study. What remains is the challenge of identifying interventions that can facilitate the achievement and maintenance of the needed level of weight loss among high-risk populations in communities at large.

The epidemic of obesity has emerged as a global phenomenon affecting millions of children and adults around the world, in both low- and middle-income countries and high-income countries.[30,56] Explanations for the genesis of this epidemic center around technological and lifestyle changes that have led to a chronic pattern of caloric intake in excess of caloric output, resulting in excess weight gain in substantial proportions of most populations.[57,58] Changes in food systems have increased the availability and marketing of high-calorie foods. Mechanization and changes in physical environments have decreased levels of routine physical activity, and the availability and popularity of sedentary leisure-time activity have also increased.[15] Within nations, populations most affected by obesity vary according to regional, social, and economic contexts and over time.[2,56,59] Findings that socially disadvantaged populations in high-income countries are at a disproportionately high risk of obesity are not confined to the United States.[60]

Widespread interest in the problem of population-wide overweight and obesity was sparked in 2001 with the publication of a report on this topic by Surgeon General David Satcher.[61] The upward trends in obesity were first observed between the National Health and Nutrition Examination Survey (NHANES) results for the 1976–80 period[62,63] and NHANES III phase I (1988–1991).[62] They were subsequently confirmed in the next round of NHANES data, for 1988–1994.[64] The increase continued between then and 1999–2000. The Centers for Disease Control and Prevention (CDC) maps of self-reported obesity prevalence by state dramatized the picture of increasing rates.[65,66] Among U.S. adults in the early 1960s, fewer than half were overweight or obese, but by the early 2000s the proportion approached 70%.[67] By 2010, over 35% of U.S. adults were obese (compared with less than 15% in the early 1960s).[68] Five percent or less of children (ages 6–11 years) and adolescents (ages 12–19 years) were obese in the mid-1960s (by definition, given the growth charts), but close to 20% were overweight by the early 2000s,[67] and 32% by 2010, when nearly 17% of children and adolescents (ages 2–19) in the United States were obese (using the same growth charts).[69]

Figure I.1 shows prevalence and trends of overweight and obesity in U.S. adults overall from the late 1980s through 2010. Health risks associated with excess body weight are graded across the continuum from overweight through severe obesity; categories of severity are defined as indicated in the figure legend. As the figure shows, overweight or obesity affected more than 70% of men and more than 60% of women in the latter period. The percentage of overweight but not obese has remained steady,

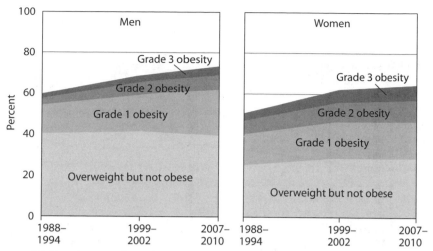

FIGURE I.1. Prevalence and trends in overweight and obesity in adults, United States, 1980s through 2010. Overweight but not obese is defined as a body mass index (BMI) ≥ 25 but < 30; grade 1 obesity, BMI ≥ 30 but < 35; grade 2 obesity, BMI ≥ 35 but < 40; grade 3 obesity, BMI ≥ 40. Source: Centers for Disease Control and Prevention/National Center for Health Statistics, Health, United States, 2012, fig. 11; data from the National Health and Nutrition Examination Survey.

while the percentage of obesity has increased. What this reflects is that, over time, people who would have been in the "healthy weight range" are shifting into the overweight category at a rate equivalent to the percentage who progress from the overweight category into the obese range. Figure I.2 shows U.S. population trends in child and adolescent obesity. Obesity prevalence in childhood and adolescence is lower than during adulthood, but it tracks into adulthood and has social and health consequences both during childhood and throughout the life course. Prevalence has approximately doubled over the past two decades.* Only in the very recent past has there been any sign of the upward trend even leveling off in national data and some localities.[24]

---

* Figures I.1 and I.2 are based on the most accurate and reliable sources of official data on overweight and obesity prevalence in the U.S. population, which come from the National Health and Nutrition Examination Survey (NHANES) conducted by the National Center for Health Statistics, a part of the CDC.[14,36] This survey obtains rigorous height and weight measurements from a probability sample of the U.S. population but provides only estimates for some racial/ethnic groups, and only at the national level. Two other national surveys, the National Health Interview Survey (NHIS) and the Behavioral Risk Factor Surveillance System, provide representative data at the national/regional and state levels, respectively, but are based on self-reported rather than measured weights and heights. Self-reported data underestimate obesity prevalence when compared with measured data for the same population. With this caveat, comparisons based on self-reported data within the same survey are informative. The NHIS provides aggregate estimates for American Indian populations and Asian Americans in addition to other racial/ethnic minority subgroups. Data for these populations have generally not been reported from NHANES due to insufficient sample sizes. It should be noted that in 2011–2012 NHANES started over-sampling non-Hispanic Asians.

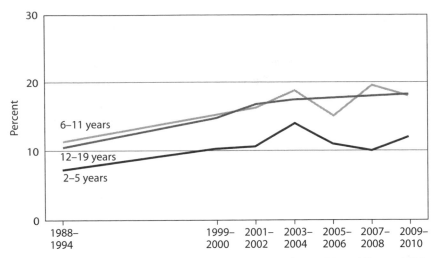

FIGURE I.2. Prevalence and trends in child and adolescent obesity, United States, 1980s through 2010. Obesity is body mass index (BMI) at or above the sex- and age-specific 95th percentile BMI cutoff points in the 2000 CDC Growth Charts. Source: Centers for Disease Control and Prevention/National Center for Health Statistics, Health, United States, 2012, fig. 10; data from the National Health and Nutrition Examination Survey.

As explained throughout this book and documented in various data sources that allow examination of obesity-related issues in high-risk and underserved populations,* these overall U.S. national data mask major variations among population subgroups. Racial, ethnic, and gender differences were noted from the start of the era of increasing body size[64] and have persisted into recent years.[24,68,69] This is compounded by the fact that, in some cases, higher levels of obesity among adults and children in racial/ethnic minority populations were observed preceding the epidemic[70,71]—that is, the baseline for the increased trajectories that followed was already higher. Amidst the early signs of success in addressing the epidemic, obesity prevalence remains high, particularly in high-risk and underserved populations, and the gaps between these populations and non-Hispanic Whites may not be closing.[15] Furthermore, within racial, ethnic, and gender groups, there are disparities among socioeconomic subgroups—in general (but not always) in the direction of greater overweight and obesity among lower-SES subgroups of any given constellation of race, ethnicity, and gender.

---

* Chapters in this book cite obesity data from a variety of sources to characterize specific populations or associations of interest. Not all data sources include or report data for the underserved populations that may be of interest, and those that do may not provide a breakdown that shows differences within groups according to gender or SES. Many surveys rely on self-reported rather than measured weight and height for calculation of BMI, but there are other representative surveys that have weight and height measurements. We encourage readers to be mindful of such variability in data sources.

Taking a Life-Course Perspective

Obesity may have its onset and be addressed through interventions at any point along the life course. In this book, we see this reflected in the many chapters that focus on particular age groups. The evidence of population-wide increases in obesity in childhood and adolescence has motivated a strong focus on interventions in childhood and adolescence and has had a particularly important role in compelling public health actions to address the obesity epidemic.[15,72,73] Besides the fact that weight patterns established early in life tend to persist, the striking trajectory of increased obesity prevalence in children fostered the acceptance that structural factors in children's environments (rather than genetic factors, for example) were involved in the causal pathways; thus, relying solely on individually oriented approaches would not solve the problem. This is also true for obesity in adults, but given that children do not control their environments and most people recognize a societal responsibility to protect children, the need for environmental changes is easier to recognize and accept. Advantages of intervening in childhood include the potential to establish parental and child behaviors conducive to healthy weight-related aspects of physical and mental development early on, thus avoiding social and health consequences of obesity during childhood and lowering the risk of adult obesity and its consequences.[72]

A focus on childhood obesity is not enough, however. Gradually, it has become clear that achieving healthy diets, exercise habits, and weight across the population will require taking into account the whole life course, from gestation through adulthood.[74–76] For women, the reproductive years are especially critical because of the heightened risk of maternal diabetes during and after pregnancy and the effects of maternal diabetes on obesity risk in the offspring.[77] The population health burden of obesity is greatest during middle age and older adulthood, when the full picture of chronic diseases emerges. Intervention during adulthood can therefore have immediate returns in terms of cost savings and prevention of disease progression.[78] Intervention with parents can improve their own weight control profiles as well as have an indirect benefit for their children through effects on home food availability, child feeding practices, and role modeling and support for healthy eating and physical activity behaviors.

Interventions for Obesity Prevention and Treatment

Typical approaches to obesity treatment and prevention have been designed to change individual behaviors, but an increasing number of initiatives around the country seek to address structural factors.[15,17,18,30,72,78–92] Structural factors associated with minority status or low SES are in the pathway that leads to obesity disparities and need to be understood when designing interventions. Consistent with this, some chapters in this volume address the working and living environments of people in underserved U.S. communities, as they affect and are affected by the epidemic of overweight and obesity. Underserved populations can disproportionately suffer from problems of overweight and obesity in numerous realms, including loss of wages, safety, and employability; increased medical costs and the increased danger of a lack of care once an individual develops the disease sequelae enumerated above (due to the impeded access to care systematically experienced by underserved populations). Structural factors may limit access to healthy food or opportunities to be physically active or may limit the ability to benefit from interventions for other reasons.[60,93–96] Instances where recent rates of obesity have risen at a faster rate in racial/ethnic minority than White populations, such as in Black and Latino children,[97] suggest a greater impact on children in these populations of the societal changes driving the epidemic. Whether or not explicitly considered, these structural issues are implicit considerations in any discussion of ways to address obesity-related disparities.

Structural and individual factors interact. Thus, the need to give more attention to structural factors does not obviate the need to determine what types of interventions will work to change individual behaviors. In fact, studies on this issue should take place in a range of contexts. Ethnic and other factors specific to particular populations must enter into the design of such interventions. The hope is that the effectiveness of behavioral interventions will improve as the contexts in which they are implemented are made more favorable from a structural perspective. The reports from the field in this volume bring fresh ideas to bear on the question of how best to intervene for healthy weight promotion in particular communities and local contexts.

Evidence

This book includes 31 chapters written by a diverse set of authors. The chapters are organized by type of contribution. Part I consists of 6 literature reviews (systematic or narrative, depending on the literature available) that provide detailed overviews on specific populations in need; part II includes 4 commentaries; and part III consists of 21 reports from the field.

The content of these chapters addresses the why, what, and how of interventions across the spectrum of underserved populations, both adult and child/adolescent. They relate to both prevention and treatment and to individually and community-oriented interventions in settings as diverse as early childhood care centers, adult workplaces, and mobile markets. Some address structural variables and some employ community-based participatory research methods. Several relate to Latino populations, Black populations, or both, and some to American Indian and Native Hawaiian communities and rural communities. The reviews and commentaries provoke thinking about conceptual, methodological, and policy issues. Perhaps most novel for a book about obesity, there are also chapters that consider how obesity affects and can be addressed in populations that fall outside the safety net, such as people who are homeless, who have mental or physical disabilities, or who are incarcerated. A chapter on the history of the U.S. military experience with weight control provides insights on approaches within this and other highly controlled settings, as well as implications post-discharge. Taken together, the contents of this book should help to crystallize the importance of taking a full view of the context (both historical and current) when considering such issues as obesity in ethnic minority, low-SES, and other underserved populations. It should also serve to refute the spoken or implicit assumptions sometimes made about why disparities exist and whether they *can* be eliminated. We are on the optimistic side: we think they can.

New Directions

What is at the root of the obesity epidemic and what can be done about it? The pathways at the population level are well worked out, both in the United States and globally, as many of the influences are global.[58,98–100] Big-picture forces involved in shaping population energy balance play critical roles.[2,58,98–102] Importantly for the motivation of this volume, many of the pathways or environments involve structural factors that may be a lot less favorable in underserved communities and thus the anchors for patterns of high risk.

How to intervene structurally,* and at what level,† are questions that provoke complex debates, especially in the areas of economics, public policy, and law, and are the subject of ongoing natural experiments.[2,58,98–117] However, the focus here is on people directly affected by the obesity epidemic, rather than on how to remedy these macro-level forces. The reason for this focus is pragmatic: clinicians, community advocates, and policymakers who work directly with and on behalf of underserved populations that suffer conditions associated with obesity and overweight must continue efforts to improve outcomes while larger, systems-level debates are being resolved. Our hope is that the knowledge imparted by the literature reviews, the insights offered in the commentaries, and the practical experiences recounted in the reports from the field provide insights and tools that can help improve outcomes in the interim. In no way does this diminish the importance of on-going and possible interventions across broader swaths of society by means of environmental and policy interventions. Indeed, in a wiser day and age we may be able to tame or effectively work around the factors that have given rise to and perpetuate the obesity epidemic. Until then, though, underserved populations need immediate help in reducing the prevalence of obesity and related diseases and achieving healthy weights. We hope this book provides that help.

---

* For example, one might intervene to fight overweight and obesity by improving access to affordable and healthy food, by decreasing access to unhealthy food, by promoting physical activity and making it feasible for all, by levying taxes, by subsidizing healthy choices, by positive social marketing, by regulating the marketing of food to children and others, by changing policies in entitlement programs, by legislation or statute, or by litigation.[2,98–117]

† For example, any or all of the following might constitute the social juncture at which one would direct interventions designed to fight overweight and obesity: individuals, neighborhoods, cultural groups, municipalities, larger political entities, or regions.[2,98–117]

Acknowledgments

The editors gratefully acknowledge the generous support of the Aetna Foundation, which underwrote the creation of this volume. They are especially grateful to Dr. Gillian Barclay and Ms. Sharon Ions at the Foundation for their steadfast support.

The staff required to coordinate and edit the volume, and the costs of production, were supplied by the Foundation in the form of a grant to create a volume that would advance the fight against obesity and overweight in underserved communities in the United States. No authors or editors received funds from the Foundation in the form of salary or stipends.

References

1. Wang Y, Beydoun MA. The obesity epidemic in the United States—gender, age, socioeconomic, racial/ethnic, and geographic characteristics: a systematic review and meta-regression analysis. Epidemiol Rev. 2007;29:6–28. Epub 2001 May 17.
2. Kumanyika SK, Obarzanek E, Stettler N, et al. Population-based prevention of obesity: the need for comprehensive promotion of healthful eating, physical activity, and energy balance. A scientific statement from American Heart Association Council on Epidemiology and Prevention, Interdisciplinary Committee for Prevention (formerly the Expert Panel on Population and Prevention Science). Circulation. 2008 Jul 22;118(4):428–64. Epub 2008 Jun 30.
3. Anderson SE, Whitaker RC. Prevalence of obesity among US preschool children in different racial and ethnic groups. Arch Pediatr Adolesc Med. 2009 Apr;163(4):344–8.
4. Kimbro RT, Brooks-Gunn J, McLanahan S. Racial and ethnic differentials in overweight and obesity among 3-year-old children. Am J Public Health. 2007 Feb;97(2):298–305. Epub 2006 Dec 28.
5. Singh GK, Kogan MD, van Dyck PC. A multilevel analysis of state and regional disparities in childhood and adolescent obesity in the United States. J Community Health. 2008 Apr;33(2):90–102.
6. Singh GK, Kogan MD, Yu SE. Disparities in obesity and overweight prevalence among U.S. immigrant children and adolescents by generational status. J Community Health. 2009 Aug;34(4):271–81.
7. May AL, Freedman D, Sherry B, et al. Obesity—United States, 1999–2010. MMWR Surveill Summ. 2013 Nov 22;62 Suppl 3:120–8.
8. Ogden CL, Lamb MM, Carroll MD, et al. Obesity and socioeconomic status in adults: United States, 2005–2008. NCHS Data Brief. 2010 Dec;(50):1–8.
9. Ogden CL, Lamb MM, Carroll MD, et al. Obesity and socioeconomic status in children and adolescents: United States, 2005–2008. NCHS Data Brief. 2010 Dec;(51):1–8.
10. Schoenborn CA, Adams PF, Peregoy JA. Health behaviors of adults: United States, 2008–2010. Vital Health Stat. 2013 May;10(257). Available at: http://www.cdc.gov/nchs/data/series/sr_10/sr10_257.pdf.
11. WHO Expert Consultation. Appropriate body-mass index for Asian populations and its implications for policy and intervention strategies. Lancet. 2004 Jan 10;363(9403):157–63.
12. McLaren L. Socioeconomic status and obesity. Epidemiol Rev. 2007;29:29–48. Available at: http://bvs.per.paho.org/texcom/nutricion/29.pdf.

13. Wang Y. Disparities in pediatric obesity in the United States. Adv Nutr. 2011 Jan;2(1):23–31. Epub 2011 Jan 10.

14. Befort CA, Nazir N, Perri MG. Prevalence of obesity among adults from rural and urban areas of the United States: findings from NHANES (2005–2008). J Rural Health. 2012 Fall;28(4)392–7. Epub 2012 May 31.

15. Institute of Medicine. Accelerating progress in obesity prevention: solving the weight of the nation. Washington, DC: Institute of Medicine, 2012. Available at: http://www.iom.edu/~/media/Files/Report%20Files/2012/APOP/APOP_insert.pdf.

16. Institute of Medicine. Evaluating obesity prevention efforts: a plan for measuring progress. Washington, DC: Institute of Medicine, 2012. Available at: http://www.iom.edu/~/media/Files/Report%20Files/2013/Evaluating-Obesity-Prevention-Efforts/EPOP_rb.pdf.

17. Davis AM, James RL. Model treatment programs. In: Jelalian E, Steele RG, eds. Handbook of childhood and adolescent obesity. New York, NY: Springer, 2008.

18. Barlow SE, Expert Committee. Expert committee recommendations regarding the prevention, assessment, and treatment of child and adolescent overweight and obesity: summary report. Pediatrics. 2007 Dec;120 Suppl 4:S164–92.

19. Artinian NT, Fletcher GF, Mozaffarian D, et al. Interventions to promote physical activity and dietary lifestyle changes for cardiovascular risk factor reduction in adults. A scientific statement from the American Heart Association. Circulation. 2010 Jul 27;122(4):406–41. Epub 2010 Jul 12.

20. Jensen MD, Ryan DH, Apovian CM, et al. 2013 AHA/ACC/TOS guideline for the management of overweight and obesity in adults: a report of the American College of Cardiology/American Heart Association Task Force on Practice Guidelines and the Obesity Society. J Am Coll Cardiol. 2013 Nov 7 [Epub ahead of print].

21. Braveman P. A health disparities perspective on obesity research. Prev Chronic Dis. 2009 Jul;6(3)A91. Epub 2009 Jun 15.

22. Farmer P. Pathologies of power: health, human rights, and the new war on the poor. Berkeley, CA: University of California Press, 2003.

23. Breiner H, Parker L, Olson S. Creating equal opportunities for a healthy weight. Washington, DC: Institute of Medicine, 2013.

24. Ogden CL, Carroll MD, Kit BK, et al. Prevalence of childhood and adult obesity in the United States, 2011–2012. JAMA. 2014 Feb 26;311(8):806–14.

25. Pan L, Blanck HM, Sherry B, et al. Trends in the prevalence of extreme obesity among US preschool-aged children living in low-income families, 1998–2010. JAMA. 2012 Dec 26;308(24):2563–5.

26. Centers for Disease Control and Prevention. Obesity in K-8 students—New York City, 2006–07 to 2010–11 school years. MMWR Morb Mortal Wkly Rep. 2011 Dec 16;60(49):1673–8.

27. Kolbo JR, Zhang L, Molaison EF, et al. Prevalence and trends in overweight and obesity among Mississippi public school students, 2005–2011. J Miss State Med Assoc. 2012 May;53(5):140–6.

28. Madsen KA, Weedn AE, Crawford PB. Disparities in peaks, plateaus, and declines in prevalence of high BMI among adolescents. Pediatrics. 2010 Sep;126(3):434–42. Epub 2010 Aug 16.

29. World Health Organization. Obesity: preventing and managing the global epidemic. Report of a WHO consultation. Geneva, Switzerland: World Health Organization, 2000.

30. Centers for Disease Control and Prevention. Defining overweight and obesity. Atlanta, GA: Centers for Disease Control and Prevention, 2012. Available at: http://www.cdc.gov/obesity/adult/defining.html.

31. Flegal KM, Graubard BI, Williamson DF, et al. Excess deaths associated with underweight, overweight, and obesity. JAMA. 2005 Apr 20;293(15):1861–7.

32. Finkelstein EA, Trogdon JG, Cohen JW, et al. Annual medical spending attributable to obesity: payer- and service-specific estimates. Health Aff (Millwood). 2009 Sep–Oct;28(5):w822–31. Epub 2009 Jul 27.

33. Ogden CL, Yanovski SZ, Carroll MD, et al. The epidemiology of obesity. Gastroenterology. 2007 May;132(6):2087–102.

34. National Institute of Diabetes and Digestive and Kidney Diseases (NIDDK). Understanding adult overweight and obesity. Bethesda, MD: NIDDK, National Institutes of Health, 2008. Available at: http://win.niddk.nih.gov/publications/PDFs/understandingobesityrev.pdf.

35. Narayan KM, Boyle JP, Thompson TJ, et al. Lifetime risk for diabetes mellitus in the United States. JAMA. 2003 Oct 8;290(14):1884–90.

36. Must A, Spadano J, Coakley EH, et al. The disease burden associated with overweight and obesity. JAMA. 1999 Oct 27;282(16):1523–9.

37. Polednak AP. Estimating the number of U.S. incident cancers attributable to obesity and the impact on temporal trends in incidence rates for obesity-related cancers. Cancer Detect Prev. 2008;32(3):190–9. Epub 2008 Sep 13.

38. National Cancer Institute. Obesity and cancer risk. Bethesda, MD: National Cancer Institute, 2012. Available at: http://www.cancer.gov/cancertopics/factsheet/Risk/obesity.

39. Centers for Disease Control and Prevention. Vital signs: asthma prevalence, disease characteristics, and self-management education: United States, 2001–2009. MMWR Morb Mortal Wkly Rep. 2011 May 6;60(17):547–52.

40. Newson RB, Jones M, Forsberg B, et al. The association of asthma, nasal allergies and positive skin prick tests with obesity, leptin and adiponectin. Clin Exp Allergy. 2014 Feb;44(2):250–60.

41. Akinbami LJ, Moorman JE, Garbe PL, et al. Status of childhood asthma in the United States, 1980–2007. Pediatrics. 2009 Mar;123 Suppl 3:S131–45.

42. Ahmad N, Biswas S, Bae S, et al. Association between obesity and asthma in US children and adolescents. J Asthma. 2009 Sep;46(7):642–6.

43. Liu P, Kieckhefer GM, Gau B. A systematic review of the association between obesity and asthma in children. J Adv Nurs. 2013 Jul;69(7):1446–65. Epub 2013 Apr 8.

44. Tavasoli S, Eghtesadi S, Heidarnazhad H, et al. Central obesity and asthma outcomes in adults diagnosed with asthma. J Asthma. 2013 Mar;50(2):180–7. Epub 2012 Dec 5.

45. Bandini LG, Curtin C, Hamad C, et al. Prevalence of overweight in children with developmental disorders in the continuous National Health and Nutrition Examination Survey (NHANES) 1999–2002. J Pediatr. 2005 Jun;146(6):738–43.

46. Chen AY, Kim SE, Houtrow AJ, et al. Prevalence of obesity among children with chronic conditions. Obesity (Silver Spring). 2010 Jan;18(1):210–3. Epub 2009 Jun 11.

47. Latner JD, Stunkard AJ. Getting worse: the stigmatization of obese children. Obes Res. 2003 Mar;11(3):452–6.

48. Ellis S, Rosenblum K, Miller A, et al. Meaning of the terms "overweight" and "obese" among low-income women. J Nutr Educ Behav. 2013 Oct 14 [Epub ahead of print].

49. Puhl RM, Luedicke J, Grilo CM. Obesity bias in training: attitudes, beliefs, and observations among advanced trainees in professional health disciplines. Obesity (Silver Spring). 2014 Apr 22;(4):1008–15. Epub 2013 Dec 4.

50. Hilbert A, Braehler E, Haeuser W, et al. Weight bias internalization, core self-evaluation, and health in overweight and obese persons. Obesity (Silver Spring). 2014 Jan;22(1):79–85. Epub 2013 Sep 10.

51. Huang DY, Lanza HI, Anglin MD. Association between adolescent substance use and obesity in young adulthood: a group-based dual trajectory analysis. Addict Behav. 2013 Nov;38(11): 2653–60. Epub 2013 Jul 3.

52. Huang DY, Lanza HI, Wright-Volel K, et al. Developmental trajectories of childhood obesity and risk behaviors in adolescence. J Adolesc. 2013 Feb;36(1):139–48. Epub 2012 Nov 28.

53. HEALTHY Study Group, Foster GD, Linder B, et al. A school-based intervention for diabetes risk reduction. N Engl J Med. 2010 Jul 29;363(5):443–53. Epub 2010 Jun 27.

54. Beckles GL, Zhu J, Moonesinghe R, et al. Diabetes—United States, 2004 and 2008. MMWR Surveill Summ. 2011 Jan 14;60 Suppl:90–3.

55. National Diabetes Information Clearinghouse. Diabetes prevention program. Bethesda, MD: National Diabetes Information Clearinghouse, 2008. Available at: http://diabetes.niddk .nih.gov/dm/pubs/preventionprogram/#results.

56. Finucane MM, Stevens GA, Cowan MJ, et al. National, regional, and global trends in body-mass index since 1980: systematic analysis of health examination surveys and epidemiological studies with 960 country-years and 9.1 million participants. Lancet. 2011 Feb 12;377(9765): 557–67. Epub 2011 Feb 3.

57. Kumanyika S, Jeffery RW, Morabia A, et al. Obesity prevention: the case for action. Int J Obes Relat Metab Disord. 2002 Mar;26(3):425–36.

58. Swinburn BA, Sacks G, Hall KD, et al. The global obesity pandemic: shaped by global drivers and local environments. Lancet. 2011 Aug 27;378(9793):804–14.

59. Molarius A, Seidell JC, Sans S, et al. Educational level, relative body weight, and changes in their association over 10 years: an international perspective from the WHO MONICA Project. Am J Public Health. 2000 Aug;90(8):1260–8.

60. Kumanyika S, Taylor WC, Grier SA, et al. Community energy balance: a framework for contextualizing cultural influences on high risk of obesity in ethnic minority populations. Prev Med. 2012 Nov;55(5):371–81. Epub 2012 Jul 16.

61. U.S. Department of Health and Human Services. Surgeon General's call to action to prevent and decrease overweight and obesity. Washington, DC: U.S. Department of Health and Human Services, 2001. Available at: http://www.surgeongeneral.gov/topics/obesity.

62. Kuczmarski RJ. Prevalence of overweight and weight gain in the United States. Am J Clin Nutr. 1992 Feb;55(2 Suppl):495–502S.

63. Gortmaker SL, Dietz WH Jr, Sobol AM, et al. Increasing pediatric obesity in the United States. Am J Dis Child. 1987 May;141(5):535–40.

64. Flegal KM, Carroll MD, Kuczmarski RJ, et al. Overweight and obesity in the United States: prevalence and trends, 1960–1994. Int J Obes Relat Metab Disord. 1998 Jan;22(1):39–47.

65. Mokdad AH, Serdula MK, Dietz WH, et al. The spread of the obesity epidemic in the United States, 1991–1998. JAMA. 1999 Oct 27;282(16):1519–22.

66. Mokdad AH, Serdula MK, Dietz WH, et al. The continuing epidemic of obesity in the United States. JAMA. 2000 Oct 4;284(13):1650–1.

67. National Center for Health Statistics. Health, United States, 2007 with chartbook on trends in the health of Americans. Hyattsville, MD: National Center for Health Statistics, Centers for Disease Control and Prevention, 2007. Available at: http://www.cdc.gov/nchs/data/hus /hus07.pdf.

68. Flegal KM, Carroll MD, Kit BK, et al. Prevalence of obesity and trends in the distribution of body mass index among US adults, 1999–2010. JAMA. 2012 Feb 1;307(5):491–7.

69. Ogden CL, Carroll MD, Kit BK, et al. Prevalence of obesity and trends in body mass index among US children and adolescents, 1999–2010. JAMA. 2012 Feb 1;307(5):483–90. Epub 2012 Jan 17.

70. Kumanyika SK. Obesity in minority populations: an epidemiologic assessment. Obes Res. 1994 Mar;2(2):166–82.

71. Kumanyika S. Ethnicity and obesity development in children. Ann N Y Acad Sci. 1993 Oct 29;699:81–92.

72. Koplan JP, Liverman CT, Kraak VI, eds. Preventing childhood obesity: health in the balance. Washington, DC: Institute of Medicine, National Academies Press, 2005.

73. White House Task Force on Childhood Obesity. Solving the problem of childhood obesity within a generation. Washington, DC: Executive Office of the President, 2010. Available at: http://www.letsmove.gov/sites/letsmove.gov/files/TaskForce_on_Childhood_Obesity _May2010_FullReport.pdf.

74. Owen CG, Martin RM, Whinchup PH, et al. Effect of infant feeding on the risk of obesity across the life course: a quantitative review of published evidence. Pediatrics. 2005 May;115(5): 1367–77.

75. Gillman MW, Ludwig DS. How early should obesity prevention start? N Engl J Med. 2013 Dec 5;369(23):2173–5. Epub 2013 Nov 13.

76. Friedman SL, Wachs T, eds. Measuring environment across the life span: emerging methods and concepts. Washington, DC: American Psychological Association Press, 1999.

77. Ferrara A, Hedderson MM, Albright CL, et al. A pragmatic cluster randomized clinical trial of diabetes prevention strategies for women with gestational diabetes: design and rationale of the Gestational Diabetes' Effects on Moms (GEM) study. BMC Pregnancy Childbirth. 2014 Jan 15;14:21.

78. Seidell JC, Nooyens AJ, Visscher TL. Cost effective measures to prevent obesity: epidemiological basis and appropriate target groups. Proc Nutr Soc. 2005 Feb;64(1):1–5.

79. Kumanyika S. Preventive medicine and diet-related diseases: searching for impact. Prev Med. 2012 Dec;55(6):542–3. Epub 2012 Sep 17.

80. Office of the Surgeon General. The Surgeon General's vision for a healthy and fit nation. Rockville, MD: Office of the Surgeon General, 2010.

81. Waters E, de Silva-Sanigorski A, Hall BJ, et al. Interventions for preventing obesity in children. Cochrane Database Syst Rev. 2011 Dec 7;(12):CD001871.

82. Dobbins M, Husson H, DeCorby K, et al. School-based physical activity programs for promoting physical activity and fitness in children and adolescents aged 6 to 18. Cochrane Database Syst Rev. 2013 Feb 28;2:CD007651.

83. Centers for Disease Control and Prevention. CDC: saving lives and protecting people 24/7. Atlanta, GA: Centers for Disease Control and Prevention, 2012. Available at: http://www .cdc.gov/features/CDC24-7.

84. Whitlock EP, Williams SB, Gold R, et al. Screening and interventions for childhood overweight: a summary of evidence for the US Preventive Services Task Force. Pediatrics. 2005 Jul;116(1): e125–44.

85. Kumanyika S. Obesity, health disparities, and prevention paradigms: hard questions and hard choices. Prev Chronic Dis. 2005 Oct;2(4):A02. Epub 2005 Sep 15.

86. Branscum P, Sharma M. A systematic analysis of childhood obesity prevention interventions targeting Hispanic children: lessons learned from the previous decade. Obes Rev. 2011 May;12(5):e151–8. Epub 2010 Oct 26.

87. Spear BA, Barlow SE, Ervin C, et al. Recommendations for treatment of child and adolescent overweight and obesity. Pediatrics. 2007 Dec;120 Suppl 4:S254–88.

88. Kimokoti RW, Millen BE. Diet, the global obesity epidemic, and prevention. J Am Diet Assoc. 2011 Aug;111(8):1137–40.

89. Polhamus B, Thompson D, Dalenius K, et al. Pediatric Nutrition Surveillance 2004 report. Atlanta, GA: Centers for Disease Control and Prevention, 2006. Available at: http://www .cdc.gov/pednss/pdfs/PedNSS_2004_Summary.pdf.

90. Flynn MA, McNeil DA, Maloff B, et al. Reducing obesity and related chronic disease risk in children and youth: a synthesis of evidence with "best practice" recommendations. Obes Rev. 2006 Feb;7 Suppl 1:7–66.

91. Monasta L, Batty GD, Macaluso A, et al. Interventions for the prevention of overweight and obesity in preschool children: a systematic review of randomized controlled trials. Obes Rev. 2011 May;12(5):e107–18.

92. Skouteris H, McCabe M, Swinburn B, et al. Parental influence and obesity prevention in pre-schoolers: a systematic review of interventions. Obes Rev. 2011 May;12(5):315–28.

93. Gordon-Larsen P, Nelson MC, Page P, et al. Inequality in the built environment underlies key health disparities in physical activity and obesity. Pediatrics. 2006 Feb;117(2):417–24.

94. Taylor WC, Carlos Poston WS, Jones L, et al. Environmental justice: obesity, physical activity, and healthy eating. J Phys Act Health. 2006;3(Suppl 1):S30–54.

95. Grier SA, Kumanyika SK. The context for choice: health implications of targeted food and beverage marketing to African Americans. Am J Public Health. 2008 Sep;98(9):1616–29. Epub 2008 Jul 16.

96. Lovasi GS, Hutson MA, Guerra M, et al. Built environments and obesity in disadvantaged populations. Epidemiol Rev. 2009;31:7–20. Epub 2009 Jul 9.

97. Freedman DS, Khan LK, Serdula MK, et al. Racial and ethnic differences in secular trends for childhood BMI, weight, and height. Obesity (Silver Spring). 2006 Feb;14(2):301–8.

98. Cutler DM, Glaeser EL, Shapiro JM. Why have Americans become more obese? J Econ Perspect. 2003 Summer;17(3):93–118.

99. Dietz WH. Reversing the tide of obesity. Lancet. 2011 Aug 27;378(9793):744–6.

100. Gortmaker SL, Swinburn BA, Levy D, et al. Changing the future of obesity: science, policy, and action. Lancet. 2011 Aug 27; 378(9793):838–47.

101. Brownell KD, Warner KE. The perils of ignoring history: Big Tobacco played dirty and millions died. How similar is Big Food? Milbank Q. 2009 Mar;87(1):259–94.

102. Sharma LL, Teret SP, Brownell KD. The food industry and self-regulation: standards to promote success and to avoid public health failures. Am J Public Health. 2010 Feb;100(2): 240–6. Epub 2009 Dec 17.

103. Brownell KD, Koplan JP. Front-of-package nutrition labeling—an abuse of trust by the food industry? N Engl J Med. 2011 Jun 23;364(25):2373–5.

104. Brownell KD. Thinking forward: the quicksand of appeasing the food industry. PLoS Med. 2012;9(7):e1001254. Epub 2012 Jul 3.

105. Kumanyika SK, Parker L, Sim LJ, eds. Bridging the evidence gap in obesity prevention: a framework to inform decision making. Washington, DC: National Academies Press, 2010.

106. Kumanyika SK, Whitt-Glover MC, Gary TL, et al. Expanding the obesity research paradigm to reach African American communities. Prev Chronic Dis. 2007 Oct;4(4):A112. Epub 2007 Sep 15.

107. Kumanyika SK. Environmental influences on childhood obesity: ethnic and cultural influences in context. Physiol Behav. 2008 Apr 22;94(1):61–70. Epub 2007 Nov 22.

108. Gutierrez G. A theology of liberation: history, politics, and salvation. Maryknoll, NY: Orbis Books, 1988.

109. Levenstein H. Paradox of plenty: a social history of eating in modern America. New York, NY: Oxford University Press, 1994.

110. Ludwig DS, Nestle M. Can the food industry play a constructive role in the obesity epidemic? JAMA. 2008 Oct 15;300(15):1808–11.

111. Yach D, Khan M, Bradley D, et al. The role and challenges of the food industry in addressing chronic disease. Global Health. 2010 May 28;6:10.

112. Long MW, Leung CW, Cheung LW, et al. Public support for policies to improve the nutritional impact of the Supplemental Nutrition Assistance Program (SNAP). Public Health Nutr. 2014 Jan;17(1):219–24. Epub 2012 Dec 6.

113. Ludwig DS, Blumenthal SJ, Willett WC. Opportunities to reduce childhood hunger and obesity: restructuring the Supplemental Nutrition Assistance Program (the Food Stamp Program). JAMA. 2012 Dec 26;308(24):2567–8.

114. Leung CW, Hoffnagle EE, Lindsay AC, et al. A qualitative study of diverse experts' views about barriers and strategies to improve the diets and health of Supplemental Nutrition Assistance Program (SNAP) beneficiaries. J Acad Nutr Diet. 2013 Jan;113(1):70–6.

115. Willett WC, Stampfer MJ. Current evidence on healthy eating. Annu Rev Public Health. 2013;34:77–95. Epub 2013 Jan 7.

116. Leung CW, Blumenthal SJ, Hoffnagle EE, et al. Associations between Food Stamp participation with dietary quality and obesity in children. Pediatrics. 2013 Mar;131(3):463–72. Epub 2013 Feb 25.

117. Hill JO, Catenacci V, Wyatt HR. Obesity: overview of an epidemic. Psychiatr Clin North Am. 2005 Mar;28(1):1–23, vii.

Bibliography

The following are other works consulted during the preparation of this introduction. Many are cited in chapters of this book.

Adams P, Gravely M, Doria J. West Virginia diabetes strategic plan 2002–2007. Charleston, WV: West Virginia Department of Health and Human Resources, 2007. Available at: http://www.wvdiabetes.org/Portals/12/Diabetes%20Plan.pdf.

Aguiar EJ, Morgan PJ, Collins CE, et al. Efficacy of interventions that include diet, aerobic and resistance training components for type 2 diabetes prevention: a systematic review with meta-analysis. Int J Behav Nutr Phys Act. 2014 Jan 15;11(1):2.

BeLue R, Francis LA, Colaco B. Mental health problems and overweight in a nationally representative sample of adolescents: effects of race and ethnicity. Pediatrics. 2009 Feb;123(2):697–702.

Berenson GS, Srinivasan SR, Bao W, et al. Association between multiple cardiovascular risk factors and atherosclerosis in children and young adults: the Bogalusa Heart Study. N Engl J Med. 1998 Jun 4;338(23):1650–6.

Biro FM, Wien M. Childhood obesity and adult morbidities. Am J Clin Nutr. 2010 May;91(5): 1499–505S.

Brooks DR, Mucci LA. Support for smoke-free restaurants among Massachusetts adults, 1992– 1999. Am J Public Health. 2001 Feb;91(2):300–3.

Brownson RC, Baker EA, Houseman RA, et al. Environmental and policy determinants of physical activity in the United States. Am J Public Health. 2001 Dec;91(12):1995–2003.

Carver A, Timperio A, Crawford D. Playing it safe: the influence of neighbourhood safety on children's physical activity. A review. Health Place. 2008 Jun;14(2):217–27. Epub 2007 Jun 27.

Casagrande SS, Whitt-Glover MC, Lancaster KJ, et al. Built environment and health behaviors among African Americans: a systematic review. Am J Prev Med. 2009 Feb;36(2);174–81.

Cassaza K, Fontaine KR, Astrup A, et al. Myths, presumptions, and facts about obesity. N Engl J Med. 2013 Jan 31;368(5):446–54.

Cassel J. The contribution of the social environment to host resistance. Am J Epidemiol. 1976 Aug;104(2):107–23.

Centers for Disease Control and Prevention. Adult obesity facts. Atlanta, GA: Centers for Disease Control and Prevention, 2012. Available at: http://www.cdc.gov/obesity/data/adult.html.

———. Behavioral Risk Factor Surveillance System (BRFSS) annual survey data 2001–2011. Atlanta, GA: Centers for Disease Control and Prevention, 2011. Available at: http://www .cdc.gov/brfss/technical_infodata/surveydata.htm.

———. Differences in prevalence of obesity among Black, White, and Hispanic adults—United States, 2006–2008. MMWR Morb Mortal Wkly Rep. 2009 Jul 17;58(27):740–4.

———. Healthy People 2010: final review. Atlanta, GA: Centers for Disease Control and Prevention, 2011.

———. Obesity prevalence among low-income, preschool-aged children—United States, 1998– 2008. MMWR Morb Mortal Wkly Rep. 2009 Jul 24;58(28):769–73.

———. Racial/ethnic disparities in self-rated health status among adults with and without disabilities—United States, 2004–2006. Atlanta, GA: Centers for Disease Control and Prevention, 2007.

———. Vital signs: obesity among low-income, preschool-aged children—United States, 2008– 2011. MMWR Morb Mortal Wkly Rep. 2013 Aug 9;62(31):629–34.

Chang VW, Lauderdale DS. Income disparities in body mass index and obesity in the United States, 1971–2002. Arch Intern Med. 2005 Oct;165(18):2122–8.

Clarke PJ, O'Malley PM, Johnston LD, et al. Differential trends in weight-related health behaviors among American young adults by gender, race/ethnicity and socioeconomic status: 1984–2006. Am J Public Health. 2009 Oct;99(10):1893–901.

Cohen L, Davis R, Lee V, et al. Addressing the intersection: preventing violence and promoting healthy eating and active living. Oakland, CA: Prevention Institute, 2010. Available at: http:// preventioninstitute.org/press/highlights/404-addressing-the-intersection.html.

Cooley-Strickland M, Quille TJ, Griffin RS, et al. Community violence and youth: affect, behavior, substance use, and academics. Clin Child Fam Psychol Rev. 2009 Jun;12(2):127–56.

Cossrow N, Falkner B. Race/ethnic issues in obesity and obesity-related comorbidities. J Clin Endocrinol Metab. 2004 Jun;89(6):2590–4.

Dietz WH. Health consequences of obesity in youth: childhood predictors of adult disease. Pediatrics. 1998 Mar;101(3 Pt 2):518–25.

Drewnowski A, Rehm CD, Solet D. Disparities in obesity rates: analysis by ZIP code area. Soc Sci Med. 2007 Dec;65(12):2458–63.

Ellaway A, Macintyre S. Does where you live predict health related behaviours? A case study in Glasgow. Health Bull (Edinb). 1996 Nov;54(6):443–6.

Ellis LJ, Lang R, Shield JP, et al. Obesity and disability—a short review. Obes Rev. 2006 Nov;7(4): 341–5.

Ezzati M, Friedman AB, Kulkarni SC, et al. The reversal of fortunes: trends in county mortality and cross-county mortality disparities in the United States. PLoS Med. 2008 Apr 22;5(4):e66.

Farley TA, Meriwether RA, Baker ET, et al. Safe places to promote physical activity in inner-city children: results from a pilot study of an environmental intervention. Am J Public Health. 2007 Sep;97(9):1625–31.

Flegal KM, Carroll MD, Ogden CL, et al. Prevalence and trends in obesity among U.S. adults, 1999–2008. JAMA. 2010 Jan 20;303(3):235–41.

Franzini L, Elliott MN, Cuccaro P, et al. Influences of physical and social neighborhood environments on children's physical activity and obesity. Am J Public Health. 2009 Feb;99(2):271–8. Epub 2008 Dec 4.

Freedman DS, Dietz WH, Srinivasan SR, et al. The relation of overweight to cardiovascular risk factors among children and adolescents: the Bogalusa Heart Study. Pediatrics. 1999 Jun 1;103(6 Pt 1):1175–82.

French SA, Jeffery RW, Story M. Pricing and promotion effects on low-fat vending snack purchases: the CHIPS Study. Am J Public Health. 2001 Jan;91(1):112–7.

French SA, Story M, Jeffery RW. Environmental influences on eating and physical activity. Annu Rev Public Health. 2001;22:309–35.

Guadamuz TE, Lim SH, Marshal MP, et al. Sexual, behavioral, and quality of life characteristics of healthy weight, overweight, and obese gay and bisexual men: findings from a prospective cohort study. Arch Sex Behav. 2012 Apr;41(2):385–9. Epub 2011 Oct 25.

Guo SS, Wu W, Chumlea WC, et al. Predicting overweight and obesity in adulthood from body mass index values in childhood and adolescence. Am J Clin Nutr. 2002 Sep;76(3):653–8.

Gutierrez G. A theology of liberation: history, politics, and salvation. Maryknoll, NY: Orbis Books, 1988.

Halpern P. Obesity and American Indians / Alaska Natives. Washington, DC: U.S. Department of Health and Human Services, 2007.

Ham SA, Ainsworth BE. Disparities in data on Healthy People 2010 physical activity objectives collected by accelerometry and self-report. Am J Public Health. 2010 Apr 1;100 Suppl 1: S263–8.

Han JC, Lawlor DA, Kimm SY. Childhood obesity. Lancet. 2010 May 15;375(9727):1737–48.

Hedley AA, Ogden CL, Johnson CL, et al. Prevalence of overweight and obesity among US children, adolescents, and adults, 1999–2002. JAMA. 2004 Jun 16;291(23):2847–50.

Hill JO, Peters JC. Environmental contributions to the obesity epidemic. Science. 1998 May 29;280(5368):1371–4.

Hill JO, Wyatt HR, Melanson EL. Genetic and environmental contributions to obesity. Med Clin North Am. 2000 Mar;84(2):333–46.

Hooks B. Sisters of the yam: Black women and self-recovery. Cambridge, MA: South End Press, 1993.

Huang TT, Drewnosksi A, Kumanyika SK, et al. A systems-oriented multilevel framework for addressing obesity in the 21st century. Prev Chronic Dis. 2009 Jul;6(3):A82. Epub 2009 Jun 15.

Iannotti RJ, Wang J. Trends in physical activity, sedentary behavior, diet, and BMI among US adolescents, 2001–2009. Pediatrics. 2013 Oct;132(4):606–14. Epub 2013 Sep 16.

James WP, Nelson M, Ralph A. Socioeconomic determinants of health. the contribution of nutrition to inequalities in health. BMJ. 1997 May 24;314(7093):1545–9.

Jun HJ, Corliss HL, Nichols LP, et al. Adult body mass index trajectories and sexual orientation: the Nurses' Health Study II. Am J Prev Med. 2012 Apr;42(4):348–54.

Kenney MK, Wang J, Iannotti RJ. Residency and racial/ethnic differences in weight status and lifestyle behaviors among US youth. J Rural Health. 2014 Winter;30(1):89–100. Epub 2013 Jun 25.

Kerr J. Designing for active living among adults. San Diego, CA: San Diego State University, Active Living Research, 2008. Available at: https://folio.iupui.edu/bitstream/handle/10244/621/Active_Adults.pdf.

Kersh R. The politics of obesity: a current assessment and look ahead. Milbank Q. 2009 Mar;87(1):295–316.

Kirk SF, Penney TL, McHugh TL. Characterizing the obesogenic environment: the state of the evidence with directions for further research. Obes Rev. 2010 Feb;11(2):109–17.

Krieger N. A glossary for social epidemiology. J Epidemiol Community Health. 2001 Oct;55(10):693–700.

Kumanyika SK, Espeland MA, Bahnson JL, et al. Ethnic comparison of weight loss in the Trial of Nonpharmacologic Interventions in the Elderly. Obes Res. 2002 Feb;10(2):96–106.

Kumanyika SK, Gary TL, Lancaster KJ, et al. Achieving healthy weight in African-American communities: research perspectives and priorities. Obes Res. 2005 Dec;13(12):2037–47.

Kumanyika SK, Morssink CB. Bridging domains in efforts to reduce disparities in health and health care. Health Educ Behav. 2006 Aug;33(4):440–58.

Kumanyika SK, Shults J, Fassbender J, et al. Outpatient weight management in African Americans: the Healthy Eating and Lifestyle Program (HELP) study. Prev Med. 2005 Aug;41(2):488–502.

Kumanyika SK, Wadden TA, Shults J, et al. Trial of family and friend support for weight loss in African American adults. Arch Intern Med. 2009 Oct;169(19):1795–804.

Larson NI, Story MT, Nelson MC. Neighborhood environments: disparities in access to healthy foods in the U.S. Am J Prev Med. 2009 Jan;36(1):74–81.

Le A, Judd SE, Allison DB, et al. The geographic distribution of obesity in the US and the potential regional differences in misreporting of obesity. Obesity (Silver Spring). 2014 Jan;22(1)300–6. Epub 2013 Jun 13.

Leddy MA, Schulkin J, Power ML. Consequences of high incarceration rate and high obesity prevalence on the prison system. J Correct Health Care. 2009 Oct;15(4):318–27.

Lees E, Taylor WC, Hepworth JT, et al. Environmental changes to increase physical activity: perceptions of older urban ethnic minority women. J Aging Phys Act. 2007 Oct;15(4):425–38.

Lindsay RS, Cook V, Hanson RL, et al. Early excess weight gain of children in the Pima Indian population. Pediatrics. 2002 Feb;109(2):E33.

McLaren L, Hawe P. Ecological perspectives in health research. J Epidemiol Community Health. 2005 Jan;59(1):6–14.

McLean N, Griffin S, Toney K, et al. Family involvement in weight control, weight maintenance and weight-loss interventions: a systematic review of randomised trials. Int J Obes Relat Metab Disord. 2003 Sep;27(9):987–1005.

McTigue KM, Garrett JM, Popkin BM. The natural history of the development of obesity in a cohort of young U.S. adults between 1981 and 1998. Ann Intern Med. 2002 Jun;136(12):857–64.

Mooney C. Cost and availability of healthy food choices in a London health district. J Hum Nutr Diet. 1990 Apr;3(2):111–20.

Moy KL, Sallis JF, David KJ. Health indicators of Native Hawaiian and Pacific Islanders in the United States. J Community Health. 2010 Feb;35(1):81–92.

Mozaffarian D, Hao T, Rim EB, et al. Changes in diet and lifestyle and long-term weight gain in women and men. N Engl J Med. 2011 Jun 23;364(25):2392–404.

National Center for Health Statistics. Pediatric Nutrition National Surveillance: summary of trends in growth and anemia indicators by race/ethnicity children aged < 5 years. Atlanta, GA: Centers for Disease Control and Prevention, 2010.

———. Prevalence of overweight and obesity among adults: United States, 1999–2000. Hyattsville, MD: National Center for Health Statistics, 2002.

New York City Department of Health and Mental Hygiene. Community health survey profiles: Take Care Highbridge and Morrisania, the Bronx. New York, NY: New York City Department of Health and Mental Hygiene, 2006. Available at: http://www.nyc.gov/html/doh/downloads /pdf/data/2006chp-106.pdf.

———. Community health survey profiles: Take Care Central Bronx. New York, NY: New York City Department of Health and Mental Hygiene, 2006. Available at: http://www.nyc.gov /html/doh/downloads/pdf/data/2006chp-105.pdf.

Ogden CL, Carroll MD. Prevalence of obesity among children and adolescents: United States, trends 1963–1965 through 2007–2008. Atlanta, GA: Centers for Disease Control and Prevention, National Center for Health Statistics, 2010.

Ogden CL, Carroll MD, Curtin LR, et al. Prevalence of high body mass index in US children and adolescents, 2007–2008. JAMA. 2010 Jan 20;303(3):242–9.

Ogden CL, Carroll MD, Curtin LR, et al. Prevalence of overweight and obesity in the United States, 1999–2004. JAMA. 2006 Apr 5;295(13):1549–55.

Ogden CL, Carroll MD, Flegal KM. High body mass index for age among US children and adolescents, 2003–2006. JAMA. 2008 May 28;299(20):2401–5.

Ogden CL, Flegal KM, Carroll MD, et al. Prevalence and trends in overweight among US children and adolescents, 1999–2000. JAMA. 2002 Oct 9;288(14):1728–32.

Pollack KM. An injury prevention perspective on the childhood obesity epidemic. Prev Chronic Dis. 2009 Jul;6(3):A107. Epub 2009 Jun 15.

Powell LM, Slater S, Chaloupka FJ, et al. Availability of physical activity-related facilities and neighborhood demographic and socioeconomic characteristics: a national study. Am J Public Health. 2006 Sep;96(9):1676–80. Epub 2006 Jul 27.

Powell LM, Wada R, Krauss RC, et al. Ethnic disparities in adolescent body mass index in the United States: the role of parental socioeconomic status and economic contextual factors. Soc Sci Med. 2012 Aug;75(3):469–76.

Robinson T. Applying the socio-ecological model to improving fruit and vegetable intake among low-income African Americans. J Community Health. 2008 Dec;33(6):395–406.

Roman CG, Chalfin A. Fear of walking outdoors: a multilevel ecologic analysis of crime and disorder. Am J Prev Med. 2008 Apr;34(4):306–12.

Ross CE, Mirowsky J. Neighborhood disadvantage, disorder, and health. J Health Soc Behav. 2001 Sep;42(3):258–76.

Rossen LM, Pollack KM. Making the connection between zoning and health disparities. Environ Justice. 2012 Jun;5(3):119–27.

Rubalcave LN, Teruel GM, Thomas D, et al. The healthy migrant effect: new findings from the Mexican Family Life Survey. Am J Public Health. 2008 Jan;98(1):78–84.

Salbe AD, Weyer C, Lindsay RS, et al. Assessing risk factors for obesity between childhood and adolescence: birth weight, childhood adiposity, parental obesity, insulin, and leptin. Pediatrics. 2002 Aug;110(2 Pt 1):299–306.

Seach KA, Dharmage SC, Lowe AJ, et al. Delayed introduction of solid feeding reduces child overweight and obesity at 10 years. Int J Obes (Lond). 2010 Oct;34(10):1475–9.

Singh GK, Kogan MD, van Dyck PC, et al. Racial/ethnic, socioeconomic, and behavioral determinants of childhood and adolescent obesity in the United States: analyzing independent and joint associations. Ann Epidemiol. 2008 Sep;18(9):682–95.

Singh GK, Siahpush M, Hiatt RA, et al. Dramatic increases in obesity and overweight prevalence and body mass index among ethnic-immigrant and social class groups in the United States, 1976–2008. J Community Health. 2011 Feb;36(1):94–110.

Slater SJ, Ewing R, Powell LM, et al. The association between community physical activity settings and youth physical activity, obesity, and body mass index. J Adolesc Health. 2012 Nov;47(5):496–503. Epub 2010 May 26.

Sorof J, Daniels S. Obesity and hypertension in children: problem of epidemic proportions. Hypertension. 2002 Oct;40(4):441–7.

Swinburn B, Egger G, Raza F. Dissecting obesogenic environments: the development and application of a framework for identifying and prioritizing environmental interventions for obesity. Prev Med. 1999 Dec;29(6 Pt 1):563–70.

Syme SL. Foreword. In: Berkman LF, Kawachi I, eds. Social epidemiology. New York, NY: Oxford University Press, 2000.

Taylor WC, Floyd MF, Whitt-Glover MC, et al. Environmental justice: a framework for collaboration between public health and parks and recreation fields to study disparities in physical activity. J Phys Act Health. 2007;4 Suppl 1:S50–63.

Taylor WC, Franzini L, Olvera N, et al. Environmental audits of friendliness toward physical activity in three income levels. J Urban Health. 2012 Feb 1 [Epub ahead of print].

Taylor WC, Hepworth JT, Lees E, et al. Obesity, physical activity, and the environment: is there a legal basis for environmental injustices? Environ Justice. 2008 Mar;1(1):45–8.

Taylor WC, Sallis JF, Lees E, et al. Changing social and built environments to promote physical activity: recommendations from low income, urban women. J Phys Act Health. 2007 Jan;4(1):54–65.

West Virginians for Affordable Health Care. Early deaths: West Virginians have some of the shortest life expectancies in the United States. Charleston, WV: West Virginians for Affordable Health Care, 2008. Available at: http://appvoices.org/images/uploads/2011/07/WV-early -deaths-_2008.pdf.

Whitaker RC, Wright JA, Pepe MS, et al. Predicting obesity in young adulthood from childhood and parental obesity. New Engl J Med. 1997 Sep 25;337(13):869–73.

White J, Jago R. Prospective associations between physical activity and obesity among adolescent girls: racial differences and implications for prevention. Arch Pediatr Adolesc Med. 2012 Jun 1; 166(6):522–7.

Wilde PE, Peterman JN. Individual weight change is associated with household food security status. J Nutr. 2006 May;136(5):13.

PART I **LITERATURE REVIEWS**

CHAPTER 1

The Potential of Early Childhood Education as a Successful Obesity Intervention

David E. Frisvold, PhD, and Animesh Giri, PhD

There has been a substantial rise in the prevalence of obesity in the United States in recent decades among adults and children of all ages. Among children, the prevalence of obesity was 16.9% in 2009–10, where *obese* is defined as having a body mass index (BMI) greater than or equal to the 95th percentile of the historical (primarily derived from the 1970s) sex- and age-in-months-specific BMI distribution.[1] The prevalence of obesity has increased from 6.5% to 18.0% among children ages 6–11 years and from 5.0% to 18.4% among children ages 12–19 during the past 30 years.[1,2] Given that the obesity rate for school-aged children has more than tripled in recent decades, many public policies naturally focus on reducing or reversing the rise in childhood obesity by attempting to change the school environment for grades K–12. For example, state legislation attempts to increase physical activity by requiring students to participate in physical education classes in school.[3] However, the increase in childhood obesity is evident even among younger children. The prevalence of obesity for children ages 2–5 years rose from 5.0% in 1976–80 to 12.1% in 2009–10.[1,2] Thus, many children are already obese on entering the public school system, and public interventions at earlier ages might be necessary to stem the rise in childhood obesity.[4] In particular, given that children spend increasing amounts of their time in childcare settings and early childhood education (ECE) programs, it is important to understand the relationship between attendance in these settings and childhood obesity and to understand whether further interventions in these programs are required to prevent and reduce obesity.[5]

This chapter reviews the literature on the impact of ECE programs on childhood obesity to examine whether such programs have been effective. Our review focuses on interventions for children prior to the start of kindergarten and, while examining the impact for all children, particularly emphasizes interventions targeting low-income children. Although the review includes a variety of ECE and childcare programs, we

David E. Frisvold is an assistant professor of economics at the University of Iowa. Animesh Giri earned his PhD in economics from Emory University.

focus primarily on the Head Start program, which is one of the largest and most-researched ECE programs targeting low-income children.[6,7]

Given that a primary reason for ECE is to improve school readiness, not to affect obesity, it is important to begin with a discussion of why such programs might reduce or prevent obesity. Early childhood education programs may influence obesity through the *direct* benefits of program attendance, which may depend on the social context of the program, or through *indirect* effects on household resources, including the reduced costs of childcare for children attending subsidized programs.[8,9] Further, the benefits depend on parents' responses to their children's participation; for example, parents may change the amount or type of foods provided at home.[9] Thus, the overall impact of participation in ECE is the net result of the direct effect of the program, the indirect effect on household resources, and the indirect augmenting or diminishing effect of changes in parents' behavior.

Early childhood education programs may have a direct impact on childhood obesity because of the timing of these programs and their specific characteristics. The preschool ages are an important period in the development of food preferences.[10] Further, the behaviors of preschoolers related to dietary intake and physical activity, along with the preschool environment, can explain more of the variation in BMI and physical activity than do parents' weight and demographic characteristics.[11,12] For preschool-aged children, recommended obesity prevention activities include exposing children to a variety of foods and flavors, encouraging the development of preferences for healthy foods and appropriate parental feeding practices, monitoring weight gain, and providing nutrition education to parents and children.[13] Early childhood education programs that adopt these practices are likely to be most effective in preventing obesity.

Early childhood education programs may also be effective in preventing obesity because of the social context underlying these programs. Programs that provide a structured environment can reduce the opportunities to consume unhealthy snacks and watch television, which may be particularly relevant for children in low-income neighborhoods with limited access to healthy foods or safe play areas outside ECE programs.[14]

The primary focus of ECE programs is not to reduce obesity, and the majority of childhood obesity prevention policies are targeted toward public school children in grades K–12, but in recent years there has been increased attention to the potential for ECE and childcare policies to affect obesity. For example, in 2004, the Office of Head Start began the I Am Moving, I Am Learning initiative to increase physical activity and improve nutrition among Head Start children, and this initiative expanded to Head Start centers nationwide in 2007.[15] In that year, the New York City Department of Health and Mental Hygiene enacted new regulations designed to affect obesity by increasing the amount of physical activity, limiting the amount of screen time, limiting the consumption of sugar-sweetened beverages, and improving nutrition.[16] Additionally, the latest reauthorization of the Head Start Act, the Improving Head

Start for School Readiness Act of 2007, addresses the potential for Head Start to affect childhood obesity and encourages new initiatives within the program to prevent and reduce obesity (H.R. 1429, P.L. 110–134). This period of increased awareness of the potential relationship between ECE programs and obesity has also been a period of uncertainty about the future of such programs, given the tightening of state budgets. Thus, understanding the conclusions of the existing research literature is both timely and relevant for policymakers considering the expansion of or modifications to ECE programs and how such changes might affect childhood obesity. There have already been multiple reviews of the literature on the impact of ECE interventions;[5,17–19] but the review here includes more recent studies, emphasizes interventions in the United States, and focuses on the impact on childhood obesity.

After describing the methodology that we used to conduct this literature review and the search criteria, we summarize, first, the literature examining the effect of the Head Start program and supplemental interventions within the Head Start program on childhood obesity, and then the literature examining the effect of other ECE programs. We conclude with a discussion of the implications of this research, some comments on the usefulness of the existing research to guide policymakers, and an outline of important areas of future research.

Methods

To conduct a systematic and thorough review of the literature, we searched four databases: PubMed, EconLit, Educational Resources Information Center (ERIC), and Web of Science. In each of the four databases we conducted a preliminary search for potentially relevant articles by searching combinations of the following keywords: *Head Start*, *obesity*, *overweight*, *body mass index*, *preschool*, *early childhood education*, *childcare centers*, and *pre-kindergarten*. We individually examined each of these articles, which were judged relevant if they involved early childhood interventions in health or education with consequent changes to children's weight or BMI. Inclusion criteria were: peer-reviewed; published between January 1990 and March 2012; written in English; and reporting interventions focusing on 2- to 4-year-olds at Head Start, preschool, or childcare centers. Although we examined articles from such a wide time frame, those that satisfied the complete criteria for inclusion were all published after 2000. Outcomes included the reporting of child anthropometric characteristics and physical activity and/or dietary behavioral changes. We included in the review those articles that provided causal estimates of specific interventions using randomized controlled trials or natural experiment designs. Additional qualitative and quantitative studies comparing anthropometric data for children attending different types of childcare programs were also examined to get a better understanding of the literature but were not included in the review. Exclusion criteria were: studies involving interventions at kindergarten and beyond; interventions focusing on parents' behaviors; and interventions in countries other than the United States. As a result, all federal-level interventions—except for Head Start—were excluded from the analysis, including the National School Lunch Program and the School Breakfast Program. The articles included in the review, with the exception of those on Head Start, document and evaluate interventions at the state, county, community, or school level.

We focus on articles published in recent years in peer-reviewed journals and emphasize those with a more rigorous methodology that aim to determine the causal effect of ECE interventions on obesity. Thus, we exclude studies that examine the determinants of childhood obesity among children within an ECE program but do not focus on the impact of the program. Additionally, we emphasize quantitative analyses over qualitative analyses of characteristics of ECE programs that might influence obesity.

We also exclude reports from the large literature that describe the prevalence of childhood obesity among children attending the Head Start program. These studies suggest that the prevalence of obesity among Head Start participants varies across regions and over time.[16,20-25] National estimates of the prevalence of obesity among children entering the Head Start program are 15.7%, from the Head Start Family and Child Experiences Survey data in 2006, and 19.1%, from the Early Childhood Longitudinal Study, Birth Cohort data in 2005.[8,26] In contrast, the prevalence of obesity for all children ages 2–5 nationwide was 12.4% during these years.[27] Thus, the prevalence of obesity in the Head Start population is high; however, these descriptive studies do not reflect the impact of the program on obesity; instead, the estimates either represent the prevalence of obesity among participants on entering Head Start (which is measured within the first 45 days) or reflect the disadvantaged background of Head Start participants. In this review, we emphasize studies that focus on determining the causal effect of program participation and, at a minimum, include demographic and family characteristics as explanatory variables in regression analyses.

Additionally, given the focus on articles published in peer-reviewed journals, we do not include articles from working paper series that are not yet published. This excludes a study by Carneiro and Ginja[28] that implements a regression discontinuity design based on the eligibility criteria for participation in the Head Start program and a study by Frisvold[29] that implements an instrumental variables approach based on the differential supply of the program across communities. It is important to note that both studies implement credible research designs with non-experimental data and find that Head Start participation leads to a persistent reduction in obesity throughout adolescence.

A total of 11 articles were studied closely for this chapter, reflecting the current state of the literature. We divide these articles into two groups. The first includes studies examining the role of Head Start and supplemental interventions within Head Start in the prevention of childhood obesity. The second group includes articles that look at the impact of other center-based childcare programs.

Head Start and Supplemental Interventions

The primary ECE program available to low-income children is Head Start, which provided services to 904,153 children in 2009 and has served more than 27 million children since the program began in 1965.[30] The Head Start program provides education, nutrition, physical and mental health, and social services to children and their families. The primary participants in the program are 3- and 4-year-old children from households with incomes below the poverty line. In 2009, 39.9% of the participants were White, 30.0% were Black / African American, 16.7% reported their race as "other," 7.8% were multiracial, 4.0% were American Indian or Alaska Native, 1.7% were Asian, and 0.6% were Hawaiian / Pacific Islander; 35.9% of participants were of Hispanic or Latino ethnicity.[30] In comparison, for all children in the United States in 2009, 74.1% were White, 15.3% were Black / African American, 4.7% were Asian, 4.7% were multiracial, 1.5% were American Indian or Alaska Native, and 0.3% were Hawaiian / Pacific Islander; 22.7% were of Hispanic ethnicity.[31]

The Head Start program entails federal performance standards that guide nutrition practices and emphasize the development of gross motor skills. The nutrition guidelines are consistent with the recommendations of the American Dietetic Association;[32] however, the Head Start program offers flexibility to local communities in the implementation of the federal standards. A survey of the obesity prevention practices of nearly all Head Start programs nationwide in 2008 demonstrated that most programs engaged in practices that exceeded the minimum federal standards for healthy eating and physical activity.[33] The barriers to implementing further activities to reduce or prevent obesity among Head Start participants, as identified by program administrators, include a lack of time in the daily schedule to engage in gross motor activity and a lack of money to provide healthier meals and purchase new equipment.[34]

In table 1.1 we list the reviewed articles related to Head Start participation, beginning with those that focus on the impact of Head Start attendance, and then focusing on articles examining the impact of interventions within the Head Start program. Only three articles directly examine the impact of Head Start participation. Lumeng et al.[35] compare changes in BMI z-scores during the academic year and the summer for 1,914 Head Start participants in 14 Head Start centers in Michigan from 2001 through 2006. This temporal comparison allows the authors to test whether children's BMI z-scores fell during the Head Start year and rose during the summer, when children were not attending Head Start. Among all children in the sample, BMI z-scores fell by −0.07 (95% CI = −0.28 to 0.14), rose during the summer by 0.62 (95% CI = −0.005 to 1.23), and fell during the second year by −0.82 (95% CI = −1.50 to −0.13). This relationship was predominantly driven by the presence of non-White females and children who began Head Start obese.

Bucholz et al.[36] compare the dietary intake of Head Start participants with that of children attending preschool or day care, children who previously attended preschool or day care, and children who did not attend any preschool or day care, using data

Table 1.1.   Literature on the impact of Head Start and supplemental interventions within Head Start on obesity

Study	Program/intervention	Data	Design	Results
Lumeng et al. (2010)[35]	Head Start	Children in 14 HS centers in south central Michigan, 2001–6 Sample size = 1,914	Multivariate regression	BMI z-scores fell by −0.07 (95% CI = −0.28 to 0.14) during the 1st year, rose during summer by 0.62 (95% CI = −0.005 to 1.23), and fell during 2nd year by −0.82 (95% CI = −1.50 to −0.13). The BMI z-scores of minority girls increased at a yearly rate of 1.69 during the summer and decreased at a rate of −1.36 during the 2nd academic year.
Bucholz et al. (2011)[36]	Head Start	NHANES 1999–2004; sample includes all children 3–5 years old from low-income families with dietary intake data Sample size = 950	Multivariate logistic regression	Children in HS were between 3.1 and 9.6 times more likely to not meet vitamins B-1 to B-3 requirements than non-HS children and past-preschoolers. They were also 1.83 times more likely to not meet calcium requirements than no-preschoolers.
Frisvold and Lumeng (2011)[8]	Full-day vs. half-day Head Start	Administrative data from HS centers in Michigan, 2002–6 Sample size = 1,833.	Difference-in-differences regression; examines the impact of a change in the supply of full-day classes due to changes in funding	Full-day classes decreased obesity by 3.9 percentage points relative to half-day classes.

Fitzgibbon et al. (2005)[37]	Hip-Hop to Health Jr.; Head Start centers randomly assigned to either intensive health intervention (dietary/ physical activity) or general health intervention; both interventions had a parent component	12 HS centers serving mainly African American children, Sept. 1999–June 2002 Baseline sample size: T = 197, C = 212; post-intervention: T = 179, C = 183; 1-year follow-up: T = 143, C = 146; 2-year follow-up: T = 146, C = 154	Randomized controlled trial	No significant change in BMI or BMI z-scores in the post-intervention period. Significant decreases in BMI z-scores in 1st and 2nd year follow-up (year 1: 95% CI = −0.35 to −0.03; year 2: 95% CI =−0.25 to −0.03). No significant changes in secondary outcomes, including TV viewing, food content, and exercise.
Fitzgibbon et al. (2006)[38]	Hip-Hop to Health Jr.	12 HS centers serving mainly Latino children; fall 2001–winter 2003 Baseline sample size: T = 202, C = 199; post-intervention: T = 196, C = 187; 1-year follow-up: T = 176, C = 160; 2-year follow-up: T = 171, C = 160	Randomized controlled trial	No significant differences between treatment and control groups for primary or secondary outcomes in post-treatment, 1st year follow-up, or 2nd year follow-up.

Abbreviations: BMI, body mass index; C, control group; CI, confidence interval; HS, Head Start; NHANES, National Health and Nutrition Examination Survey; T, treatment group.

from the National Health and Nutrition Examination Survey 1999–2004. The authors restrict the sample to 3- to 5-year-old children from households below 200% of the federal poverty line, for a final sample size of 950 children. The authors use multivariate logistic regression analysis and control for differences in demographics, socioeconomic characteristics, and health-related variables. The results suggest that Head Start participants were between 3.1 and 9.6 times more likely to not meet the Recommended Dietary Allowances for vitamins B-1 to B-3 compared with non–Head Start participants and past-preschoolers, and they were 1.83 times more likely to not meet the calcium requirements than no-preschoolers.

Frisvold and Lumeng[8] examine the impact of attending a full-day compared with a half-day Head Start class for 1,532 children in Michigan. The authors compare the changes in obesity for full-day participants over the course of the year to the changes in obesity for half-day participants, and they find that full-day Head Start attendance reduced obesity by 3.9 percentage points, or 25%. At the beginning of the year, 17% of children were obese in both the full-day and half-day groups; by the end of the year, 16% of half-day children were obese, and 12% of full-day children were obese. To examine the possibility that selection on unobservable characteristics biases the estimates, the authors examine the variation in the supply of full-day program slots that was affected by the elimination of a state-provided full-day expansion grant, using an instrumental variables approach. The results of this natural experiment design confirm the estimates of a reduction of obesity during the year of approximately 4 percentage points due to attending a full-day Head Start program.

Additional research examines the impact of supplemental interventions within the Head Start program that are designed by researchers to reduce and prevent obesity within this population. Hip-Hop to Health Jr. is a 14-week intervention that was conducted in Chicago between September 1999 and June 2002 in 12 Head Start programs serving predominantly African American children and between fall 2001 and winter 2003 in 12 Head Start programs serving predominantly Latino children.[37,38] In the program, Head Start centers were paired based on class size and were randomly assigned to an intensive intervention involving nutrition education and periods of physical activity or a general health intervention that did not focus on dietary or physical activity. Both intervention arms had a parent component. Among Head Start centers serving African American children,[37] there was no statistically significant decrease in BMI z-scores following the intervention (−0.02; 95% CI = −0.13 to 0.08). However, one year after the intervention, the treatment group had experienced less weight gain than the control group, for a greater decrease in BMI z-score of −0.19 (95% CI = −0.35 to −0.03). Two years after the intervention, the BMI z-score of the treatment group remained −0.14 (95% CI = −0.25 to −0.03) less than that of the control group. There were no statistically significant differences in physical activity or diet between the treatment and control groups. When the Hip-Hop to Health Jr. intervention was implemented in Head Start centers serving predominantly Latino children, there were no statistically significant impacts on BMI following the intervention or at the one- and two-year follow-up examinations.[38]

In summary, there are only three studies that examine the influence of Head Start participation on obesity or related questions and satisfy the requirements for inclusion in this review. The two studies using data from Michigan[8,35] suggest that participation in Head Start reduces childhood obesity and that further attendance in the program through a full-day class has an even greater impact. Although the aggregate statistics in Michigan are not different from national estimates for Head Start participants,[8] the study using national data[36] finds that Head Start participants are less likely to consume a diet that satisfies the guidelines of Recommended Dietary Allowances.

These studies are not without limitations. Lumeng et al.[35] compare changes in weight among the same individuals over time but are not able to examine whether similar changes occur among non–Head Start participants. Thus, causal inference is limited by the potential that seasonal trends influenced these patterns. Bucholz et al.[36] compare the diet of Head Start participants with that of low-income nonparticipants. Although the authors use multivariate logistic regression to statistically control for individual and family background characteristics, these estimates are unlikely to represent causal relationships, given the limited covariates and the significant differences in the family characteristics of each group of children; this suggests that there are likely to be significant differences in unobserved characteristics that would bias the estimates. For example, Head Start participants in the sample were more likely than the children in other groups to be non-Hispanic Black and to have mothers who were pregnant as teenagers. This concern applies more generally to most studies that simply adjust for observed individual and family characteristics through multivariate regression methods to determine the impact of ECE in general and Head Start in particular. Head Start administrators often offer admission to applicants with the most disadvantaged backgrounds, which can bias estimates of the impact of the program toward finding a negative or null impact.[29] Frisvold and Lumeng[8] provide credible estimates of the impact of full-day classes, but further replication is needed to understand the external validity and the mechanisms determining their results.

The Hip-Hop to Health Jr. intervention was a randomized controlled trial that demonstrates the potential that modifications to the Head Start program could further enhance the program's benefits.[37] However, additional research on this supplemental intervention could help illuminate why the program was more effective in centers predominantly serving African American children than those serving Latino children, why the program influenced BMI but not diet or physical activity, and whether an enhanced focus on nutrition education and physical activity comes at the cost of a reduction in cognitive or social outcomes or enhances outcomes in these other domains.

Overall, these results suggest that the Head Start program and supplemental interventions within the program may be helpful in stemming the rise in obesity, even though there may be barriers to reducing or preventing obesity among Head Start participants.[34] We now turn to the literature on other ECE programs in an attempt to understand whether the results for Head Start generalize to other settings, which can help inform the mechanisms and social contexts in which ECE programs might be most successful.

Other Early Childhood Education Programs

Working parents have a multitude of childcare types that they can choose for their children, both from the private market and from informal settings. More than 80% of children spend time in nonparental childcare facilities.[39] Education program interventions to prevent obesity at these childcare centers are relatively few. One article in our review estimates the causal impact of an intervention to reduce children's TV viewing at 8 preschools and childcare centers in New York,[40] while another examines the impact of a physical activity and nutrition education intervention at 18 preschools in Chicago.[41] Additional reports in the literature focus on the impact of the type of childcare, the extent of attending a childcare center (the number of daily or weekly hours spent at a center), and childcare subsidies on childhood obesity status. We begin with a review of the studies that focus on existing childcare programs and then turn to studies of supplemental interventions within the preschool setting (see table 1.2).

Maher et al.[39] examine the impact of the type of primary childcare attended. Using Early Childhood Longitudinal Study, Kindergarten Class of 1998–99 (ECLS-K) data and logistic regression analysis controlling for a variety of individual and family background characteristics, the authors find that children in family, friend, and neighbor care were 22% more likely to be obese than children in parental care. However, this was not true for all children; Latino children in parental care had a 15.7% probability of being obese, compared with a 14.9% probability for those in family, friend, and neighbor care and an 11.4% probability for those in Head Start.

Whereas Maher et al.[39] examine the influence of all forms of childcare attended for at least 10 hours per week, Lumeng et al.[42] estimate whether the duration of exposure to center-based care is related to obesity later in life, between the ages of 6 and 12. Using data from the Panel Study of Income Dynamics and multivariate logistic regression, Lumeng et al. find an association between limited childcare attendance (0–15 hours per week) and a decreased risk of obesity relative to no childcare (adjusted odds ratio = 0.56; 95% CI = 0.34 to 0.93). The authors find no statistically significant relationship between childcare attendance for at least 15 hours per week and being obese at 6–12 years of age.

Instead of directly examining attendance at center-based care, Herbst and Tekin[43,44] estimate the influence of receiving a childcare subsidy on obesity. Using ECLS-K data restricted to children living with single unmarried mothers, Herbst and Tekin present a multivariate regression analysis that compares children within the same county and find that children who received a childcare subsidy had a BMI that was 1.7% greater in the fall of kindergarten, were 5.2 percentage points more likely to

Table 1.2. Literature on the impact of pre-kindergarten programs and other early childhood education programs on obesity

Study	Program/intervention	Data	Design	Results
Maher et al. (2008)[39]	Types of primary childcare include (> 10 hr/wk): (1) parent care; (2) family, friend, and neighbor care at home; (3) family care outside the child's home; (4) HS; (5) center care (day care, nursery school, preschool, or kindergarten)	ECLS-K Sample size = 15,691	Multivariate logistic regression	Children in family, friend, and neighbor care were 1.9 percentage points more likely to be obese than children in parent care. Latino children in parent care had a 15.7% probability of being obese, compared with a 14.9% probability for those in family, friend, and neighbor care, and an 11.4% probability for those in HS.
Lumeng et al. (2005)[42]	Center-based childcare	Panel Study of Income Dynamics, 1997 Sample size = 1,244, children ages 6–12	Multivariate logistic regression	Limited childcare attendance (<15 hr/wk) decreased the odds of obesity (adjusted odds ratio = 0.56). No significant relationship between extensive use of childcare (> 15 hr/wk) and obesity.
Herbst and Tekin (2011)[43]	Childcare subsidies	ECLS-K; sample = children living with unmarried mothers and children not attending HS Sample size = 3,113	Multivariate regression and quantile regression	Childcare subsidy receipt was associated with a 1.7% increase in children's fall-of-kindergarten BMI, and a 5.2 and 3.1 percentage point increase in the likelihood of being overweight and obese, respectively.

(continued)

Table 1.2. (continued)

Study	Program/intervention	Data	Design	Results
Herbst and Tekin (2012)[44]	Childcare subsidies	ECLS-K; sample = low-SES children Sample size = 9,231	Instrumental variables regression; instrument = physical distance from the child's home to the nearest public human services agency	Children receiving a childcare subsidy in the year before kindergarten entered school with a BMI 3.5% higher than that of nonrecipients and were 11.9 percentage points more likely to be overweight and 4.8 percentage points more likely to be obese.
Dennison et al. (2004)[40]	Preschool and day-care centers; education-based intervention to reduce TV viewing	16 centers in rural New York, 2000–2001 Sample size: T = 8 centers, 90 children; C = 8 centers, 73 children	Randomized controlled trial	TV viewing decreased 3.1hr/wk in the treatment group and increased 1.6 hr/wk in the control group. No significant changes in growth.
Fitzgibbon et al. (2011)[41]	Hip-Hop to Health Jr. in Chicago Public Schools	18 preschools serving mainly African American children Baseline sample size: T = 325, C = 293; post-intervention: T = 309, C = 280	Randomized controlled trial	No change in BMI or diet in the post-intervention period. Significant increases in MVPA of 7.46 min/day (95% CI = 1.41 to 13.51)

Abbreviations: BMI, body mass index; C, control group; ECLS-K, Early Childhood Longitudinal Study, Kindergarten; HS, Head Start; MVPA, moderate-to-vigorous physical activity; SES, socioeconomic status; T, treatment group.

be overweight, and were 3.1 percentage points more likely to be obese than children who had not received a subsidy. Based on their quantile regression estimates, the authors conclude that childcare subsidies increase BMI only among children in the upper end of the BMI distribution. Further, the authors conclude that the increase in obesity is due to attendance in center-based care, as opposed to the increase in maternal employment resulting from childcare subsidies. Children in center-based care had BMIs that were 3.8% higher and rates of overweight and obesity that were 6.8 and 7.6 percentage points higher, respectively.

Herbst and Tekin[44] estimate the causal impact of childcare subsidies on obesity and overweight status among children, using instrumental variables regression. The authors use the accessibility of public human services agencies (measured by the physical distance from home to the nearest agency) as an instrument for the utilization of childcare subsidies. Using ECLS-K data, the study finds that children receiving a childcare subsidy in the year before kindergarten entered school with a BMI 3.5% higher than that of nonrecipients. Additionally, subsidized children were 11.9 percentage points more likely to be overweight and 4.8 percentage points more likely to be obese.

Dennison et al.[40] report the findings from a randomized controlled trial involving an intervention to reduce children's TV viewing in 16 preschool centers in rural, upstate New York mostly serving White children. The intervention included seven 20-minute weekly sessions, each of which had components for the children, the day care staff, and parents. Day care staff were encouraged to take part in the sessions, which promoted reading and introduced students to alternative activities they could participate in at home instead of watching television. Children made "no television" signs and were encouraged to involve their parents in completing their activities at home. The authors estimate a decrease in mean weekly TV/video viewing of 3.1 hours per week among children in the intervention group, compared with an increase of 1.6 hours per week among those in the control group. The study finds no significant differences, however, in the growth of children in the intervention and control groups.

Fitzgibbon et al.[41] describe the impact of introducing the Hip-Hop to Health Jr. intervention in preschool classrooms in the Chicago Public Schools serving predominantly African American children. This randomized controlled trial demonstrated that children receiving the 14-week intervention, which emphasizes physical education and nutrition education, increased their moderate-to-vigorous physical activity, but there was no effect on dietary outcomes or BMI at the conclusion of the intervention. Results from one and two years post-intervention are not yet available.

Overall, these studies suggest that preschool and childcare attendance contributes to the rise in obesity, but supplemental interventions within preschools provide promising results. The negative results for childcare attendance with respect to obesity are not uniform for all children, however; beneficial impacts were found for Latino children[39] and children attending childcare part-time.[42] Like the studies of the Head Start program, these studies are not without limitations. All studies do not explicitly account for the varying length of time children spend in these programs. The studies that use multivariate regression assume that attendance in different ECE or childcare programs is random, conditional on the observed individual and family characteristics. The studies that use instrumental variables techniques or a randomized controlled trial provide estimates with a high degree of internal validity but face questions about the external validity of the estimates and the mechanisms underlying the results.

Discussion and Conclusions

Despite the increasing amount of time that children spend in childcare or ECE programs, and despite the rise in obesity, only a small number of studies have examined the importance of these programs in *preventing and reducing* childhood obesity. Based on the design of the program, including its nutrition and physical activity components, Head Start has the potential to affect obesity significantly by completely changing the child's environment for a large portion of each day at an important stage in child development; however, we found only three articles that focused specifically on the impact of participating in the Head Start program. Given the size and significance of the program, the lack of research addressing obesity is unfortunate. In particular, the Head Start Impact Study, the recent randomized trial of Head Start participation mandated by Congress, examined a variety of childhood outcomes but did not examine the impact on obesity. The Head Start Act of 2007 requested that the secretary of health and human services report on the program's efforts to prevent obesity; however, there is little research on this topic.[15] That said, two of the three articles on Head Start that we reviewed support the conclusion that Head Start is an effective program in stemming the rise in obesity. Clearly, additional research is needed to better understand how Head Start influences childhood obesity and how changes to the program—either through changes in federal guidelines or through centers' deciding to increase opportunities for physical activity or improving dietary offerings—can alter the program's impact.

Additional interventions have focused on the potential to prevent or reduce obesity within the Head Start population. However, if participation in the Head Start program itself is already having an effect on obesity, the impact of further interventions within the program may be muted because both the treatment and control groups receive a benefit from Head Start itself. Nonetheless, the results from the Hip-Hop to Health Jr. intervention demonstrate that it is possible to generate a persistent impact on obesity.

In contrast to the somewhat promising results among Head Start and supplementary interventions within the program, the results for childcare settings and other ECE programs are largely negative (as summarized in table 1.2). However, the evaluations of supplemental interventions within preschools point to positive improvements in obesity-related behaviors. Thus, changes within childcare settings and preschools, such as the regulations adopted in New York City,[16] may be needed to further stem the rise in obesity among young children.

As it stands, the existing body of research is insufficient to guide public policy. The most important questions to answer in this line of research are: do ECE programs lead to a persistent reduction in obesity, and, if so, why, and which design is most effective? The current research finds that participation in the Head Start program leads to a short-term reduction in obesity, but childcare attendance does not. Potential reasons for the differences in these results are that Head Start centers follow guidelines related to physical activity and nutrition, which are generally absent from the broader childcare industry, and that the Head Start program is intended for children from disadvantaged backgrounds, which includes poverty but also a broader array of sources of disadvantage. Further understanding of why some ECE and childcare settings are effective in preventing or reducing obesity and others are not remains an important area for future research. Some of the most promising areas for future study include the following:

1. Determine whether ECE programs have a persistent impact. Two unpublished working papers suggest that Head Start participation has a persistent effect through adolescence.[28,29] An important step to further address this issue would be to include measures of height and weight in any subsequent waves of the Head Start Impact Study, the randomized controlled trial of the impact of the opportunity to participate in Head Start.

2. Determine the influence on obesity of the rise in states' pre-kindergarten programs. An important change in ECE and childcare in recent years has been the introduction and expansion of states' pre-kindergarten programs. However, we did not find any research that has examined the impact of participating in these programs.

3. Determine the impact of community, environmental, and social contexts on the effectiveness of the program. Replicating the study of the same program in different communities can help to address this issue to understand why and how early childhood interventions can be effective. For example, the Hip-Hop to Health Jr. intervention was effective in predominantly African American neighborhoods in Chicago,[37] but not in predominantly Latino neighborhoods.[38] The impact of the intervention may depend on access to healthy foods and opportunities for exercise in the surrounding neighborhoods.

4. Determine how the structure of the program influences its effectiveness. Head Start and other preschool programs may prepare meals at the center or contract food preparation to an outside agency. Programs may be administered through community action agencies, public schools, nonprofit agencies, for-profit agencies, or churches. Programs differ in the training and characteristics of staff. Additional research on these topics is needed to understand how to enhance the effectiveness of these programs.

5. Determine whether Head Start and other ECE attendance influences obesity-related behaviors at home. Programs vary in the extent of parental

involvement, and programs that are able to positively influence physical activity and diet in the home environment are likely to be the most effective.

These areas of future research are not independent, and additional insights on these topics will help to determine the programmatic and social mechanisms through which ECE programs can be most effective. In a period when a high proportion of children are obese on entering the public school system, further research along these lines is important for guiding future policy efforts in preventing and reducing obesity.

LESSONS LEARNED
- Early childhood education programs have the potential to reduce childhood obesity.
- Few high-quality studies are available to draw definitive conclusions.
- The available evidence suggests that Head Start participation reduces obesity.
- Childcare and other preschool attendance may contribute to the rise in obesity, but supplemental interventions within preschools provide promising results.

References

1. Ogden CL, Carroll MD, Kit BK, et al. Prevalence of obesity and trends in body mass index among US children and adolescents, 1999–2010. JAMA. 2012 Feb 1;307(5):483–90.
2. Ogden CL, Flegal KM, Carroll MD, et al. Prevalence and trends in overweight among US children and adolescents, 1999–2000. JAMA. 2002 Oct 9;288(14):1728–32.
3. Cawley J, Frisvold D, Meyerhoefer C. The impact of physical education on obesity among elementary school children. Presented at: National Bureau of Economic Research Health Economics Program Meeting, Boston, MA, Apr 2012.
4. Davis K, Christoffel KK. Obesity in preschool and school-age children: treatment early and often may be best. Arch Pediatr Adolesc Med. 1994 Dec;148(12):1257–61.
5. Story M, Kaphingst KM, French S. The role of schools in obesity prevention. Future Child. 2006 Spring;16(1):109–42.
6. Currie J. Early childhood education programs: what do we know? J Econ Perspect. 2000;15(2): 213–38.
7. Ludwig J, Phillips D. The benefits and costs of Head Start. Soc Policy Rep. 2007;21(3): 3–18.
8. Frisvold DE, Lumeng JC. Expanding exposure: can increasing the daily duration of Head Start reduce childhood obesity? J Hum Resour. 2011 Mar 20;46(2):373–402.
9. Behrman JR, Cheng Y, Todd PE. Evaluating preschool programs when length of exposure to the program varies: a nonparametric approach. Rev Econ Stat. 2004 Feb;86(1):108–32.
10. Birch LL. Development of food preferences. Annu Rev Nutr. 1999;19:41–62.
11. Klesges RC, Klesges LM, Eck LH, et al. A longitudinal analysis of accelerated weight gain in preschool children. Pediatrics. 1995 Jan;95(1):126–30.
12. Pate RR, Pfeiffer KA, Trost SG, et al. Physical activity among children attending preschools. Pediatrics. 2004 Nov;114(5):1258–63.

13. Deckelbaum RJ, Williams CL. Childhood obesity: the health issue. Obes Res. 2001;9: 239–43S.
14. Morland K, Wing S, Diez Roux A. The contextual effect of the local food environment on residents' diets: the atherosclerosis risk in communities study. Am J Public Health. 2002 Nov;92(11):1761–7.
15. Office of Head Start. Report to Congress on Head Start efforts to prevent and reduce obesity in children. Washington, DC: U.S. Department of Health and Human Services, 2008. Available at: http://eclkc.ohs.acf.hhs.gov/hslc/mr/rc/Head_Start_Efforts_to_Prevent_and_Reduce _Obesity_in_Children.pdf.
16. New York City Department of Health and Mental Hygiene, Board of Health. Notice of adoption of amendments to Article 47 of the New York City health code. New York, NY: New York City Department of Health and Mental Hygiene, 2009. Available at: http://www.nyc.gov /html/doh/downloads/pdf/public/notice-adoption-hc-art47-0308.pdf.
17. D'Onise K, Lynch JW, Sawyer MG, et al. Can preschool improve child health outcomes? A systematic review. Soc Sci Med. 2010 May;70(9):1423–40.
18. Almond D, Currie J. Human capital development before age five. In: Ashenfelter O, Card D, eds. Handbook of labor economics, vol 4. Amsterdam, NL: North Holland, 2010.
19. Nixon CA, Moore HJ, Douthwaite W, et al. Identifying effective behavioral models and behavior change strategies underpinning preschool- and school-based obesity prevention interventions aimed at 4–6-year-olds: a systematic review. Obes Rev. 2012 Mar;13 Suppl 1:106–17.
20. Wiecha JL, Casey VA. High prevalence of overweight and short stature among Head Start children in Massachusetts. Public Health Rep. 1994 Nov–Dec;109(5):767–73.
21. Derrickson J, Tanaka D, Novotny R. Heights and weights of Head Start preschool children in Hawaii. J Am Diet Assoc. 1997 Dec;97(12):1424–6.
22. Hernandez B, Uphold CR, Graham MV, et al. Prevalence and correlates of obesity in pre-school children. J Pediatr Nurs. 1998 Apr;13(2):68–76.
23. Stolley MR, Fitzgibbon ML, Dyer A, et al. Hip-Hop to Health Jr., an obesity prevention program for minority preschool children: baseline characteristics of participants. Prev Med. 2003 Mar;36(3):320–9.
24. Hu WT, Foley TA, Wilcox RA, et al. Childhood obesity among Head Start enrollees in south-eastern Minnesota: prevalence and risk factors. Ethn Dis. 2007 Winter;17(1):23–8.
25. Piziak V, Morgan-Cox M, Tubbs J, et al. Elevated body mass index in Texas Head Start children: a result of heredity and economics. South Med J. 2010 Dec;103(12):1219–22.
26. West J, Tarullo L, Aikens N, et al. Beginning Head Start: study design and data tables for FACES 2006 baseline report. Washington DC: Office of Planning, Research and Evaluation, Administration for Children and Families, U.S. Department of Health and Human Services, 2008. Available at: http://www.acf.hhs.gov/programs/opre/hs/faces/reports/beginning_hs _tables/beginning_hs_tables.pdf.
27. Ogden CL, Carroll MD, Flegal KM. High body mass index for age among US children and adolescents, 2003–2006. JAMA. 2008;299(20):2401–5.
28. Carneiro P, Ginja R. Preventing behavior problems in childhood and adolescence: evidence from Head Start. Chicago, IL: National Opinions Research Center at the University of Chicago, 2008.
29. Frisvold D. Head Start participation and childhood obesity. Emory University working paper, 2011.

30. Office of Head Start. 2010 Head Start program fact sheet fiscal year 2010. Washington, DC: Administration for Children and families, U.S. Department of Health and Human Services, 2010. Available at: http://eclkc.ohs.acf.hhs.gov/hslc/mr/factsheets/fHeadStartProgr.htm.

31. Federal Interagency Forum on Child and Family Statistics. America's children in brief: key national indicators of well-being, 2012. Washington, DC: U.S. Government Printing Office, 2012. Available at: http://www.childstats.gov/pdf/ac2012/ac_12.pdf.

32. Briley ME, Roberts-Gray C. Position of the American Dietetic Association: nutrition standards for childcare programs. J Am Diet Assoc. 1999;99(8):981–8.

33. Whitaker RC, Gooze RA, Hughes CC, et al. A national survey of obesity prevention practices in Head Start. Arch Pediatr Adolesc Med. 2009 Dec;163(12):1144–50.

34. Hughes CC, Gooze RA, Finkelstein DM, et al. Barriers to obesity prevention in Head Start. Health Aff (Millwood). 2010 Mar–Apr;29(3):454–62.

35. Lumeng JC, Kaciroti N, Frisvold D. Changes in body mass index z score over the course of the academic year among children attending Head Start. Acad Pediatr. 2010 May–Jun;10(3): 179–86.

36. Bucholz EM, Desai MM, Rosenthal MS. Dietary intake in Head Start vs non–Head Start preschool-aged children: results from the 1999–2004 National Health and Nutrition Examination Survey. J Am Diet Assoc. 2011 Jul;111(7):1021–30.

37. Fitzgibbon ML, Stolley MR, Schiffer L, et al. Two-year follow-up results for Hip-Hop to Health Jr.: a randomized controlled trial for overweight prevention in preschool minority children. J Pediatr. 2005 May;146(5):618–25.

38. Fitzgibbon ML, Stolley MR, Schiffer L, et al. Hip-Hop to Health Jr. Latino preschool children. Obesity (Silver Spring). 2006 Sep 9;14(9):1616–25.

39. Maher EJ, Li G, Carter L, et al. Preschool child care participation and obesity at the start of kindergarten. Pediatrics. 2008 Aug;122(2):322–30.

40. Dennison BA, Russo TJ, Burdick PA, et al. An intervention to reduce television viewing by preschool children. Arch Pediatr Adolesc Med. 2004 Feb;158(2):170–6.

41. Fitzgibbon ML, Stolley MR, Schiffer LA, et al. Hip-Hop to Health Jr. Obesity Prevention Effectiveness Trial: postintervention results. Obesity (Silver Spring). 2011 May;19(5):994–1003.

42. Lumeng JC, Gannon K, Appugliese D, et al. Preschool child care and risk of overweight in 6- to 12-year-old children. Int J Obes (Lond). 2005 Jan;29(1):60–6.

43. Herbst CM, Tekin E. Child care subsidies and childhood obesity. Rev Econ Household. 2011 Sep;9(3):349–78.

44. Herbst CM, Tekin E. The geographic accessibility of child care subsidies and evidence on the impact of subsidy receipt on childhood obesity. J Urban Econ. 2012;71:37–52.

CHAPTER 2

Latino Childhood Obesity

Amelie Ramirez, DrPH, Kipling Gallion, MA, and Cliff Despres, BS

High body mass index (BMI) is an increasing public health concern in the United States. As noted in chapter 1, children have not escaped this trap: the U.S. Centers for Disease Control and Prevention (CDC) estimates that approximately 17% of children aged 2–19 years are obese, which represents nearly a tripling in just one generation.[1–3] Not only are they at risk for immediate health effects such as high blood pressure, but children with a high BMI also have an increased likelihood of becoming obese during adulthood and are thereby at greater risk of developing associated conditions such as diabetes, cardiovascular disease, and cancers.

Latino youths are disproportionally affected by overweight and obesity, with epidemiological evidence pointing to significant increases in the numbers of Latino children and adolescents who have a high BMI compared with their non-Hispanic counterparts. The negative effects of overweight and obesity for Latino children are significant and of great general concern, given that Latinos are the most populous and rapidly growing ethnic minority in the United States. In 2010, Latinos numbered approximately 50.5 million, or 16% of the total U.S. population; this number had grown by 43% since the year 2000.[4] Thus, as this population continues to grow in the coming years, the negative health effects conferred on the Latino community by overweight and obesity will affect the nation as a whole, with greater health care costs and higher rates of disability, as well as a decreased ability for Latinos to form part of the workforce, among other issues.

In this chapter we provide an overview of the problem of overweight and obesity among Latino youths and address considerations for intervention strategies. We describe several intervention approaches that have been evaluated specifically in the Latino youth community and conclude with a discussion of the need for a clear research agenda to address this significant issue in the coming years. To gather evidence on

Amelie Ramirez is a professor and director of the Institute for Health Promotion Research in the School of Medicine at the University of Texas Health Science Center at San Antonio (UTHSC-SA). Kipling Gallion is an assistant professor and deputy director of the Institute for Health Promotion Research at UTHSC-SA. Cliff Despres is the communication director at the Institute for Health Promotion Research at UTHSC-SA.

these subjects, we conducted a literature review using the search term *Latino child-hood obesity* in databases including PubMed and Web of Science; other reference sources included U.S. government websites (CDC and Department of Health and Human Services). Due to the changing and time-sensitive nature of this topic, our review was limited to studies published since 2000.

The Epidemiology and Extent of Overweight and Obesity among Latino Youths

Numerous studies have detailed the disproportionate prevalence of obesity in the Latino community. Given the scope of this brief review, only national data are addressed in any detail; however, we also include some references to several smaller-scale studies.

One of the key epidemiological findings on Latino childhood obesity comes from a 2012 study conducted by Ogden and colleagues.[5] This analysis estimated the BMI among children and adolescents, using data from the 2009–10 National Health and Nutrition Examination Survey (NHANES). Conducted by the CDC, NHANES combines both interviews and physical examinations, using complex, multistage probability samples of the U.S. civilian, non-institutionalized population.

Results of this analysis are presented in figure 2.1. Overall, among children aged 2–19 years, the prevalence of combined overweight (≥ 85th percentile BMI) and obesity (≥ 95th percentile BMI) was 31.8% (95% CI = 29.8 to 33.7); the prevalence of obesity alone was 16.9% (95% CI = 15.4 to 18.4). Hispanic individuals had among the highest prevalence of combined overweight and obesity (39.1%; 95% CI = 36.9 to 41.4) and of obesity alone (21.2%; 95% CI = 19.5 to 23.0). Non-Hispanic Blacks had a similar prevalence of combined overweight and obesity (39.1%; 95% CI = 35.5 to 42.8) and a slightly higher prevalence of obesity alone (24.3%; 95% CI = 20.5 to 28.6). In contrast, non-Hispanic Whites had a lower prevalence of both combined overweight and obesity (27.9%; 95% CI = 25.1 to 31.0) and obesity alone (14.0%; 95% CI = 11.7 to 16.7). This report also contained a comparative analysis of trends in obesity prevalence among children and adolescents between 1999–2000 and 2009–10. The analysis revealed that over this 12-year period, Mexican American males (considered separately from Hispanics) had the highest odds of being obese compared with their non-Hispanic White counterparts (odds ratio = 1.81; 95% CI = 1.56 to 2.09).

Anderson and Whitaker performed a cross-sectional secondary data analysis of 4-year-old children enrolled in the Early Childhood Longitudinal Study, Birth Cohort, a nationally representative sample of children born in the United States in 2001.[6] Of the 8,550 children included in this analysis, 54.0% were non-Hispanic White, 24.1% were Hispanic, and 15.6% were non-Hispanic Black, with the remaining racial/ethnic groups including Asian, American Indian/Alaskan Native, and Pacific Islander. The overall prevalence of obese BMI (≥ 95th percentile) was 18.4%, and this prevalence differed significantly ($p < .001$) by racial/ethnic group. The prevalence of obese BMI among Hispanic 4-year-olds was 22.0% (95% CI = 19.5 to 24.5), which was exceeded only by that for American Indians/Native Alaskans (31.2%;

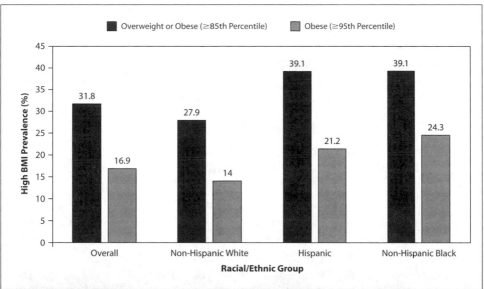

	Overall	Non-Hispanic White	Hispanic	Non-Hispanic Black
Overweight or Obese (≥85th Percentile)				
Males	33.0	30.1	39.6	36.9
Females	30.4	25.6	38.6	41.3
Obese (≥95th Percentile)				
Males	18.6	16.1	23.4	24.3
Females	15.0	11.7	18.9	24.3

FIGURE 2.1. Prevalence (percent) of high body mass index (BMI) among children and adolescents (ages 2–19 years) during 2009–10, by race/ethnicity and sex. Source: Data adapted from Ogden et al. (2012).[5]

95% CI = 24.6 to 37.8). The prevalence was higher than that reported among non-Hispanic Blacks (20.8%; 95% CI = 17.8 to 23.7), non-Hispanic Whites (15.9%; 95% CI = 14.3 to 17.5), and Asians (12.8%; 95% CI = 10.0 to 15.6).

Other epidemiological studies, based on data from national surveys and projects, have also been reported on the topic of overweight and obesity among Latino youths. Fuentes-Afflick and Hessol[7] reported on follow-up results from the Latino Health Project, a prospective study of pregnant Latinas, which showed that nearly half (42.8%) of the children in this study met the criteria for overweight (≥ 85th percentile) BMI. Lutfiyya and colleagues[8] performed a multivariate analysis of cross-sectional data collected in 2003–4 from the National Survey of Children's Health. A multivariate logistic regression analysis showed that Hispanic children aged 5–18 had an odds ratio of 1.298 (95% CI = 1.293 to 0.303) for being overweight and/or obese compared with White children. Kimbro and colleagues[9] analyzed data collected between 1999 and 2003 in the Fragile Families and Child Wellbeing Survey, a national survey that followed a birth cohort of new parents (mainly unwed) and their children. The authors calculated that compared with White children, Hispanic children had a more than threefold greater risk of being overweight or at risk for overweight (adjusted odds ratio = 3.44; 95% CI = 1.42 to 8.35; $p < .01$).

Other smaller studies provide further evidence supporting the significant and disparate nature of Latino childhood obesity.[10–14] A discussion of these smaller-scale studies, which focus primarily on small regional datasets, is outside the scope of this review.

While these epidemiological studies differ greatly in design, in study population, and even in their definition of overweight and obesity, together they provide evidence that high BMI is a rising and significant concern among Latino youths. In nearly all cases, Latino children show a disproportionate prevalence of overweight and/or obesity compared with their non-Hispanic White counterparts. These data, taken together with the fact that Latinos constitute the fastest-growing minority in the United States, suggest that childhood obesity in this community is a problem of significant public health concern.

As the prevalence of overweight and obesity grows among Latino youths, so does the risk of a lifetime of adverse health conditions. This increased risk of chronic health concerns is well documented in several studies. For example, Narayan and colleagues[15] used data compiled during 1984–2000 in the National Health Interview Survey to estimate the lifetime risk for developing diabetes mellitus in the United States. These authors found that Hispanics had the highest estimated lifetime risk for diabetes (45.4% for males and 52.5% for females) compared with non-Hispanic Blacks and Whites. BeLue and colleagues showed in a population-based study of 35,184 youths (ages 12–17 years) that Hispanics who were overweight were far more likely than their non-overweight counterparts to experience depression or anxiety, feelings of worthlessness or inferiority, behavioral issues, and bullying by their peers.[16] Obesity has also been linked with an increased risk for the development of certain cancers, including esophageal carcinoma, pancreatic cancer, colorectal cancer, breast cancer (postmenopausal), endometrial cancer, kidney cancer, and cancers of the thyroid and gallbladder.[17] Other chronic health issues associated with high BMI and obesity include cardiovascular disease, asthma, type 2 diabetes, liver disease, and sleep apnea.

Considerations for Intervention Strategies

Before addressing the intervention strategies, it is important to consider some of the factors that affect the development of overweight and obesity among Latino youths. The risk for Latino children of becoming overweight or obese is multifactorial. The factors range from unmodifiable ones, such as underlying biological characteristics, to modifiable factors, such as children's living and economic setting and food habits. McArthur and colleagues[18] found that many at-risk behaviors are pervasive among immigrant Hispanic households, including frequent television watching and keeping unhealthy snack foods readily available. Even speaking Spanish at home was found to independently increase the risk for obesity among Latino school children in San Francisco.[19] Additionally, society contributes to this risk, with media and advertising having a strong influence on the development of obesity in this community. Further complicating matters, significant differences exist among the risk factors for Latino children of Mexican family origin and Latino children of Central or South American origin.[19] Here we examine some of the risk factors that should be considered when developing strategies for intervention, organizing them into social and economic factors, parental/familial factors (including parents' perceptions), food habits, media and marketing, and genetic or biological factors. Finally, we identify several barriers to effective interventions for Latino youths.

Social and Economic Considerations

Among Latino families, low income and education are important risk factors determining overweight or obesity in children. When data from the kindergarten class (1998–99) of the Early Childhood Longitudinal Study were examined for change in BMI through fifth grade, a weakly negative association was found between parents' education and growth in BMI for children of Hispanic immigrants, but no such association was found among children of native (U.S.-born) Hispanic families.[20] Compared with non-Hispanic White children in kindergarten, Hispanic kindergarteners had significantly higher BMI across all levels of parental education except for the lowest level (parents not high school graduates), where there was no difference between the two groups. This same trend in higher BMI among Hispanic kindergarten children was also apparent across all family income levels. Interestingly, at the highest level of family income, BMI was higher among children of Hispanic immigrants than among children from native Hispanic families. The effect of income on BMI was strongly negative when education was controlled for.

A cross-sectional analysis of the Viva La Familia study was conducted to determine dietary intake among Hispanic children (ages 4–19 years) from families of low socioeconomic status living in Houston.[21] The proportion of energy intake from most food categories was largely similar between the overweight and non-overweight children. However, overweight children consumed a significantly lower proportion of cold cereal and white milk; the proportion of energy from snack chips was higher specifically among overweight girls. Overweight children consumed a higher number of servings of vegetables, meats, fats, and beverages than non-overweight children. Overweight girls ate fewer servings of fruit than non-overweight girls. When adjusted for age, the overall energy intake was higher among overweight children than among non-overweight children. Absolute amounts of carbohydrates (in girls only), proteins, and fats were all higher among overweight than among non-overweight children.

Increased acculturation to the U.S. lifestyle has been pinpointed as an important risk factor for overweight and obesity among Latino youths. A study that included 1,385 Hispanic adolescents (sixth- and seventh-graders) from Southern California reported that acculturation to the United States was significantly associated with a lower frequency of physical activity and an increased frequency of fast-food consumption, both considered obesity-related behaviors.[22] More-acculturated Latino families have less healthy dietary behaviors than less-acculturated families.[23] For example, families with a higher acculturation level are more likely to eat away from home at least weekly.

Parental/Familial Factors

Parents and other family members play an important part in role modeling and controlling the types and amounts of food eaten by their children. A comprehensive review of the literature found that 86% of 19 studies demonstrated at least one significant association between parental feeding style and child outcome.[24] Focus groups of Latina mothers identified both family role modeling and psychosocial stressors as causative factors of obesity.[25] One study found that a higher frequency of family meals slightly increased the risk for obesity among Hispanic boys in low-education households; the same association was not apparent for Hispanic girls in similar households.[26] Family meals decreased the risk of obesity in non-Hispanic White and non-Hispanic Black boys.

Parents' perceptions of healthy behaviors are also an important factor in determining the physical activity of their children. In many Latino households, parents often put a decreased emphasis on physical activity, and foreign-born Latino parents are less likely than U.S.-born parents to encourage and support physical activity. The effects of this were evident in a cross-sectional analysis of data from the 2003 National Survey of Children's Health.[27] In this analysis, immigrant Hispanic children were far more likely than U.S.-born White children with U.S.-born parents to be physically inactive (22.5% vs. 9.5%). Further, more than twice as many of these immigrant Hispanic children as native Asian children did not participate in sports (67% vs. 30.2%). This study also demonstrated that immigrant Latino children were less physically active than even native Latinos.

Parents' perceptions about whether their children are overweight and/or obese have an important role in furthering or curbing a child's high BMI. When parents incorrectly perceive their overweight or obese child as being of normal weight, they may not be as receptive to weight loss interventions and, indeed, may continue to promote diet and lifestyles that contribute to the high BMI. Several investigators have sought to define parental perceptions regarding overweight and obesity in the Latino community. When asked about their children's weight, 75.8% of Latina mothers recruited from a predominantly Latino San Francisco community reported that the child's weight was fine or normal; however, 42.8% of these children were classified as overweight (≥ 85th percentile).[7] Only 9.3% of the mothers described their child's weight as too high, and 15% classified their child's weight as too low. Children whose weight was perceived to be too high by their mothers were more than 11-fold more likely to indeed be overweight (adjusted odds ratio = 11.88; 95% CI = 2.37 to 59.60; $p = .003$) than children whose weight was perceived as normal.

Guerrero and colleagues[25] conducted a survey of 24 low-income, Spanish-speaking, Mexican-descent mothers of preschool-aged children (ages 2–5) who received health care at a large free clinic in the West Los Angeles area. The authors aimed to better understand the mothers' definitions and perceptions of health, obesity, and physicians' weight assessments. Most mothers (80%) accurately perceived their own weight; of the 13 mothers who were overweight or obese, 94% correctly perceived their status as overweight. In contrast, only 58% of the mothers correctly perceived their child's weight, and this number dropped to less than half (42%) for mothers of overweight children. During follow-up focus groups, four major topics emerged in the area of maternal perceptions of children's weight. The first topic dealt with definitions of health and overweight, which mothers overwhelmingly discussed in terms of the child's ability to function. The mothers defined an overweight child as one who is less active, with declining physical abilities, and who tires easily. The second topic related to the role of health professionals in assessing child health and obesity. Overall, the mothers agreed that the judgment of these health professionals could be useful for helping to determine a child's weight, especially when it is not made obvious by physical function. The third topic concerned the etiology of childhood obesity, with mothers identifying factors that contributed to overweight and obesity (such as a high-fat diet, eating out, lack of exercise, and poor role models). The fourth topic dealt with parental interventions for prevention and management of childhood obesity. None of the focus group participants identified increased physical activity as an effective intervention; instead, the common theme was controlling the type and amount of food children consumed. In an ensuing discussion, many mothers reported disagreement among family members about the food consumed by young children in the home.

Latina mothers may unconsciously promote excess weight in their children. In an assessment of low-income Latina mothers that showed participants a series of body images, the mothers thought that children with a BMI in either the 50th or 75th percentile were actually too thin to be attractive or healthy.[28] In addition, these mothers considered children with a BMI in the 97th percentile to be only barely too large. Interestingly, the perception of excess weight as being preferable was limited to their children, as the mothers desired a thin figure for themselves. Latina mothers feel the family and cultural pressures to have a "chubby child" despite knowing the health and social consequences of overweight.[29]

After conducting a focus group of Latina mothers, authors of one study concluded that based on the mothers' difficulties in acknowledging their children's overweight status, as well as a strong cultural influence on the mother's association between health and weight, a traditional nutrition counseling paradigm might not be effective for these women.[30] Instead, a reframed strategy may be required to address the belief system and cultural framework of Latino families.

Several investigators have sought to define parental perceptions of overweight and obesity in the Latino community.[31–35] Intriguingly, these studies have not revealed a conclusive approach by which parents generally view their children's weight; instead, they have highlighted the various views on high BMI that exist throughout the culture. Overall, these studies make it clear that many Latino parents incorrectly perceive their overweight or obese children as being of normal or healthy weight. Many of these misperceptions can be traced to a cultural understanding of what a healthy weight is, while others are simply due to lack of awareness or education. Comparison of these studies is complicated by the disparate study populations, as well as by the differing thresholds used to define overweight and obesity in children. Because of the important role of parents in influencing the diet and lifestyle patterns of children, their misconceptions about excess weight may play a key role in the rising incidence of overweight and obesity among Latino youths.

Food Habits

The intake of energy-dense foods, nutrient-poor foods, and sugar-sweetened beverages is clearly associated with overweight and obesity, regardless of race/ethnicity. For example, both BMI and frequency of obesity increase with each additional serving of sugar-sweetened drink consumed.[36] Longitudinal studies have overwhelmingly demonstrated a positive association between obesity development and sugar-sweetened beverage consumption.[37] Cross-sectional studies have further shown links between being overweight in childhood and buying lunch at school, eating supper while watching television or without family supervision, consuming less energy at breakfast or more at dinner, and missing breakfast.

One survey examined the relationship between away-from-home eating, children's dietary intake, and children's and adults' weight status in a predominantly Mexican American population.[23] This study probed deeply into types of away-from-home eating, differentiating these events as eating at the home of a relative, neighbor, or friend versus eating at a restaurant. Nearly half (45.9%) of families reported consuming away-from-home foods at a restaurant (any type) at least once weekly, and just over one-third (37.5%) reported doing so at the home of a relative, neighbor, or friend. Children who ate away from home at least once weekly consumed higher amounts of sugar-sweetened beverages and sweet or savory snacks and less water than children who ate away from home less frequently. Childhood overweight (defined in this study as ≥ 95th percentile BMI) was 5% more prevalent in families who ate away from home (either at the home of a relative, neighbor, or friend or at a restaurant) at least once a week than in those who did not. In an exploratory empirical study, 43% of parents of Hispanic children reported consuming fast food one or more times per week, twice the percentage of parents of non-Hispanic White children (21%).[38] The only other racial/ethnic group that exceeded this frequency was African Americans (44%).

Less access to healthful foods is also an important risk factor for Latino children. Grocery stores are less abundant in low-income minority neighborhoods, while fast-food and convenience stores are more predominant.[39–41] *Tiendas*, or small Latino grocery stores, often provide less access to affordable and healthy dairy and meat products than do non-Latino grocery stores.[42] For example, one gallon of skim milk was significantly costlier in *tiendas* than in non-Latino grocery stores ($3.29 vs. $2.69 [in U.S. dollars]; $p = .005$). Lean (7%) ground beef was available in only one *tienda*, versus 10 non-Latino grocery stores ($p = .01$). However, produce of the same quality and price was available in both settings. In Latino households, food insecurity and unreliable access to sufficient food occurs at a markedly high frequency (26.9%) compared with households overall (14.7%) or White non-Hispanic households (11.0%).[43]

Poor eating habits are also prevalent among Latino children. In one study, use of the Eating in Emotional Situations Questionnaire determined that eating in emotional situations was a common occurrence among low-income Latino fourth-graders.[44] The questionnaire evaluates certain eating activities, such as emotion-driven consumption (e.g., eating when lonely) and context-driven consumption (e.g., eating after receiving a bad grade). Approximately half of the surveyed children reported eating in at least 3 of 11 types of emotional situations (when stressed, when sad, and when bored). More than a quarter (28%) of the children reported eating in at least 6 of the 11 types of emotional situations. An observational study of food practices among Latino families in a low-income Brooklyn, New York, neighborhood found that these families relied on everyday food practices to provide coping measures to their children.[45] The authors of this study concluded that these practices were so ingrained in the family that they formed the "sociocultural roots of childhood obesity," as they drove both food choices and food-related activities.

Influence of Media and Marketing

The impact of media, advertising, and marketing on the risk of overweight and obesity among youths is an increasing focus of study. Television watching has been clearly linked to the development of excess weight in children. This problem is a particular concern among Latinos, as these children tend to spend a greater amount of time watching television. For example, one study showed that a higher proportion of Mexican American children (ages 8–16 years) than non-Hispanic White children watched three or more hours of television daily (53% vs. 37%).[46] The same study showed that fewer Mexican American children than their non-Hispanic White counterparts were physically active on five or more days of the week (49.9% vs. 61.1%). Television watching was associated with obesity, as the highest prevalence of obesity was found among those children who watched the greatest number of hours of television. Accordingly, the unadjusted prevalence of obesity was 16.3 per 100 individuals among Mexican American children, higher than that observed among non-Hispanic White children, at 11.8 per 100 individuals. A meta-analysis confirmed a statistically significant relationship between television viewing and excess weight in children of all races/ethnicities, although the analysis suggested that this association was not especially clinically relevant.[47] Matheson and colleagues[48] provided one explanation for the association between higher BMI and television watching, showing that in a population of predominantly Latino fifth-graders, $18.3\% \pm 19.9\%$ and $26.4\% \pm 29.8\%$ of the total daily energy was consumed during television viewing on weekdays and weekends, respectively. Between 58.2% and 76.0% of these children consumed food while watching television, depending on whether it was a weekday or the weekend. Most of this food consisted of snacks, not full meals. The authors suggested that because these children consume a substantial proportion of their daily food intake while watching television, this may be an important behavior to target for modification.

Latino youths are avid consumers of media. A Kaiser Family Foundation study that focused on the role of media in the lives of adolescents (ages 8–18 years) reported that Hispanic adolescents consumed about 4 more hours of media daily (13 hours) than non-Hispanic White adolescents (8 hours 36 minutes).[49] This increased use held true across all types of media except print, including television (5 hours 21 minutes vs. 3 hours 36 minutes), music/audio (3 hours 8 minutes vs. 1 hour 56 minutes), computers (1 hour 49 minutes vs. 1 hour 17 minutes), video games (1 hour 35 minutes vs. 56 minutes), and movies (33 minutes vs. 13 minutes). Additionally, this study found that the total daily media exposure among Hispanic adolescents grew rapidly over the past decade (8 hours 19 minutes in 1999, 8 hours 52 minutes in 2004, and 13 hours in 2009), while this growth was less robust among non-Hispanic Whites (6 hours 56 minutes in 1999, 7 hours 58 minutes in 2004, and 8 hours 36 minutes in 2009). This study did not consider the impact of more recent types of media, including the Internet, smartphones, and social media. The roles of these media types among Latino youths were evaluated in a Yahoo!-sponsored white paper,[50] which noted that Hispanics are major users of technology, consuming more media than the general population. This is exemplified by the percentage of Hispanics who have a cellphone (90%, vs. 79% of the general population) and use text messaging (66% vs. 38%).

Because of their robust media use, Latinos are considered an especially important target market for the fast-food and soft drink industries. Low-income Latino neighborhoods have a disproportionately high density of outdoor advertisements for high-calorie, low-nutrient foods and beverages.[51] Notably, approximately 5% of the $4.2 billion spent on advertising by fast-food companies in 2009 specifically appeared on Spanish-language television,[52] where children are the primary target of fast-food advertisers—with one study finding that 31% of food and drink commercials on U.S. Spanish-language channels target children.[53] The extent of advertising targeted to Latino youths is not limited to television. Fast-food companies have greatly expanded the number and sophistication of websites and web marketing efforts targeted to Latino youths.[52,54] Advertising has now extended to social media platforms, furthering the reach of these companies.

Biological Factors

While many of the risk factors for overweight and obesity among Latino youths are modifiable, some are genetic or biological. Several published studies have begun to elucidate some of the biological factors that may increase risk among Latinos.[55-61] However, since much of this research remains to be validated in large trials, an in-depth analysis is outside the scope of this review.

Barriers to Effective Interventions

Among youths overall, many barriers exist to preventing and managing overweight and obesity effectively. The Latino community suffers from additional barriers related to perceptions and practices particular to the culture. The demanding work schedule of parents has often been cited as a barrier to preventing and managing high BMI and, indeed, is cited as a cause of obesity. Having to work long hours limits the amount of time that parents are home to encourage healthy food options and the consumption of healthful meals. Lack of physical activity, one contributor to overweight and obesity, is a particular barrier among Latino households. Many Latino parents and grandparents put little emphasis on the importance of participating in regular sports or physical activities, and often they feel that it is a waste of time. In addition, some of the lack of physical activity is attributed to the expense and lack of availability of safe, local recreation facilities.[62] Neighborhood safety concerns, especially prevalent in some low-income Latino communities, can also decrease the amount of physical activity among Latino children. In fact, a perception of inadequate police protection was found to correlate with increased television viewing as well as higher BMI levels in Latino families.[63]

Health care settings may also be barriers to effective weight management interventions in Latino communities. A focus group–based study conducted in the Denver area found that health care providers felt ambivalent toward their role in addressing obesity among Mexican American infants.[64] Hispanic parents are far more likely than non-Hispanic White parents to rate the quality of overweight counseling they received during a child's primary care visit as poor or fair (odds ratio = 2.78).[65] In addition, some Latino parents feel that their health care providers do not provide high-quality advice on physical activity and weight issues.[66]

Promising Intervention Approaches

A large number of strategies have been explored to prevent or decrease overweight and obesity among American youths. One of the most recent of these is the large national Let's Move! campaign, a comprehensive initiative to solve the problem of obesity within a generation by putting children on healthier paths during their earliest months and years. In contrast, there is a paucity of interventions designed to address this issue in the Latino community. Here we summarize data from the few published studies that have focused specifically on Latino youths, providing the reader with a framework to determine what has been done and what research remains to be done.

A systematic review of nine different health education and promotion interventions for Hispanic children found that among the most successful shared characteristics were the following: including older children at a higher risk for obesity, a central parental component, theoretical underpinnings, delivery by a dedicated staff, and long duration.[67] However, because only four of the nine studies included in this review had significant findings, it is obvious that more interventions for Latino children and adolescents are necessary.

Promotoras and *curanderos* are two types of community health workers specifically active in Latino communities. *Promotoras* are minimally trained lay workers who provide basic health education and advice.[68] These workers, often volunteers, are generally from the target community. In their interactions with Latinos, *promotoras* strongly consider linguistic and cultural factors in their presentations and discussions.[69] One study evaluated *promotora* visits as a potential intervention for childhood obesity and related outcomes among Mexican American mothers and children (kindergarten through second grade).[70] The combined use of regular *promotora* visits and a monthly newsletter positively modified the risk for childhood obesity. After a two-year follow-up, significant improvements were noted in parenting strategies, parental support, and parent-mediated family behaviors. Other health care workers, called *curanderos*, are sometimes consulted as an alternative to routine health care in the greater Southwest region of the United States. *Curanderos* often heavily rely on elements from nature to frame explanations for a particular condition and/or components of treatment. Thus, a study by Clark and colleagues[71] concluded that *curanderos* incorporate the socially marginalized experiences of Latinos as an essential element of obesity management. These authors speculated that traditional physicians and clinicians may find it difficult to work readily with *curanderos* but acknowledged that these community health workers could serve as collaborators in childhood obesity interventions.*

Crespo and colleagues[72] reported on the results of a randomized controlled comparison conducted in 13 Latino elementary schools. Interventions were conducted by *promotoras*, and children were between kindergarten and second grade. Children and families were randomized to one of four intervention arms: individual and family level only; school or community level only; combined individual/family and school/community levels; or no intervention. Unfortunately, null results were reported, with

---

* For more on the importance of *promotoras/promotores* and *curanderos* in providing care to Latino communities, see chapters 6 and 15–17.

no significant effects on the children's BMI attributed to any intervention. However, family-level intervention was associated with improvements in some obesity-related child behaviors, such as fruit and vegetable consumption.

The Healthier Options for Public Schoolchildren (HOPS) intervention was designed to maintain children at a healthy weight and improve their health status and academic achievement.[73] This intervention had several components, including modified dietary offerings, nutrition/lifestyle educational curricula, physical activity, and wellness projects. The study reported significant improvements in BMI, blood pressure, and academic scores among low-income Hispanic children with the HOPS intervention.

A randomized controlled trial evaluated an intensive lifestyle-based weight management program delivered to Mexican American children in Houston schools.[74] Children received either an instructor-led or a self-help intervention. Those who received the instructor-led intervention achieved significantly greater decreases in BMI than those who received the self-help intervention; this difference was observed at both one and two years. Other changes experienced by participants in the instructor-led intervention group included improvements in body composition (measured by triceps skinfold), total cholesterol, and triglycerides.

Interventions need not be formalized or delivered in a school- or community-based format to be successful. For example, one long-term study showed that significant decreases in visceral fat levels among overweight Latino adolescents were associated with an increase in dietary fiber intake.[75] When Latino adolescents decreased their total dietary fiber intake, they exhibited significant increases in visceral fat compared with those who had increased their total dietary fiber (21% vs. −4%; $p = .02$). Separately, a secondary analysis of a randomized controlled trial found that overweight Latino adolescents who decreased their added sugar intake experienced improvements in glucose tolerance.[76] In this study, Latino adolescents who increased their fiber intake achieved BMI improvements compared with those who did not increase fiber intake (−2% vs. 2%; $p = .01$); a similar trend was observed in visceral adipose tissue levels (−10% vs. no change; $p = .03$). Physical activity, even in the absence of weight loss, can provide health benefits to overweight Latino youths.[77-79] A randomized controlled trial showed that among Mexican American children (ages 10–14 years), an intensive individualized intervention could significantly reduce BMI more than a self-help intervention.[80] This study followed up on the children at three and six months, finding significantly greater decreases in BMI in the intensive individualized intervention group at both time points.

Research Agenda

Overall, while some improvements in managing overweight and obesity among Latino youths have been achieved, they are at best small and incremental. This, combined with a relative paucity of research data on Latino childhood obesity, limits the

Table 2.1. Key research areas, and priorities within each area, identified as important for the development and implementation of evidence-based, culturally appropriate obesity interventions for Latino youths

Research Area 1: Society
1. Policies that subsidize accessibility of healthy foods to improve diet among Latino families
2. Programs to influence state and local legislation at different levels regarding physical activity and healthy foods available to children
3. Policies that make playgrounds, schools, parks, and recreational facilities available for physical activity for Latino children and families on non-school days
4. Policies to improve nutrition and physical activity education in the media and in community settings
5. Policies that provide health care access for screening and treatment of childhood obesity

Research Area 2: Community
1. Built-environment policies involving collaborations with multiple stakeholders to promote physical activity
2. Collaborations among community, schools, and families to generate after-school opportunities for children to be more physically active
3. Community participatory processes that encourage Latino families to discuss their needs and define action strategies
4. Policies that limit the sale of unhealthy foods and drinks in public institutions
5. Neighborhood safety influence on outdoor recreation and physical activity

Research Area 3: School
1. Health, nutrition, and active physical education classes as part of the school curriculum
2. Collaborations among community, schools, and families to generate after-school opportunities for children to be more physically active
3. Community participatory processes that encourage Latino families to discuss their needs and define action strategies
4. Policies that limit the sale of unhealthy foods and drinks in public institutions
5. Neighborhood safety influence on outdoor recreation and physical activity

Research Area 4: Family
1. Engaging Latino families as advocates of childhood obesity prevention initiatives at the community and school levels
2. Collaborations among community, schools, and families to generate after-school opportunities for children to be more physically active
3. Community participatory processes that encourage Latino families to discuss their needs and define action strategies
4. Policies that limit the sale of unhealthy foods and drinks in public institutions
5. Neighborhood safety influence on outdoor recreation and physical activity

Research Area 5: Individual
1. Programs making physical activity more attractive than watching TV or playing video games
2. Collaborations among community, schools, and families to generate after-school opportunities for children to be more physically active
3. Community participatory processes that encourage Latino families to discuss their needs and define action strategies
4. Policies that limit the sale of unhealthy foods and drinks in public institutions
5. Neighborhood safety influence on outdoor recreation and physical activity

Source: Adapted from Ramirez et al. (2011).[81]
Note: Numbers refer to priority rankings within each research area. These research priorities are described as the basis of the National Latino Childhood Obesity Research Agenda.

development and implementation of evidence-based, culturally appropriate child-hood obesity interventions. In response, several ongoing efforts are now focused on developing effective interventions for this particular population. Salud America!, the Robert Wood Johnson Foundation Research Network to Prevent Obesity among Latino Children, has been instrumental in identifying research priorities and providing a framework and resources to stimulate research and collaboration among investigators, providers, community leaders, and policymakers. This program has led to the development of the first-ever National Latino Childhood Obesity Research Agenda.[81] The agenda has identified five main areas of research, and a survey of key stakeholders ranked particular research priorities in each of these areas (see table 2.1). Based on the research priorities from the National Latino Childhood Obesity Research Agenda, Salud America! has awarded funding to several pilot grantee research projects.[82]

Conclusions

Widespread evidence conclusively shows that overweight and obesity are public health issues of particular importance in Latino communities. Latino youths are among the hardest hit, with a frequency of overweight or obesity rivaling or exceeding that of White and Black youths. The consequences of childhood obesity among Latinos are numerous; particularly critical are those that can lead to detrimental health effects later in life, such as diabetes and cardiovascular disease.

Many factors are responsible for the development of obesity among Latino children and adolescents and can be traced back to social and familial circumstances, as well as recently identified biological factors. Other factors include poor food habits, lack of physical activity, economic disparities, and advertising and media campaigns directed at Latino youths. Parental perceptions seem to be of particular importance, with many studies showing that Latino parents often do not correctly identify overweight or obesity in their children. Indeed, the impact of family on the health of Latino youths remains an important area of future research, as this represents a critical target for intervention. Another necessary area for more research encompasses barriers to implementing healthy activities in Latino households, such as long parental work hours, the small emphasis placed by Latino parents and grandparents on physical activity, and lack of access to affordable physical activity programs.

While several interventions have been attempted, none have reported significant success. The incorporation of *promotoras* and *curanderos* represents one promising strategy with unique benefits in the Latino community, but even this is associated with certain barriers. The success of the design and implementation of future interventions will depend primarily on further research into the cultural and social underpinnings that explain the rising prevalence of overweight and obesity among Latino youths and demonstrate the effectiveness of tools to fight it.

LESSONS LEARNED
See table 2.1.

References

1. Ogden CL, Flegal KM, Carroll MD, et al. Prevalence and trends in overweight among US children and adolescents, 1999–2000. JAMA. 2002 Oct 9;288(14):1728–32.
2. Ogden CL, Carroll MD, Curtin LR, et al. Prevalence of overweight and obesity in the United States, 1999–2004. JAMA. 2006 Apr 5;295(13):1549–55.
3. Ogden CL, Carroll MD, Flegal KM. High body mass index for age among US children and adolescents, 2003–2006. JAMA. 2008 May 28;299(20):2401–5.
4. Humes KR, Jones NA, Ramirez RR. Overview of race and Hispanic origin: 2010 (C2010BR-02). Washington, DC: U.S. Census Bureau, 2011. Available at: http://www.census.gov/prod/cen2010/briefs/c2010br-02.pdf.
5. Ogden CL, Carroll MD, Kit BK, et al. Prevalence of obesity and trends in body mass index among US children and adolescents, 1999–2010. JAMA. 2012 Feb 1;307(5):483–90.
6. Anderson SE, Whitaker RC. Prevalence of obesity among US preschool children in different racial and ethnic groups. Arch Pediatr Adolesc Med. 2009 Apr;163(4):344–8.
7. Fuentes-Afflick E, Hessol NA. Overweight in young Latino children. Arch Med Res. 2008 Jul;39(5):511–8.
8. Lutfiyya MN, Garcia R, Dankwa CM, et al. Overweight and obese prevalence rates in African American and Hispanic children: an analysis of data from the 2003–2004 National Survey of Children's Health. J Am Board Fam Med. 2008 May–Jun;21(3):191–9.
9. Kimbro RT, Brooks-Gunn J, McLanahan S. Racial and ethnic differentials in overweight and obesity among 3-year-old children. Am J Public Health. 2007 Feb;97(2):298–305.
10. Warner ML, Harley K, Bradman A, et al. Soda consumption and overweight status of 2-year-old Mexican-American children in California. Obesity (Silver Spring). 2006 Nov;14(11):1966–74.
11. Nelson JA, Chiasson MA, Ford V. Childhood overweight in a New York City WIC population. Am J Public Health. 2004 Mar;94(3):458–62.
12. Margellos-Anast H, Shah AM, Whitman S. Prevalence of obesity among children in six Chicago communities: findings from a health survey. Public Health Rep. 2008 Mar–Apr;123(2):117–25.
13. Eichner JE, Moore WE, Perveen G, et al. Overweight and obesity in an ethnically diverse rural school district: the Healthy Kids Project. Obesity (Silver Spring). 2008 Feb;16(2):501–4.
14. Cole TJ, Bellizzi MC, Flegal KM, et al. Establishing a standard definition for child overweight and obesity worldwide: international survey. BMJ. 2000 May 6;320(7244):1240–3.
15. Narayan KM, Boyle JP, Thompson TJ, et al. Lifetime risk for diabetes mellitus in the United States. JAMA. 2003 Oct 8;290(14):1884–90.
16. BeLue R, Francis LA, Colaco B. Mental health problems and overweight in a nationally representative sample of adolescents: effects of race and ethnicity. Pediatrics. 2009 Feb;123(2):697–702.
17. National Cancer Institute. Obesity and cancer risk. Bethesda, MD: National Cancer Institute, 2012. Available at: http://www.cancer.gov/cancertopics/factsheet/Risk/obesity.
18. McArthur LH, Anguiano R, Gross KH. Are household factors putting immigrant Hispanic children at risk of becoming overweight: a community-based study in eastern North Carolina. J Community Health. 2004 Oct;29(5):387–404.
19. Wojcicki JM, Schwartz N, Jiménez-Cruz A, et al. Acculturation, dietary practices and risk for childhood obesity in an ethnically heterogeneous population of Latino school children in the San Francisco Bay area. J Immigr Minor Health. 2012 Aug;14(4):533–9.

20. Balistreri KS, Van Hook J. Socioeconomic status and body mass index among Hispanic children of immigrants and children of natives. Am J Public Health. 2009 Dec;99(12): 2238–46.
21. Wilson TA, Adolph AL, Butte NF. Nutrient adequacy and diet quality in non-overweight and overweight Hispanic children of low socioeconomic status: the Viva la Familia Study. J Am Diet Assoc. 2009 Jun;109(6):1012–21.
22. Unger JB, Reynolds K, Shakib S, et al. Acculturation, physical activity, and fast-food consumption among Asian-American and Hispanic adolescents. J Community Health. 2004 Dec;29(6):467–81.
23. Ayala GX, Rogers M, Arredondo EM, et al. Away-from-home food intake and risk for obesity: examining the influence of context. Obesity (Silver Spring). 2008 May;16(5):1002–8.
24. Faith MS, Scanlon KS, Birch LL, et al. Parent-child feeding strategies and their relationships to child eating and weight status. Obes Res. 2004 Nov;12(11):1711–22.
25. Guerrero AD, Slusser WM, Barreto PM, et al. Latina mothers' perceptions of healthcare professional weight assessments of preschool-aged children. Matern Child Health J. 2011 Nov;15(8): 1308–15.
26. Rollins BY, Belue RZ, Francis LA. The beneficial effect of family meals on obesity differs by race, sex, and household education: the National Survey of Children's Health, 2003–2004. J Am Diet Assoc. 2010 Sep;110(9):1335–9.
27. Singh GK, Yu SM, Siahpush M, et al. High levels of physical inactivity and sedentary behaviors among US immigrant children and adolescents. Arch Pediatr Adolesc Med. 2008 Aug;162(8):756–63.
28. Contento IR, Basch C, Zybert P. Body image, weight, and food choices of Latina women and their young children. J Nutr Educ Behav. 2003 Sep–Oct;35(5):236–48.
29. Lindsay AC, Sussner KM, Greaney ML, et al. Latina mothers' beliefs and practices related to weight status, feeding, and the development of child overweight. Public Health Nurs. 2011 Mar–Apr;28(2):107–18.
30. Crawford PB, Gosliner W, Anderson C, et al. Counseling Latina mothers of preschool children about weight issues: suggestions for a new framework. J Am Diet Assoc. 2004 Mar;104(3): 387–94.
31. Small L, Melnyk BM, Anderson-Gifford D, et al. Exploring the meaning of excess child weight and health: shared viewpoints of Mexican parents of preschool children. Pediatr Nurs. 2009 Nov–Dec;35(6):357–66.
32. Bayles B. Perceptions of childhood obesity on the Texas-Mexico border. Public Health Nurs. 2010 Jul–Aug;27(4):320–8.
33. Guendelman S, Fernald LC, Neufeld LM, et al. Maternal perceptions of early childhood ideal body weight differ among Mexican-origin mothers residing in Mexico compared to California. J Am Diet Assoc. 2010 Feb;110(2):222–9.
34. Kersey M, Lipton R, Quinn MT, et al. Overweight in Latino preschoolers: do parental health beliefs matter? Am J Health Behav. 2010 May–Jun;34(3):340–8.
35. Rich SS, DiMarco NM, Huettig C, et al. Perceptions of health status and play activities in parents of overweight Hispanic toddlers and preschoolers. Fam Community Health. 2005 Apr–Jun;28(2):130–41.
36. Ludwig DS, Peterson KE, Gortmaker SL. Relation between consumption of sugar-sweetened drinks and childhood obesity: a prospective, observational analysis. Lancet. 2001 Feb 17;357(9255):505–8.

37. Moreno LA, Rodriguez G. Dietary risk factors for development of childhood obesity. Curr Opin Clin Nutr Metab Care. 2007 May;10(3):336–41.

38. Grier SA, Mensinger J, Huang SH, et al. Fast-food marketing and children's fast-food consumption: exploring parents' influences in an ethnically diverse sample. J Public Policy Marketing. 2007 Fall;26(2):221–35.

39. Black JL, Macinko J. Neighborhoods and obesity. Nutr Rev. 2008 Jan;66(1):2–20.

40. Larson NI, Story MT, Nelson MC. Neighborhood environments: disparities in access to healthy foods in the U.S. Am J Prev Med. 2009 Jan;36(1):74–81.

41. Lovasi GS, Hutson MA, Guerra M, et al. Built environments and obesity in disadvantaged populations. Epidemiol Rev. 2009;31:7–20.

42. Emond JA, Madanat HN, Ayala GX. Do Latino and non-Latino grocery stores differ in the availability and affordability of healthy food items in a low-income, metropolitan region? Public Health Nutr. 2012 Feb;15(2):360–9.

43. Nord M, Coleman-Jensen A, Andrews M, et al. Household food security in the United States, 2009 (ERR-108). Washington, DC: Economic Research Service, U.S. Department of Agriculture, 2010. Available at: http://www.ers.usda.gov/media/122550/err108_1_.pdf.

44. Rollins BY, Riggs NR, Spruijt-Metz D, et al. Psychometrics of the Eating in Emotional Situations Questionnaire (EESQ) among low-income Latino elementary-school children. Eat Behav. 2011;12 (2):156–9.

45. Kaufman L, Karpati A. Understanding the sociocultural roots of childhood obesity: food practices among Latino families of Bushwick, Brooklyn. Soc Sci Med. 2007 Jun;64(11):2177–88.

46. Crespo CJ, Smit E, Troiano RP, et al. Television watching, energy intake, and obesity in US children: results from the third National Health and Nutrition Examination Survey, 1988–1994. Arch Pediatr Adolesc Med. 2001 Mar;155(3):360–5.

47. Marshall SJ, Biddle SJ, Gorely T, et al. Relationships between media use, body fatness and physical activity in children and youth: a meta-analysis. Int J Obes Relat Metab Disord. 2004 Oct;28(10):1238–46.

48. Matheson DM, Killen JD, Wang Y, et al. Children's food consumption during television viewing. Am J Clin Nutr. 2004 Jun;79(6):1088–94.

49. Rideout VJ, Foehr UG, Roberts DF. Generation M2: media in the lives of 8- to 18-year-olds. Menlo Park, CA: Henry J. Kaiser Family Foundation, 2010. Available at: http://www.kff.org /entmedia/upload/8010.pdf.

50. Rich L. Shiny new things: what digital adopters want, how to reach them, and why every marketer should pay attention. New York, NY: Crain Communications, 2010. Available at: http://adage.com/images/bin/pdf/shiny_new_things.pdf.

51. Yancey AK, Cole BL, Brown R, et al. A cross-sectional prevalence study of ethnically targeted and general audience outdoor obesity-related advertising. Milbank Q. 2009 Mar;87(1):155–84.

52. Harris JL, Schwartz MB, Brownell KD, et al. Fast food FACTS: evaluating fast food nutrition and marketing to youth. New Haven, CT: Yale University, Rudd Center for Food Policy and Obesity, 2010. Available at: http://fastfoodmarketing.org/media/FastFoodFACTS _Report.pdf.

53. Thompson DA, Flores G, Ebel BE, et al. Comida en venta: after-school advertising on Spanish-language television in the United States. J Pediatr. 2008 Apr;152(4):576–81.

54. Chester J, Montgomery K. Interactive food and beverage marketing: targeting children and youth in the digital age—an update. Berkeley, CA: Berkeley Media Studies Group, 2008. Available at: http://digitalads.org/documents/NPLAN_digital_mktg_memo.pdf.

55. Romeo S, Kozlitina J, Xing C, et al. Genetic variation in PNPLA3 confers susceptibility to nonalcoholic fatty liver disease. Nat Genet. 2008 Dec;40(12):1461–5.
56. Goran MI, Walker R, Le KA, et al. Effects of PNPLA3 on liver fat and metabolic profile in Hispanic children and adolescents. Diabetes. 2010 Dec;59(12):3127–30.
57. Butte NF, Cai G, Cole SA, et al. Viva la Familia Study: genetic and environmental contributions to childhood obesity and its comorbidities in the Hispanic population. Am J Clin Nutr. 2006 Sep;84(3):646–54.
58. Butte NF, Comuzzie AG, Cole SA, et al. Quantitative genetic analysis of the metabolic syndrome in Hispanic children. Pediatr Res. 2005 Dec;58(6):1243–8.
59. Cai G, Cole SA, Butte N, et al. A quantitative trait locus on chromosome 18q for physical activity and dietary intake in Hispanic children. Obesity (Silver Spring). 2006 Sep;14(9): 1596–604.
60. Cai G, Cole SA, Butte NF, et al. A quantitative trait locus on chromosome 13q affects fasting glucose levels in Hispanic children. J Clin Endocrinol Metab. 2007 Dec;92(12):4893–6.
61. Cai G, Cole SA, Haack K, et al. Bivariate linkage confirms genetic contribution to fetal origins of childhood growth and cardiovascular disease risk in Hispanic children. Hum Genet. 2007 Jul;121(6):737–44.
62. White House Task Force on Childhood Obesity. Increasing physical activity. In: Solving the problem of childhood obesity within a generation. Washington, DC: Executive Office of the President of the United States, 2010. Available at: http://www.letsmove.gov/sites/letsmove. gov/files/TaskForce_on_Childhood_Obesity_May2010_FullReport.pdf.
63. Sen B, Mennemeyer S, Gary LC. The relationship between perceptions of neighborhood characteristics and obesity among children. In: Grossman M, Mocan N, eds. Economic aspects of obesity (National Bureau of Economic Research Conference Report). Chicago, IL: University of Chicago Press, 2011.
64. Johnson SL, Clark L, Goree K, et al. Healthcare providers' perceptions of the factors contributing to infant obesity in a low-income Mexican American community. J Spec Pediatr Nurs. 2008 Jul;13(3):180–90.
65. Taveras EM, Gortmaker SL, Mitchell KF, et al. Parental perceptions of overweight counseling in primary care: the roles of race/ethnicity and parent overweight. Obesity (Silver Spring). 2008 Aug;16(8):1794–801.
66. Elder JP, Arredondo EM, Campbell N, et al. Individual, family, and community environmental correlates of obesity in Latino elementary school children. J Sch Health. 2010 Jan;80(1): 20–30.
67. Branscum P, Sharma M. A systematic analysis of childhood obesity prevention interventions targeting Hispanic children: lessons learned from the previous decade. Obes Rev. 2011 May;12(5):e151–8.
68. Ayala GX, Vaz L, Earp JA, et al. Outcome effectiveness of the lay health advisor model among Latinos in the United States: an examination by role. Health Educ Res. 2010 Oct;25(5): 815–40.
69. Viswanathan M, Kraschnewski J, Nishikawa B, et al. Outcomes of community health worker interventions (AHRQ Pub. No. 09-E014). Rockville, MD: Agency for Healthcare Research and Quality, 2009. Available at: http://www.ahrq.gov/downloads/pub/evidence/pdf /comhealthwork/comhwork.pdf.
70. Ayala GX, Elder JP, Campbell NR, et al. Longitudinal intervention effects on parenting of the Aventuras para Ninos study. Am J Prev Med. 2010 Feb;38(2):154–62.

71. Clark L, Bunik M, Johnson SL. Research opportunities with curanderos to address childhood overweight in Latino families. Qual Health Res. 2010 Jan;20(1):4–14.
72. Crespo NC, Elder JP, Ayala GX, et al. Results of a multi-level intervention to prevent and control childhood obesity among Latino children: the Aventuras para Ninos study. Ann Behav Med. 2012 Feb;43(1):84–100.
73. Hollar D, Lombardo M, Lopez-Mitnik G, et al. Effective multi-level, multi-sector, school-based obesity prevention programming improves weight, blood pressure, and academic performance, especially among low-income, minority children. J Health Care Poor Underserved. 2010 May;21(2 Suppl):93–108.
74. Johnston CA, Tyler C, Fullerton G, et al. Effects of a school-based weight maintenance program for Mexican-American children: results at 2 years. Obesity (Silver Spring). 2010 Mar;18(3):542–7.
75. Davis JN, Alexander KE, Ventura EE, et al. Inverse relation between dietary fiber intake and visceral adiposity in overweight Latino youth. Am J Clin Nutr. 2009 Nov;90(5):1160–6.
76. Ventura E, Davis J, Byrd-Williams C, et al. Reduction in risk factors for type 2 diabetes mellitus in response to a low-sugar, high-fiber dietary intervention in overweight Latino adolescents. Arch Pediatr Adolesc Med. 2009 Apr;163(4):320–7.
77. HEALTHY Study Group, Foster GD, Linder B, et al. A school-based intervention for diabetes risk reduction. N Engl J Med. 2010 Jul 29;363(5):443–53.
78. van der Heijden GJ, Toffolo G, Manesso E, et al. Aerobic exercise increases peripheral and hepatic insulin sensitivity in sedentary adolescents. J Clin Endocrinol Metab. 2009 Nov;94(11):4292–9.
79. Van Der Heijden GJ, Wang ZJ, Chu Z, et al. Strength exercise improves muscle mass and hepatic insulin sensitivity in obese youth. Med Sci Sports Exerc. 2010 Nov;42(11):1973–80.
80. Johnston CA, Tyler C, McFarlin BK, et al. Weight loss in overweight Mexican American children: a randomized, controlled trial. Pediatrics. 2007 Dec;120(6):e1450–7.
81. Ramirez AG, Chalela P, Gallion KJ, et al. Salud America!: developing a National Latino Childhood Obesity Research Agenda. Health Educ Behav. 2011 Jun;38(3):251–60.
82. Salud America!. Pilot grantees and briefs. San Antonio, TX: Salud America! The RWJF Research Network to Prevent Obesity among Latino Children, 2011. Available at: http://www.salud-america.org/sites/www.salud-america.org/files/upload/List20GranteeBriefs_0.pdf.

CHAPTER 3

Is That All There Is?

A Comprehensive Review of Obesity Prevention and
Treatment Interventions for African American Girls

Bettina M. Beech, DrPH, MPH, and Maryam M. Jernigan, PhD, MA

Data from the National Health and Nutrition Examination Survey (2009–10) indicated a flattening in the rise of the obesity epidemic among some subpopulations of children and adolescents in the United States.[1] Despite this encouraging finding, the overweight and obesity prevalence rates experienced by African American children and adolescents remain unacceptably high.[1]*

There are no significant differences in obesity prevalence between African American boys and girls, despite gender differences in behavioral and contextual risk factors for excessive weight gain. While boys tend to consume higher quantities of sugar-sweetened beverages,[2] girls are more sedentary,[3] consume higher amounts of dietary fat,[4] and experience higher levels of stress and depression[5] and poor sleep hygiene.[6] Biological and gender-related determinants may account for some of the variation in obesogenic behaviors between African American boys and girls; cultural and physiological differences have been shown to be significant factors in accounting for racial differences between African American and White girls.[7]

Racial disparities in overweight and obesity between African American and White girls are well documented,[1,8–11] as are the racial ideological beliefs that characterize the bodies of White girls as more easily controllable and regulated than the bodies of African American girls, which are seen as uncontrollable and more noncompliant.[12,13] In a recently published study using data from the National Growth and Health Study, exercise was found to be an effective weight loss mechanism for White

---

Bettina M. Beech is professor and vice chair of the Department of Social Sciences and Health Policy in the Division of Public Health Sciences, professor in the Departments of Pediatrics and Internal Medicine, and codirector of Maya Angelou Center for Health Equity at Wake Forest School of Medicine. Maryam M. Jernigan is Ruth L. Kirschstein Research Service Award Fellow in the Department of Psychiatry at the Yale University School of Medicine.

* Many chapters in this volume focus, in whole or in part, on African American (or African immigrant) populations. See chapters 7, 8, 10, 12, 18, 21, 25, 26, 29, and 31.

girls, but not for African American girls.[14] The exercise levels and caloric intakes of 1,148 (538 African American and 610 White) girls were examined at ages 12 and 14, and a strong inverse association was found between quartiles of daily accelerometer counts and body mass index (BMI) for White girls at age 14 ($p < .001$), but not for African American girls.[14] The authors hypothesized that African American girls have reduced fat oxidation rates coupled with reduced resting metabolic rates, which predisposes them to retain fat during puberty. Findings such as these have led researchers to question whether the obesity epidemic differs somehow between African American and White girls and have underscored the need for interventions specifically designed for African American girls, taking into account their characteristic biopsychosocial factors.

Obesity prevention and treatment interventions tailored for African American girls are typically designed to integrate cultural elements that are presumed to foster and reinforce obesity-preventing health behaviors. Tailoring interventions based on cultural values, norms, and experiences is believed to enhance participation and improve overall outcomes.[15] Interestingly, culturally tailored interventions targeting African American girls tend to highlight racial dimensions of culture without an explicit focus on gender. Gender, like race, is a deep structural construct influencing health behaviors.[16]

Gender is not a static construction or a single product. Rather, gender emerges from a myriad of social practices constructed within a given social environment. While sex is typically used to describe study participants, social scientists have asserted for some time that sex and gender are not interchangeable constructs. *Sex* refers to the biological facts that differentiate the physiological states and processes of males and females, whereas *gender* is a system of relations that permeates major institutions as well as group- and individual-level interactions. Gender has been used to distinguish and exaggerate differences between the sexes.[17]

The purpose of this study was to systematically review obesity prevention and treatment interventions specifically designed for African American girls 2–19 years of age, highlighting gendered elements in the interventions and associated measures. To our knowledge, this is the first review with a specific focus on gender in obesity prevention and treatment interventions developed for African American girls.*

Methods

We conducted an extensive literature search to identify intervention studies for inclusion in this review, using PubMed, Google Scholar, Cumulative Index to Nursing and Allied Health Literature (CINHAL), and PsyLit. The reference lists of eligible published studies were also scanned for additional studies. Dissertations were not included in this review. Keywords used as search terms included *African American, Black, girls, adolescents, childhood obesity, weight gain prevention, weight loss, obesity treatment,* and *inter-*

---

* For a discussion of the place of obesity prevention efforts in the larger context of the many concerns facing the African American community, see chapter 7.

vention. The review included original articles focusing on African American girls (younger than 18 years of age) that met the following inclusion criteria: (1) English language; (2) intervention studies in which African American girls constituted 50%–100% of the sample; (3) publication between 1980 and July 2011; and (4) peer-reviewed articles. We excluded (1) intervention studies that were only descriptive, without outcome data, (2) review articles, and (3) studies that provided results only in aggregate form, without race-specific outcomes. A highlight of this review was to assess the gender-related intervention components included in obesity prevention and treatment programs for African American girls. Intervention activities that specifically incorporated issues related to "femininity" or socially constructed attitudes and beliefs about girls and obesity were considered gender-related intervention components.

The quality of the studies was evaluated based on study design, measurement of the study variables, cultural tailoring, and sample representativeness. Participation and retention rates were evaluated in treatment and prevention interventions. We further evaluated the length and intensity of the interventions, the inclusion of parents/guardians, gendered elements of the intervention, gendered measures used, and study outcomes. The source of data for the outcome variables (BMI, waist circumference, percentage weight loss) was also considered.

Results

The electronic database search identified 71 articles. After removal of duplicate studies, 62 articles remained, of which 15 were excluded because they were not intervention studies or the interventions included males and females. Of the remaining 47 articles, 29 were excluded after we read the full text; 6 articles did not include outcome data categorized in terms of race and gender. Therefore, this review includes 12 articles. Characteristics of the intervention studies and brief summaries of the central findings are provided in table 3.1 (obesity treatment interventions) and table 3.2 (obesity prevention interventions). Eight of the articles focused on obesity prevention[18-25] and four on treatment interventions.[26-29] The four treatment studies were conducted in different settings (clinics, churches, university, and homes) and used different modalities (feeding study, motivational interviewing, group counseling, and the Internet). The length of the interventions ranged from 16 weeks to 2 years. In three of the four treatment studies, individuals were randomized to condition, and one used a group-randomized design.[27] Each study also incorporated active comparison conditions, in contrast to a traditional "no treatment" control group. "No treatment" control groups varied among the 12 interventions; some were weaker versions of the active intervention, while others delivered interventions not intended to have an effect on weight.[21-24] Interventions were typically delivered by African American females, with the exception of one study, in which one interventionist was a White male clinical psychologist.[21] Body mass index was the most common primary outcome of interest, although percentage body fat was also used to assess weight change over time.

Table 3.1. Obesity treatment interventions targeting African American girls

Study	Sample size and age	Theory	Study design and primary outcomes	Intervention and gendered elements	Gendered measures	Main findings
Williamson et al. (2006)[26]	57; overweight children, 11–15 years old, and their obese parents	Social cognitive theory	RCT; interactive, Internet-based behavioral therapy vs. passive, Internet-based health education intervention; 2-year intervention; BMI and % body fat	Behavioral: nutrition education and behavioral modification; website with interactive components, including links to women's health websites; counseling via asynchronous emails and feedback on program components Passive: links to a variety of health-related websites Both groups received 4 face-to-face counseling sessions	None	During the first 6 months, adolescents in the behavioral condition lost more mean body fat (SD −1.12 +0.47% vs. 0.43 + 0.47 body fat; $p < .05$) and parents lost more body weight (SD −2.43 +0.66 vs. −0.35 +0.64 kg; $p < .06$). Weight regain occurred by the 2-year follow-up assessment; outcomes did not differ between the behavioral and control intervention groups at this time point.
Resnicow et al. (2000)[27]	123; overweight children, 12–16 years old, and their parents	Social cognitive theory	GRT; 10 churches randomized to either high- or moderate-intensity obesity prevention interventions BMI at 6-month follow-up	High-intensity (20–26 sessions): weekly, behavioral, 30 minutes physical activity, low-fat, portion-controlled meal/snack, pagers used to deliver messages to the girls, motivational interviewing phone calls; kick-off retreat Moderate-intensity (6 monthly sessions): nutrition-centered topics and benefits of physical activity Parental participation in every other session in both groups No identified gendered elements in the intervention	None	Intent to treat analysis: there were no significant differences in BMI between the two groups at the 6-month or 1-year follow-up (73% of girls). However, girls in the high-intensity group who attended more than 75% of the sessions did show a decrease in BMI (0.8 units) compared with those with lower attendance, who showed an increase of 0.5 units.

Study	Sample	Theory	Design & measures	Methods	Gender	Results
Wadden et al. (1990)[28]	47; overweight children, 12–16 years old, and their mothers	Social cognitive theory	3-condition RCT; child alone (n = 19); mother and child (n = 14); and mother and child separately (n = 14) Weight, fat (kg), and BMI	16 weekly, 1-hour sessions, with 6 monthly follow-up sessions delivered in a group format Treatment: principles of WRAP using a 100-page treatment manual for girls and separate manual for mothers Weekly homework assignments and quizzes, with incentives provided for completion of assignments Both interventionists were clinical psychologists: one AA female and one White male No identified gendered elements in the intervention	None	Weight reduction: 87% of the total sample reduced BMI, 37% achieved a 5% or more reduction. Those who completed both baseline and end-of-treatment body assessments (n = 28) had an average weight loss of 1.7 kg at the 2nd measurement. There were no significant differences between the three groups; however, daughters whose mothers attended sessions more frequently lost more weight than those whose mothers attended fewer sessions.
Casazza et al. (2012)[29a]	26; overweight children, peripubertal, 9–14 years old	None mentioned	RCT; two dietary conditions with varying CHO intake BMI and weight change	16-week intervention; block randomization to one of two diets: (1) 42% of energy from CHO; (2) 55% of energy from CHO (standard) Two phases: (1) 5-week eucaloric phase; (2) 11-week hypocaloric phase All food was provided for both phases No identified gendered elements in the intervention	None	Both groups had reductions in weight/adiposity, but there were no significant differences between the two groups. Girls exposed to the low-CHO diet did have improved glucose/insulin homeostasis and lower triglycerides.

[a] This study is not designated as an obesity intervention, but the methods included techniques similar to those of obesity prevention programs, and the results did show differences in body fat.

Abbreviations: AA, African American; BMI, body mass index; CHO, carbohydrate; GRT, group randomized trial; RCT, randomized controlled trial; WRP, Weight, Reduction, and Pride.

Table 3.2. Obesity prevention interventions targeting African American girls

Study	Sample size and age	Theory	Study design and primary outcomes	Intervention and gendered elements	Gendered measures	Main findings
Stolley and Fitzgibbon (1997)[18]	65; children 7–12 years old and their mothers	Social learning theory	RCT; random assignment to treatment or attention placebo control group. Outcomes not clearly identified	Treatment group: 1-hour group sessions for 12 weeks, followed by a meeting every 3 months for 15 months; culturally adapted Know Your Body program; received nutrition lessons, food tasting, and culturally relevant music and dance. Control group: general health program conducted weekly in small groups. No identified gendered elements in the intervention	None	Treatment group decreased fat intake (< 32% Cal) and saturated fat (11.5 g) compared with pre-treatment diet of 40% of daily calories from fat and nearly 14 g of saturated fat. Daughters' behaviors changed only minimally over the 12-week intervention. No changes in body weight for the mothers were noted for treatment or control group.
Klesges et al. (2010)[19]	303; children 8–10 years old, with BMI > 25th percentile, and their parents	Social cognitive theory	RCT; random assignment to active or alternative intervention groups (girls only). BMI at 2 years	Active intervention: 90-minute weekly meetings for 14 weeks and then monthly for 20 months; practical experience with nutrition and physical activity; parents participated weekly in a combination of separate and joint sessions. Control intervention: group meeting frequency same as the active intervention; focus on self-esteem and social efficacy. Both interventions were held in community centers or YMCAs and were delivered by AA females with experience in working with children. No identified gendered elements in the intervention	Female AA preadolescent body figure silhouettes to evaluate weight satisfaction	Prevention program did not significantly reduce weight gain compared with alternative intervention group. Results showed statistically significant differences in intake of sweetened beverages, water, and vegetables, but not for physical activity. Post hoc analysis suggested an intervention effect among younger girls, when adjusted for age at 2-year follow-up.

Source	Sample	Theory	Study design/outcome	Intervention description	Additional measures	Results
Robinson et al. (2010)[20]	261; children 8–10 years old, with BMI > 25th percentile	Social cognitive theory	RCT; two-condition study, active vs. active placebo intervention BMI	2-year after-school intervention Active intervention (GEMS Jewels)–dance intervention offered 5 days/wk, 12 months/yr in local community centers; sessions included 1 hour of homework, small snack, and then 45–50 minutes of dance led by female AA college students; screen time reduction intervention including 24 lessons over the 2-year intervention designed to promote AA history and culture; AA mentors met with families in their homes to deliver each lesson Active placebo–culturally tailored, health information–based curriculum on nutrition, physical activity, and reducing cardiovascular risk No identified gendered elements in the intervention	Female AA preadolescent body figure silhouettes to evaluate weight satisfaction	No significant difference in BMI between the two groups. Secondary outcomes were decreased more among girls in the dance and screen time–reduction intervention (e.g., fasting total cholesterol, low-density lipoprotein cholesterol, hyperinsulinemia, and depressive symptoms).
Baranowski et al. (2003)[21]	80; AA girls, 8–10 years old, with BMI > 50th percentile	Social cognitive theory / Elaboration-Likelihood used for the character development and design framework	Pilot RCT study of an Internet intervention; delayed or immediate incentives provided; no control group FJV intake, physical activity, and self-efficacy	8-week Internet intervention; weekly goals were set to increase FJV and water consumption and lifestyle physical activity; activities included role modeling comics, problem solving, goal setting/review No identified gendered elements in the intervention	None	Statistically significant for pre-to-post differences noted for FJV consumption, physical activity, and FJV self-efficacy.

(continued)

Table 3.2. (continued)

Study	Sample size and age	Theory	Study design and primary outcomes	Intervention and gendered elements	Gendered measures	Main findings
Beech et al. (2003)[22a]	60; children 8–10 years old, at risk for obesity, (BMI > 25th percentile), and their parents	Social cognitive theory	Three-condition pilot RCT; two active interventions (child-targeted and parent-targeted) and control group (girls alone) Implementation measures and changes in physical activity, sugared beverage intake, and water intake	12-week intervention with 90-minute weekly sessions conducted in community centers Child-targeted: after-school intervention delivered by AA females; hip-hop dance, taste testing, food-prep activities Parent-targeted: evening sessions focused on physical activity, interactive nutrition activities, and goal setting Comparison condition: monthly sessions focused on self-esteem Girls club embedded in the intervention	Female AA preadolescent body figure silhouettes to evaluate weight satisfaction	Given lack of power and limited time frame, only changes in BMI, waist circumference, and body composition were tracked. Girls in both active intervention conditions (child-targeted and parent-targeted) showed trends toward lower BMI and waist circumference compared with the comparison condition.
Robinson et al. (2003)[23a]	61; children 8–10 years old, at risk for obesity (BMI > 25th percentile)	Social cognitive theory	Pilot RCT of an after-school dance and reduced TV time intervention Implementation measures and changes in physical activity, sugared beverage intake, and water intake	12-week intervention with 90-minute weekly sessions conducted in community centers Treatment group: attended after-school dance classes and home-based intervention to reduce screen time Control group: received newsletters and health education lectures No identified gendered elements in the intervention	Female AA preadolescent body figure silhouettes to evaluate weight satisfaction	Given lack of power and limited time frame, only changes in BMI, waist circumference, and body composition were tracked. Participants in the treatment group showed trends toward lower BMI and waist circumference and an increase in after-school physical activity while reducing screen time.

Study	Sample	Theory	Design; Outcome	Intervention	Measure	Results
Story et al. (2003)[24a]	54; girls 8–10 years old, at risk for obesity (BMI > 25th percentile), and their parents or guardians	Social cognitive theory	Two-arm parallel group RCT; BMI	12-week after-school intervention. Active group: met twice a week; focus on increased physical activity and healthy eating with a family component. Control group: 12-week intervention unrelated to nutrition and physical activity. Girls club embedded in the intervention	Female AA preadolescent body figure silhouettes to evaluate weight satisfaction	After adjusting for baseline values, follow-up BMI did not differ between the active and control groups; however, differences were in the hypothesized direction of change for most variables for the girls and their parents.
Baranowski et al. (2004)[25a]	35; girls 8 years old, at risk for obesity (BMI > 25th percentile), and their parents	Social cognitive theory	Two-arm parallel group RCT; BMI	12-week summer day camp and Internet intervention. Active group: 4-week summer day camp followed by 8-week home-based Internet intervention for girls and parents. Control group: different 4-week summer day camp and monthly home-based Internet intervention without the enrichments in the active intervention. No identified gendered elements in the intervention	Female AA preadolescent body figure silhouettes to evaluate weight satisfaction	No significant difference in BMI between groups at the end of 4 and 12 weeks. By the end of summer camp, girls with high baseline BMIs exhibited a trend ($p < .08$) toward lower BMI compared with girls with high baseline BMIs in the control group.

[a] GEMS multisite studies

Abbreviations: AA, African American; BMI, body mass index; FJV, fruit, juice, and vegetables; RCT, randomized controlled trial.

Of the eight obesity prevention interventions, six represented a single, multisite investigation (Girl's Health Enrichment Multi-site Studies, or GEMS), including four 12-week pilot studies[21-24] and two 2-year longitudinal interventions.[19,20] One of the remaining two prevention interventions was a modification of one of the GEMS pilot studies.[21] The other was a 12-week, randomized pilot intervention conducted in 1997.[18] In contrast to the treatment studies, the obesity prevention interventions were largely conducted in community settings, with one delivered via the Internet.[21] Like the treatment studies reviewed here, the prevention interventions were typically delivered by African American females, and some form of dance was the typical modality used to conduct the physical activity component of the programs.

The obesity treatment and prevention interventions also shared many features, including the theoretical frameworks used, the ages of the African American girls enrolled in the studies, the length of the interventions, and inclusion of parents/ guardians. Social cognitive theory (SCT)[30] was the dominant paradigm used across the obesity treatment and prevention interventions included in this review. This is not surprising since SCT is the most common theory used in successful behavioral change interventions targeting children.[31] Use of this model was apparent through activities involving observational learning, vicarious reinforcement of healthy behaviors, and increasing self-efficacy. African American girls who participated in these intervention studies were between 7 and 16 years of age, with younger girls represented in the prevention studies (7–12 years) and adolescents and preadolescents in the treatment studies (11–16 years). Most of the obesity prevention interventions were pilot studies; only three were full-scale studies with up to 24 months of intervention and follow-up. Lastly, with the exception of one study—a clinic-based, feeding study[29]—all of the interventions involved parents to some degree. In seven studies, parents were fully engaged in the interventions and completed outcome measures, while in others, parents were only tangentially involved. This level of parental participation is not surprising, given that familial influences on health behaviors are well documented in the literature and family-based interventions are considered the gold standard approach in the pediatric/adolescent literature.[32]

Despite being conducted exclusively with African American girls, the majority of the studies did not report the inclusion of explicit elements of the intervention that were focused on gender. Exceptions include one Internet study that provided links to women's health websites and two of the GEMS pilot studies that used a "girls' club" theme that undergirded the intervention activities. Similarly, only one gendered measure was included across the treatment and prevention interventions: body silhouettes designed for use with African American girls.

Discussion

Obesity is thought to be a complex chronic disease developing from an intricate interaction of biological, behavioral, and social influences.[33-35] The impact of these influences can vary by group, and few studies have specified how these factors interact to affect the increased prevalence of overweight and obesity. Comprehensive multidimensional approaches are needed to address obesity among African American girls; it is surprising that few intervention studies have focused explicitly on this population, particularly given the numerous descriptive studies conducted. Findings from this review highlight a significant disparity between the number of intervention studies specifically designed for African American girls and the prevalence of obesity in this population. Our extensive review of the literature, covering four databases and the span of approximately three decades, yielded only 12 studies that met our criteria for inclusion. Of these studies, few demonstrated significant differences in BMI between intervention and comparison groups or maintenance of initial weight changes at follow-up measurement visits. The lack of studies focusing on African American girls is underscored when taking into consideration a recent Cochrane review of child and adolescent obesity interventions,[36] which included 64 randomized controlled trial studies. Given the stringent criteria for the inclusion of studies in a Cochrane review, the number of published obesity studies focused on children and adolescents in general is probably much larger.

The scientists who study obesity among African American girls clearly recognize race and culture as important factors and have developed culturally responsive weight-related interventions targeting this group. Wilson[37] notes in a review of obesity studies targeting ethnic minority youths that culturally tailored interventions were found to have a positive impact on the success of programs designed to improve health behaviors and lower adiposity among these youths. However, the author also points out that few researchers defined what was meant by culturally adapted or culturally tailored treatments. Like Wilson, we found that most studies in our review used material and content that were visually representative of African Americans and/or included African American staff in some research capacity. However, cultural adaptation of treatment interventions should extend beyond superficial racial alterations of treatment protocol elements and the recruitment of people of the same race or ethnicity as subjects for research studies. Culturally tailored interventions are seen as increasingly effective when employing a systemic modification of the intervention protocol that takes into consideration a broader definition of cultural context (i.e., not solely race).[38] Effective cultural adaptation for African American girls includes the attitudes, beliefs, values, and behaviors that reflect their social, political, and ecological realities. Gender, like social class and age, is an important dimension to consider when designing interventions targeting African American girls.

Several facets of gender identification, development, and functioning have been addressed by social cognitive theory, which is widely used as a framework in obesity prevention and treatment interventions. Bandura and Bussey[39,40] proposed the Social Cognitive Theory of Gender-Role Development and Functioning to specify how gender conceptions are constructed from complex mixes of experience and how they connect with motivational and self-regulatory mechanisms that guide gender conduct. Put slightly differently, a myriad of social phenomena occurring independently across a variety of subsystems combine to generate conceptions of gender and gender roles.[40] These concepts appear to interleave quite easily with reciprocal determinism (i.e., the idea that individual behavior and the social environment influence one another) and may supply additional insights into the particular manner in which gender operates in behavioral change initiatives (such as obesity prevention and treatment interventions).

Nearly all of the studies in our review used SCT in the obesity treatment and prevention interventions targeting African American girls. None, however, also incorporated the SCT of gender development. According to Bem,[41] this neglect of gender is indicative of androcentric science, where males represent the "genderless" norm or are seen as representative of the general population. Hence, the neglect of a serious consideration of gender by researchers may have hindered the development of more efficacious obesity treatment and prevention programs targeting African American girls.

Future Directions

Disciplines such as psychology and sociology have made some progress in exploring the racial and gender concepts of African American girls.[42–47] Historically, the racialized experiences of African American girls have been conceptualized using the construct of *racial identity*.[48] Research related to racial identity in African American youths indicates that a more sophisticated racial identity status (i.e., a greater understanding of race, racial discrimination, and the use of strategies to manage such experiences)[49–51] is related to higher self-esteem,[52,53] decreased mental health problems,[54,55] and increased educational outcomes,[56,57] and is probably related to positive health outcomes.[58–60] Gender-based concepts such as gender identity are informed by an individual's beliefs about gender, gender role expectations, and gender expression.[61] Gender identity models parallel racial identity in that a more sophisticated gender identity for girls incorporates a more sophisticated understanding of the social and political connotations of gender.[43]

Although researchers have typically examined race and gender as separate entities, more recently, scholars have proposed that the identity development of African American girls and women,[42] which is central to their positive mental and physical development, is better understood through a recognition of the intersections between race and gender.[42,44–47] African American girls contend with what is called the *double jeopardy* phenomenon. They exist in a society that historically devalues racial/ethnic minorities regardless of gender and disempowers girls regardless of their racial background. As essential cultural components, race and gender identities, developed positively, yield traits that are protective[47,62] against negative psychological and social forces and that contribute to positive physical health outcomes. Yet, few health intervention researchers have extended their definitions of culturally adapted treatment beyond the consideration of race to include gender.

Strengths and Limitations

To our knowledge, this is the first review that examines the inclusion of gendered intervention elements and measures in obesity prevention and intervention studies. A noted strength of this study is the comprehensiveness of the review. However, our review yielded few obesity prevention and treatment intervention studies specifically designed for African American girls and even fewer that explicitly reported any use of gender constructs in the development, assessment, or prevention and treatment of obesity in these girls. We also recognize a clear limitation of our study. Although we carefully reviewed the published intervention descriptions, the intervention protocols could have included additional gender components that were not described in the articles. However, such an omission would speak to the relatively low priority assigned to gender-related issues. To the best of our ability, we attempted to provide information as reported by the original research studies. Inconsistencies in the language used across studies to identify outcomes (see tables 3.1 and 3.2) and the lack of relevant demographic information created additional challenges throughout the review and our interpretation of the findings.

Conclusions

This review of the literature highlights the paucity of obesity intervention studies targeting African American girls. This finding is disquieting given the reverberating calls for the development of interventions and programs to address obesity among this group. The conditions of overweight and obesity in African American girls place them at increased risk for the eventual onset of type 2 diabetes, cardiovascular disease, and other health problems associated with higher mortality rates.[11] In addition to risks for adverse physical health outcomes, African American girls face negative psychological, social, and emotional consequences of obesity that often continue into adulthood and decrease their quality of life.[63]

Based on findings from this review and the consistently high rate of overweight and obesity among African American girls, the need for effective prevention and interventions to address health concerns remains critical. Understanding the social-ecological pathways by which larger societal forces (e.g., race and gender), psychosocial factors, and environments affect obesity for African American girls is a necessity for addressing and preventing future health disparities and facilitating the development of effective treatment programs.

We propose that future interventions targeting African American girls explicitly integrate race- and gender-based constructs throughout the treatment protocols (e.g., theoretical model, recruitment strategies, implementation, and evaluation), while simultaneously considering age and social class. In an effort to facilitate progress in this area, more research is needed specifying research questions that investigate the overall and gendered biological, psychological, and social parts of African American girls' lives that influence or contribute to the development and maintenance of obesity.

This will allow researchers to develop and implement more effective prevention and intervention programs and to increase positive primary outcomes related to overweight and obesity for African American girls. Such a shift in paradigm will allow the elucidation of broader cultural and gendered experiences and an exploration of the heterogeneity among African American girls.

LESSONS LEARNED

- Despite high obesity prevalence rates, few obesity prevention and treatment interventions specifically designed for African American girls were found in the scientific literature.
- Effective, scalable, and cost-effective interventions are critically needed to reduce the obesity prevalence rates among African American girls.
- Existing obesity-related interventions for African American girls often include cultural adaptations; however, specific gender-based constructions are frequently absent.
- Future obesity-related interventions for African American girls specifically designed to address the intersection of race and gender may improve participation and weight-related outcomes.

References

1. Ogden CL, Carroll MD, Kit BK, et al. Prevalence of obesity and trends in body mass index among U.S. children and adolescents, 1999–2010. JAMA. 2012 Feb 1;307(5):483–90. Epub 2012 Jan 17.
2. Brener ND, Merlo C, Eaton D, et al. Beverage consumption among high school students—United States 2010. Atlanta, GA: Centers for Disease Control and Prevention, 2011.
3. Taylor WC, Yancey AK, Leslie J, et al. Physical activity among African American and Latino middle school girls: consistent beliefs, expectations, and experiences across two sites. Women Health. 1999;30(2):67–82.
4. Di Noia J, Schinke SP, Contento IR. Dietary fat intake among urban African American adolescents. Eat Behav. 2008 Apr;9(2):251–6. Epub 2007 Aug 3.
5. Dockray S, Susman EJ, Dorn LD. Depression, cortisol reactivity, and obesity in childhood and adolescence. J Adolesc Health. 2009 Oct;45(4):344–50. Epub 2009 Aug 3.
6. Spilsbury JC, Storfer-Isser A, Drotar D, et al. Effects of the home environment on school-aged children's sleep. Sleep. 2005 Nov;28(11):1419–27.
7. Kimm SY, Barton BA, Obarzanek E, et al. Obesity development during adolescence in a biracial cohort: the NHLBI Growth and Health Study. Pediatrics. 2002 Nov;110(5):e54.
8. Bethell C, Simpson L, Stumbo S, et al. National, state, and local disparities in childhood obesity. Health Aff (Millwood). 2010 Mar–Apr;29(3):347–56.
9. Delva J, Johnston LD, O'Malley PM. The epidemiology of overweight and related lifestyle behaviors: racial/ethnic and socioeconomic status differences among American youth. Am J Prev Med. 2007 Oct;33(4 Suppl):S178–86.
10. Hudson CE. An integrative review of obesity prevention in African American children. Issues Compr Pediatr Nurs. 2008 Oct–Dec;31(4):147–70.

11. Wang Y, Beydoun MA. The obesity epidemic in the United States—gender, age, socioeconomic, racial/ethnic, and geographic characteristics: a systematic review and metaregression analysis. Epidemiol Rev. 2007 May 17;29(1):6–28.

12. Collins PH. The sexual politics of Black womanhood. In: Bent PD, Moran EG, eds. Violence against women: the bloody footprints. Newbury Park, CA: Sage Publications, 1993.

13. Thomas AJ, Witherspoon KM, Speight SL. Toward the development of the Stereotypic Roles for Black Women Scale. J Black Psychol. 2004 Aug 1;30(3):426–42.

14. White J, Jago R. Prospective associations between physical activity and obesity among adolescent girls: racial differences and implications for prevention. Arch Pediatr Adolesc Med. 2012 Jun 1;166(6):522–7.

15. Kreuter MW, Lukwago SW, Bucholtz DC, et al. Achieving cultural appropriateness in health promotion programs: targeted and tailored approaches. Health Educ Behav. 2003 Apr;30(2):133–46.

16. Resnicow K, Baranowski T, Ahluwahlia JS, et al. Cultural sensitivity in public health. Ethn Dis. 2009 Winter;9(1):10–21.

17. Lorber J. Paradoxes of gender. New Haven, CT: Yale University Press, 1994.

18. Stolley MR, Fitzgibbon ML. Effects of an obesity prevention program on the eating behavior of African-American mothers and daughters. Health Educ Behav. 1997 Apr;24(2): 152–64.

19. Klesges RC, Obarzanek E, Kumanyika S, et al. The Memphis Girls Health Enrichment Multisite Studies (GEMS): an evaluation of the efficacy of a two-year obesity prevention intervention in African-American girls. Arch Pediatr Adolesc Med. 2010 Nov;164(11):1007–14.

20. Robinson TN, Matheson DM, Kraemer HC, et al. Stanford GEMS: a randomized controlled trial of culturally tailored dance and reducing screen time to prevent weight gain in low-income African American girls. Arch Pediatr Adolesc Med. 2010 Nov;164(11):995–1004.

21. Baranowski T, Baranowski JC, Cullen KW, et al. The Fun, Food, and Fitness Project (FFFP): the Baylor GEMS pilot study. Ethn Dis. 2003 Winter;13(1 Suppl 1):S30–9.

22. Beech BM, Klesges RC, Kumanyika SK, et al. Child- and parent-targeted interventions: the Memphis GEMS pilot study. Ethn Dis. 2003 Winter;13(1 Suppl 1):S40–53.

23. Robinson TN, Killen JD, Kraemer HC, et al. Dance and reducing television viewing to prevent weight gain in African-American girls: the Stanford GEMS pilot study. Ethn Dis. 2003 Winter;13(1 Suppl 1):S65–77.

24. Story M, Sherwood NE, Himes JH, et al. An after-school obesity prevention program for African-American girls: the Minnesota GEMS pilot study. Ethn Dis. 2003 Winter;13(1 Suppl 1): S54–58.

25. Baranowski T, Klesges LM, Cullen KW, et al. Measurement of outcomes, mediators, and moderators in behavioral obesity prevention research. Prev Med. 2004 May;38 Suppl:S1–13.

26. Williamson DA, Walden HM, White MA, et al. Two-year internet based randomized controlled trial for weight loss in African-American girls. Obesity (Silver Spring). 2006 Jul;14(7): 1231–43.

27. Resnicow K, Yaroch AL, Davis A, et al. GO GIRLS!: results from a nutrition and physical activity program for low-income overweight African American adolescent females. Health Educ Behav. 2000 Oct;27(5):616–31.

28. Wadden TA, Stunkard AJ, Rich L, et al. Obesity in black adolescent girls: a controlled clinical trial of treatment by diet, behavior modification, and parental support. Pediatrics. 1990 Mar;85(3):345–52.

29. Casazza K, Cardel M, Dulin-Keita A, et al. Reduced carbohydrate diet to improve metabolic outcomes and decrease adiposity in obese peripubertal African American girls. J Pediatr Gastroenterol Nutr. 2012 Mar;54(3):336–42.

30. Bandura A. Social cognitive theory of self-regulation. Organ Behav Hum Decis Process. 1991;50:248–87.

31. Lytle L, Achterberg C. Changing the diet of America's children: what works and why? J Nutr Educ. 1995 Sep;27(5):250–60.

32. Institute of Medicine. Preventing childhood obesity: health in the balance. Washington, DC: Institute of Medicine, 2005.

33. Simen-Kapeu A, Veugelers PJ. Should public health interventions aimed at reducing childhood overweight and obesity be gender-focused? BMC Public Health. 2010 Jun 14;10:340.

34. Sweeting HN. Gendered dimensions of obesity in childhood and adolescence. Nutr J. 2008 Jan 14;7:1.

35. Krieger N. Genders, sexes, and health: what are the connections—and what does it matter? Int J Epidemiol. 2003 Aug;32(4):652–7.

36. Oude Luttikhuis H, Baur L, Jansen H, et al. Interventions for treating obesity in children: a review. Cochrane Database Syst Rev. 2009 Jan 21;(1):CD001872.

37. Wilson DK. New perspectives on health disparities and obesity interventions in youth. J Pediatr Psychol. 2009 Apr;34(3):231–44. Epub 2009 Feb 16.

38. Bernal G, Domenech MM. Cultural adaptations: tools for evidence-based practice with diverse populations. Washington DC: American Psychological Association, 2012.

39. Bandura A, Bussey K. On broadening the cognitive, motivational, and sociostructural scope of theory about gender development and functioning: comment on Martin, Rubel, and Szkrybalo (2002). Psychol Bull. 2004 Sep;130(5):691–701.

40. Bussey K, Bandura A. Social cognitive theory of gender development and differentiation. Psychol Rev. 1999 Oct;106(4):676–713.

41. Bem SL. Lens of gender. New Haven, CT: Yale University Press, 1994.

42. Thomas AJ, Hacker JD, Hoxha D. Gendered racial identity of black young women. Sex Roles. 2011;64(7–8):530–42.

43. Lips HM. A new psychology of women—gender, culture, and ethnicity (2nd ed). New York, NY: McGraw-Hill, 1999.

44. Parks EE, Carter RT, Gushue GV. At the crossroads: racial and gender identity development in black and white women. J Couns Dev. 1996 Jul–Aug;74(6):624–31.

45. Shorter-Gooden K. Multiple resistance strategies: how African American women cope with racism and sexism. J Black Psychol. 2004;30:406–25.

46. Shorter-Gooden K, Washington NC. Young, black, and female: the challenge of weaving an identity. J Adolesc. 1996 Oct;19(5):465–75.

47. Ward JV, Robinson-Wood TR. Room at the table: racial and gendered realities in the schooling of black children. In: Skelton C, Fracis B, Smulyan L, eds. SAGE handbook of gender and education. London, UK: Sage Publications, 2006.

48. Cross WE, Parham TA, Helms JE. Nigrescence revisited: theory and research. In: Jones RL, ed. Advances in black psychology. Oakland, CA: Cobb & Henry, 1996.

49. Helms JE. An update of Helms' White and People of Color racial identity models. In: Potterotto JG, Casas JM, Suzuki LA, et al, eds. Handbook of multicultural counseling. Thousand Oaks, CA: Sage Publications, 1995.

50. Neblett EW, Shelton JN, Sellers RM. The role of racial identity in managing daily racial hassles. In: Philogene G, ed. Racial identity in context: the legacy of Kenneth Clark. Washington, DC: American Psychological Association Press, 2004.

51. Sellers RM. A call to arms for researchers studying racial identity. J Black Psychol. 1993 Aug;19(3):327–32.

52. Scottham KM, Cooke DY, Sellers RM, et al. Integrating process with content in understanding African American racial identity development. Self Identity. 2010; 9(1):19–40.

53. Franklin DC, Carter RT. Race related stress, racial identity and psychological health for black Americans. J Black Psychol. 2007 May;33(2):208–31.

54. Sellers RM, Linder NC, Martin PP, et al. Racial identity matters: the relationship between racial discrimination and psychological functioning in African American adolescents. J Res Adolesc. 2006 Jun;16(2):187–216.

55. Yip T, Seaton EK, Sellers RM. African American ethnic identity across the lifespan: a cluster analysis of identity status, identity content and depression among adolescents, emerging adults and adults. Child Dev. 2006 Sep–Oct;77(5):1504–17.

56. Perry JC. School engagement among urban youth of color: criterion pattern effects of vocational exploration and racial identity. J Career Dev. 2008 Jun;34(4):397–422.

57. Smalls CP, White RL, Chavous TC, et al. Racial ideological beliefs and racial discrimination experiences as predictors of academic engagement among African American adolescents. J Black Psychol. 2007 Aug;33(3):299–330.

58. Pieterse AL, Carter RT. An exploratory investigation of the relationship between racism, racial identity, perceptions of health, and health locus of control among black American women. J Health Care Poor Underserved. 2010 Feb;21(1):334–48.

59. Nicolas G, Helms JE, Jernigan MM, et al. The strengths of black children and adolescents. J Black Psychol. 2008 Aug;34(4):261–80.

60. Talleyrand R. Eating disorders in African American girls: implications for counselors. J Couns Dev. 2010 Summer;88(3):319–24.

61. Downing NE, Roush KL. From passive-acceptance to active commitment: a model for feminist identity development for women. Couns Psychol. 1985 Oct;13(4):695–709.

62. Carter RT, Parks EE. Womanist identity and mental health. J Couns Dev. 1996 Aug;74(5): 484–9.

63. Cornette RE. The emotional impact of obesity on children. New York, NY: Elsevier, 2011.

CHAPTER 4

Dietary Acculturation in U.S. Hispanic Communities

Earle C. Chambers, PhD, MPH, Margaret Pichardo, MPH, and Nichola Davis, MD

While overall obesity trends in U.S. adults remained stable from 1999 to 2010,[1] studies have noted an increase in rates of obesity among underserved racial groups, specifically, non-Hispanic Blacks and Mexican Americans.[1,2] The rise in obesity can be partly explained by an increase in consumption of an energy-dense diet with nutrient-poor foods and a decrease in leisure-time physical activity.[3] Several studies demonstrate the consumption of less healthful diets among Hispanic immigrants with increased duration of residence in the United States.[4-8] As immigrating Hispanics become more immersed in American culture, significant changes in dietary behaviors are observed, although the influence of these changes on health is unclear.

Healthy immigrant selectivity refers to the fact that Hispanic immigrants tend to be healthier than their U.S.-born counterparts,[9] even though they have greater poverty rates[10] and come from developing countries with lower standards of living than the United States.[11] One cause of this is a natural selection of healthy immigrants arriving in the United States. As these individuals assimilate into the mainstream culture, however, health and healthy behaviors decline.[12] Scholars discussing the *Hispanic paradox* have attempted to explain the initial protective cultural buffering that diminishes with assimilation, allowing immigrants to become more prone to chronic diseases the longer they live in the United States.[12,13] Among immigrants, acculturation is an important social determinant of health disparities, strongly influencing changes in health behaviors and dietary patterns after arrival in the United States.[14-16] Given that Hispanic subgroups in the United States are more prone to poverty, unhealthy lifestyles, and chronic diseases,[17] culturally sensitive research studies are essential to

Earle C. Chambers is an assistant professor in the Department of Family and Social Medicine and Department of Epidemiology and Population Health at Albert Einstein College of Medicine in the Bronx. Margaret Pichardo is a graduate student at the State University of New York–Stony Brook. Nichola Davis is an associate professor of clinical medicine in the Department of Medicine (General Internal Medicine) and Department of Clinical Epidemiology and Population Health at Albert Einstein College of Medicine.

an understanding of the complex ethnic, social, and environmental factors that influence health.[6,18–21]*

Acculturation is defined as the degree of assimilation undergone by immigrants in adopting the dominant culture's norms, values, behaviors, and attitudes into their daily lives.[13,14,17,18] How acculturation should be measured has been debated; several limitations to measuring acculturation are discussed below.[22,23] Current measures assess, at a single point in time, a person's level of assimilation into the mainstream culture by using single proxies (language, generational status, or nativity) or scales that combine a variety of proxies.[18] Acculturation scales capture a wider perspective on the acculturation experience by assessing an array of factors such as language, cultural identity, social networks, place of origin, and media preferences.[18] Despite this, scales remain limited by the "static and proxy view of acculturation,"[24 [p. 18]] which ignore the influence of other social, economic, or environmental factors that influence the acculturation process.[24] More specifically, the effects of neighborhood and environmental context (e.g., ethnic enclaves, access to healthy options), social context (e.g., racial or ethnic discrimination), and socioeconomic position[20,22,24] are usually considered independent of acculturation, even though these factors can differentially influence an individual's acculturation experience and process of change.[23] As a result, acculturation research is often unable to capture a full picture of the acculturation process of change. In addition, acculturation scales and single proxy measurements also view Hispanics as a homogeneous ethnic and cultural group,[23] ignoring the differences in native language, customs, and beliefs as well as the historical, geographic, and political links of the country of origin[22] and the "starting conditions" of the individual or population that may contribute to distinct acculturation trajectories.[23]

Under the rubric of acculturation, a change in dietary behavior due to a change in country of residence is a process known as *dietary acculturation*.[19] Predominantly, dietary acculturation refers to a process through which immigrants may retain traditional foods, adopt new ones, and/or eliminate traditional foods. Dietary acculturation is a complex, multidimensional, and multidirectional process that focuses on the dietary shifts undergone by immigrants as they assimilate into the host society.[19] This process may be influenced by factors such as dietary habits in the native country, socioeconomic status (SES), and environmental context (e.g., access to healthy food options). Dietary acculturation among Hispanics involves adopting Western diets (specifically, increasing the consumption of dietary fats, fried foods, and sugar-sweetened beverages, with variable retention of traditional dietary patterns).[25]

Through the use of a range of acculturation measurement methods, lower acculturation has been associated with a greater intake of fibers, fruits, and vegetables.[26–29] Several studies show a consistent positive trend between acculturation and higher consumption of calorically dense foods.[28–30] This difference in dietary intake can be

---

* See also chapter 2, which covers many of the points mentioned in this paragraph.

observed over one generation among Mexican American women.[26,30,31] Furthermore, a significant increase in the risk of obesity, hyperlipidemia, and smoking begins to appear at the 15 years (of residence in the United States) threshold, including body mass index (BMI) approaching the levels of U.S.-born individuals.[11] Cross-cultural dietary influences have also been observed between Hispanic subgroups.[32,33] For example, Romero-Gwynn et al.[32] were able to identify 20% of Salvadoran participants who had adopted Mexican food items such as flour tortillas, tacos, dairy cream, Mexican cheeses, and hot salsa into their core diets. The process is also known to take place in a reciprocal fashion, with individuals in the host society adopting certain staple foods, spices, and foreign flavors into their own diets.[32] These models, however, do not fully capture how underlying factors such as socioeconomics, food availability and accessibility, food taste and preference, time constraints on meal preparation, and parental and child inclinations can affect health behaviors.[28,29,34] Dietary acculturation is probably an important mediator of the increased prevalence of obesity and diet-related chronic diseases;[27] however, there is not enough consistent evidence to understand this process fully.[26,35] While several theoretical models have been created in an attempt to explain dietary acculturation, there is still a need for a theory-driven model to encompass all of the underlying factors that may contribute to this phenomenon.[15,18,36] Recent models highlight the multidimensional and bidirectional nature of this process, but little research has been done to analyze the influence of beliefs, tastes, and preferences on eating behaviors.[9,14]

Dietary acculturation has sparked recent interest in nutritional and obesity research due to the exponential growth of the foreign-born Hispanic population in the United States,[6,20] coupled with the overwhelming prevalence of chronic diseases and risk factors such as overweight and obesity. Understanding the process of dietary acculturation, the degree to which immigrants are acculturated to an American diet, and how this is related to obesity can guide the development of effective interventions and educational programs to target this population. This chapter reviews the current literature linking dietary acculturation with obesity in the Hispanic population, with a focus on differences based on nationality.

Methods

Two independent literature searches were conducted using the PubMed, Medline, PsycINFO, and Web of Science databases. Keywords entered into the searches included *acculturation*, *diet*, *obesity*, *Latinos*, *Hispanics*, *dietary trial*, *clinical trial*, and *intervention*. A total of 111 original research articles and review articles published between 2000 and 2012 met our search criteria. From these 111 articles, we selected 17 studies that examined acculturation in relation to diet and/or obesity for inclusion in this review, based on the following criteria: the study (1) focused on adults, (2) included a measure of acculturation, (3) included a measurement of BMI, (4) included a measure of dietary intake, (5) used acculturation in its analysis of diet and/or BMI; and (6) was published in English.

Results

The 17 articles included in this review represent epidemiological studies (11), qualitative studies (5), and a clinical intervention study (1). Tables 4.1 and 4.2 present detailed information on the relationship between diet, acculturation, and obesity among U.S. Hispanics. Each table presents data on BMI, dietary intake, and acculturation.

Acculturation Measures and Proxies

There is no gold standard for assessing acculturation, and studies use a variety of acculturation measurement scales.[35,37–39] Additionally, some studies include a single proxy or a combination of proxies to determine level of acculturation, such as English use; English proficiency; U.S.-born spouse; length of residence in the United States; country of origin/birth; migration status; language used to think, read, write, talk, watch TV, and/or listen to the radio; language of interview; ethnicity; and neighborhood-level factors such as linguistic isolation, poverty rate, and retail food environment.

Dietary Measurements

Each study used at least one type of dietary intake measure. Food frequency questionnaires (FFQs)[40–46] and 24-hour dietary recalls[2,4,38,47] were among the measures most commonly employed. The FFQs varied in the food items and number of items included. Some FFQs were tailored to identify consumption of Hispanic foods.[44,45] In addition to dietary intake, several studies asked about dietary behavior such as healthy dietary habits[29] and intentions to change behavior such as reducing dietary fat.[35] Other studies asked open-ended questions to evaluate stages of change of fruit and vegetable consumption,[28,48–51] perceived food quality,[28,51] food preference,[28,49–51] and barriers to healthy eating.[4,28,48,50]

Hispanic Subgroups

The following subgroups were included in the studies reviewed: Puerto Rican,[4,43,44] Dominican,[44] Cuban,[4,45] Salvadoran,[4] Guatemalan,[4] Colombian,[4] Caribbean,[45] Central American,[45] South American,[45] Mexican American,[4,37,38,40,45,52] and others/mixed ethnicities.[4] Two studies, conducted in Connecticut[42] and on the Mexican-U.S. border,[35] did not report their population's ethnicity or country of birth. One study did not specifically examine differences in diet and acculturation based on country of origin.[4]

Associations between Acculturation and Diet

Table 4.1 summarizes the epidemiological data linking acculturation, diet, and obesity. All studies included a large percentage of females, including five that included only females.[26,38,40,42,43] Using data from the National Health and Nutrition Examination Survey and the Mexican National Institute, Batis et al.[26] found that a high acculturation score (signifying greater acculturation) was positively associated with a

Table 4.1. Epidemiological studies of dietary acculturation in Hispanic communities

Study	Study sample and study design	N	Sample characteristics	Acculturation measure	Dietary measure	BMI measure	Results
Ayala et al. (2004)[38]	Secretos de la Buena Vida Trial Cross-sectional	357	100% female Mean age (yr): 39.7 ± 9.9 Income (average monthly household): $1,501–$2,000 Education[a] 100% MA	1. Acculturation Rating Scale for Mexican Americans-II (ARSMA-II): 30-item 2. Proxy: length of residence	24-hour dietary recall Barriers to healthy eating: 7 and 12 items	BMI/WHR: height, weight, waist and hip measured	1. Years in U.S.: (+) BMI and WHR; (−) Anglo orientation[d] 2. Length of residence: bicultural (≤ 13 yr): lower risk of obesity based on WHR Traditional (≥13 yr): more risk of obesity based on WHR (Isolation from Anglo culture and increased years in U.S. increases risk for obesity.) 3. Bicultural: perceived fewer barriers to low-fat foods, F&V, smaller BMI, WHR
Akresh (2007)[4]	New Immigrant Survey (NIS), 2003 Cross-sectional	2,132	54% female Mean age (yr): 38.8 ± 13.1 Income (annual household): $17,110 Education (mean, yr): 10.2 41% Mexico; 17% El Salvador; 7% Guatemala; 6% Cuba/ DR; ≤ 5% PR/Colombia; ≤ 3% other	1. Speaks English with friends or at work 2. English proficiency 3. U.S.-born spouse 4. Years in U.S.	Scale 1–10: questions about changes in diet, open-ended questions about specific foods.	Self-reported height and weight	1. Acculturation: (+) degree of dietary change 2. Speaking English at work: (+) dietary change for men 3. Spouse born in U.S.: (+) degree of dietary change for women 4. English proficiency: ∅ degree of dietary change for men and women 5. Eating more junk food and meat: (+) BMI for women 6. Coefficient measuring pre-U.S. and post-U.S. diet: (+) BMI

Study	Sample/Design	N	Sample characteristics	Acculturation measure	Dietary measure	Anthropometric	Results
Batis et al. (2011)[26]	Mexican National Institute, 1999; NHANES, 1999–2006 Cross-sectional	16,293	100% female Mean age for adult women (yr)[b]: Mexican, 32.4 ± 0.3; MAMX, 33 ± 0.4; MAUS, 32.2 ± 0.5; NHW, 35.2 ± 0.2 Income[a] Education: less than HS: Mexican, 71%; MAMX, 65.9%; MAUS, 26.3%; NHW, 11.4% 34.8% Mexican; 9.1% MAMX; 22.4% MAUS; 33.5% NHW	1. Country of birth	24-hour dietary recall	BMI from secondary data	1. Country of birth: (low acculturation = Mexico-born; high acculturation = U.S.-born subpopulations) (−) Intake of low-fat meat and fish, high-fiber bread, and lower intake of lower-fiber bread and Mexican fast food (for U.S. subgroups) (+) Dessert and salty snacks, pizza, French fries; energy of unhealthy food percentage was higher for U.S. subpopulations 2. Influence of Mexican diet is almost lost over one generation
Fitzgerald et al. (2008)[42]	Connecticut sample Case control	201	100% female Age range (yr)[b]: 35–60 Income[a] Education: 63.7% with < HS Subgroups[a]	1. Acculturation scale: self-identification, bilingual status, preferred language at home, city size and country/ territory where they grew up, length of residence in U.S.	1. Nutrition knowledge scale: 25-item; 2. FFQ: 18-item	Weight and height measured	Acculturation: (+) regular soft drinks and salty snacks, adjusting for age and BMI

(continued)

Table 4.1. (continued)

Study	Study sample and study design	N	Sample characteristics	Acculturation measure	Dietary measure	BMI measure	Results
Fitzgerald et al. (2006)[43]	Connecticut sample, 1998–99 Cross-sectional	200	100% female Mean age (yr): 28.7 ± 9.7 Household income[a] Education: 62% < HS 100% PR	Proxies: 1. Primary language spoken at home 2. Self-assessed English proficiency	1. FFQ: 14-item	Height and weight measured	Acculturation: 1. Ø Any food group intake 2. (+) Obesity (BMI) 3. Less-acculturated were 54% less likely to be obese
Ghaddar et al. (2010)[37]	Alliance for a Healthy Border, 2006–8; Arizona, California, New Mexico, Texas sample Cross-sectional	2,381	78.8% female Age range (yr)[c]: ≥18 Income: 93% < $30,000 Education: 70% no HS 99% Mexico-born	1. Short Acculturation Scale for Hispanics (SASH): 5-item scale: identifies language preferences 2. Proxies: language, country of birth	1. Weekly frequency of F&V: juice, fruits, green salad, potatoes, carrots, and vegetables 2. Healthy Habits Scale: 12-item	Height, weight, and waist-hip ratio measured	Language (low acculturation): 1. (+) Physical activity 2. (+) 14% higher F&V intake 3. (+) Healthy Habits Scale score 4. (−) BMI (unadjusted) Birthplace (low acculturation): 1. Ø Physical activity 2. (+) 17% higher F&V intake 3. (+) Healthy Habits Scale score 4. (+) BMI (unadjusted)

Study	N	Sample	Acculturation measure	Dietary measure	Anthropometric measure	Results
Gregory-Mercado et al. (2006)[40]	346	100% female; Mean age (yr): 57.5 ± 5.0; Income (household): 42% > $10,000; Education[a]; 74.8% MA; 25.1% NHW	1. Acculturation Rating Scale for MA (ARSMA): language, cultural identity, and assessment of pride in heritage	Three 24-hour dietary recalls	Height and weight measured	1. Acculturation (higher): (−) F&V intake (other comparisons use NHW as reference, with no tests within MA group); 2. Acculturation (lower): (+) BMI for women; 3. Acculturation (more): (+) BMI for MA; 4. Acculturation (lower) / NHW: shared similar consumption of F&V
Arizona Well-Integrated Screening and Evaluation for Women across the Nation (AZ WISE-WOMAN) study; Cross-sectional						
Hu et al. (2011)[35].	693	59% female; Mean age (yr): 19.6 ± 3.33; Income[a]; Education: college students; Subgroups[a]	Short Acculturation Scale for Hispanics (SASH): 1. Language 2. Media 3. Ethnic social relations	1. Stage of Change (dietary fat): evaluates intentions to reduce dietary fat 2. Stage of Change (5-A-Day): 2 items for F&V consumption	Self-reported height and weight	Acculturation: 1. Ø BMI 2. Ø Increased behavioral risks
Students from psychology classes; Mexican-U.S. border sample; Cross-sectional						

(continued)

Table 4.1. (continued)

Study	Study sample and study design	N	Sample characteristics	Acculturation measure	Dietary measure	BMI measure	Results
Hubert et al. (2005)[52]	California sample, July 2000– December 2000 Cross-sectional	901	Women, n = 380 Mean ages (yr): Community women: With BMI < 25: 33.2 ± 10.5 With BMI 25–29.9: 37.1 ± 10.7 With BMI ≥ 30: 39.8 ± 11 Community men: With BMI < 25: 30.7 ± 11 With BMI 25–29.9: 36.3 ± 11.2 With BMI ≥ 30: 38.2 ± 11.9 Labor camp men: With BMI < 25: 31 ± 7.2 With BMI 25–29.9: 33.1 ± 9.3 With BMI ≥ 30: 37.9 ± 9.9 Income (annual household) < $15,000: Community women: With BMI < 25: 32.9% With BMI 25–29.9: 36.4% With BMI ≥ 30: 42.8% Community men: With BMI < 25: 31.5% With BMI 25–29.9: 27.8% With BMI ≥ 30: 30.8%	Proxies: 1. Length of residence in U.S. 2. Generational status 3. Language spoken at home	Dietary practice: high-fat, fast food, F&V consumption, alcohol consumption	Self-reported weight and height	Acculturation: 1. Generation: (+) BMI in women only 2. Years in U.S.: (+) BMI in community sample and (−) BMI in labor camp men

Reference	Study, years, design	Sample characteristics	N	Acculturation measure	Dietary assessment	Anthropometry	Results
Lin et al. (2003)[44]	Massachusetts Hispanic Elders Study (MAHES), 1993–97 Cross-sectional	Labor camp men: With BMI <25: 73.3% With BMI 25–29.9: 67.3% With BMI ≥ 30: 64.7% 66% of community sample: born in Mexico ~98% of labor camp sample: born in Mexico % female[a] Age range (yr)[c]: 60–92 Income[a] Education[a] 54.4% PR; 16.1% DR; 29.5% NHW	825	1. Language used for speaking, reading, and writing	FFQ: 118-item	Height, weight, and waist circumference measured	Acculturation (in order of increasing score; low score = less acculturation): (–) Rice cluster (–) Sweets cluster (–) Starchy vegetables (–) Milk cluster (+) Fruit and cereal Hispanics: (–) Consuming F&V pattern
Monroe et al. (2003)[45]	Multiethnic Cohort Study (MEC) ecological study; Los Angeles sample Cross-sectional	50% female Age range (yr)[c]: 45–74 Education (yr) by number of years in U.S.: Males: Mexico-born: ≤15 years: 8 16–25 years: 7.6 ≥25 years: 8.9	32; 255	1. Generational status. 2. Birthplace. 3. Length of residence in U.S	FFQ: 180-item	BMI from study data	Acculturation: 1. Birthplace: Mexico-born: (+) energy intake 2nd gen. U.S.-born: (–) F&V for males and females; (+) monounsaturated fat intake 3rd gen. U.S. born: (+) monounsaturated fat intake 2. Ø BMI

(continued)

Table 4.1. (continued)

Study	Study sample and study design	N	Sample characteristics	Acculturation measure	Dietary measure	BMI measure	Results
			U.S.-born: 2nd gen.: 11.3 3rd gen.: 12.1 Income[a] 56.5% U.S.-born; 4.3% Mexican-born; 17.2% CA or SA; 4.4% Cuban or Caribbean				

[a] Not reported.
[b] Although the study included children, only adult information is reported.
[c] Overall mean age was not reported.
[d] (−) Anglo orientation = negative association with higher acculturation.

Abbreviations and symbols: BMI, body mass index; CA, Central American; DR, Dominican or Dominican Republic; FFQ, Food Frequency Questionnaire, with number of items; F&V, fruit and vegetables; HS, high school degree; MA, Mexican American; MAMX, Mexican American born in Mexico; MAUS, Mexican American born in the United States; NHANES, National Health and Nutrition Examination Survey; NHW, non-Hispanic White; PR, Puerto Rican or Puerto Rico; SA, South American; WHR, waist-hip ratio; (+), positive association (e.g., as acculturation increases, physical activity increases); (−), negative association (e.g., as acculturation increases, F&V consumption decreases); (∅), no association.

Table 4.2. Qualitative studies of dietary acculturation in Hispanic communities in the United States

Study	Study design	N	Sample characteristics	Acculturation measure	Dietary measure	BMI measure	Results
Cason et al. (2006)[49]	12 focus groups Pennsylvania sample	117	58.1% female Mean age (yr)[a]: 31.9 Income[b]: 46.5% $15,0001–$25,000; 18.8%, ≤ $15, 000 Education (yr): 72% ≤ 9 70.1% Mexican; 29.9% U.S, CA, DR, SA, PR	Open-ended questions asked: 1. How eating habits have changed since coming to the U.S.	1. Food choices and practices 2. Favorite foods 3. What affects food choices? 4. Food security 5. What has changed since immigration, and why? 6. Nutrition knowledge	None	1. Food choice affected by others in the household, price, and convenience 2. Foods that changed: more meats, more vegetables (some said vegetables are more expensive in U.S.) 3. With more money, participants would buy more fruits, vegetables, meats, and seafood (expensive in U.S.) 4. After immigration: ate more junk food and fast food because of convenience, and ate fewer F&V 5. Have gained weight since arriving in U.S.; have gone from preparing 3 meals/day to 1 or 2. 6. Some have a garden and grow vegetables; others can't do so because of space or landlord 7. Flavor, habit, tradition, and pleasure variously affect food choice, price, food quality, language, and difficulty identifying foods by English name

(continued)

Table 4.2. (continued)

Study	Study design	N	Sample characteristics	Acculturation measure	Dietary measure	BMI measure	Results
Hoke et al. (2006)[48]	Focus group Southwestern U.S. sample	15	100% female Mean age (yr): 44.6 ± 5.5 Income (household): 73% < $20,000 Education: 60% completed HS 100% MA	1. Acculturation Rating Scale for Mexican Americans-II (ARSMA-II)	1. Asked how eating behaviors affected personal health 2. Meaning, barriers, and consequences of healthy eating	Height and weight measured	1. Food habits established in childhood and continued through adulthood 2. Factors associated with healthy eating include stress, self-control, and eating habits of significant others
Gray et al. (2005)[50]	Focus groups Mississippi sample	35	51% female Mean age (yr): 39.8 ± 13.2 Education (mean, yr): 11.2 ± 8.6 Income[c] Phase 1: community representatives (n = 11); phase 2: focus group (n = 6) (validation); phase 3: interviews with Hispanic immigrants (n = 18) 11.4% Mexico; 2.9% PR; 2.9% El Salvador; 8.6% Chile; 5.7% Peru; 5.7% Cuba; 2.9% Honduras; 2.9% Nicaragua; 5.7% Argentina	None	1. Native food habits in comparison to U.S. food habits 2. Food purchasing and who usually prepares meals 3. Influences on food choices 4. Meaning of healthy eating 5. Perceived differences in food between countries	None	1. Work and time were the most influential factors on food choices, resulting in convenience foods gaining importance 2. Decreased time spent preparing traditional meals

| Himmel-green et al. (2007)[51] | Project PAN Florida sample Focus groups | 18 | 83.3% female Mean age (yr): 37 ± 11.9 Education: 55% postsecondary Income[c] 67% Colombia; 33% Cuba, Mexico, and Peru | Proxies: 1. Language use 2. Proficiency in spoken and written English 3. Interviews (n = 10) about pre- and post-migration daily lives | Described changes since coming to the U.S.: 1. Diets 2. Food habits 3. Lifestyle | Self-reported body weight increase since arrival | 1. 85.7% were more sedentary in U.S. 2. 71.4% had less time for food preparation 3. 76.5% relied more on fast food 4. 66.7% increase in processed food intake, soda (66.1%), artificial juice (55.6%), sweets (46.7%), and increased weight (82.4%) 5. Decreased time for cooking and relied more on processed foods and soda 6. Decreased physical activity and social interaction 7. Loss of traditional soups "from scratch" 8. 40% of participants concerned about child preference for American foods and loss of control over child's eating habits 9. Pizza and hamburgers seemed to be high-status foods, increased consumption of these items in native countries |

(continued)

Table 4.2. (continued)

Study	Study design	N	Sample characteristics	Acculturation measure	Dietary measure	BMI measure	Results
Sussner et al. (2008)[28]	6 focus groups with individual interviews on subsample Boston sample	51	100% female Mean age (yr)[a]: 32 Income: 47% ≤ $20,000 41% CA; 33% DR; 8% SA; 6% Mexico; 4% U.S.; 2% Spain	Marin acculturation scale: 12-item: language and media use, ethnic social relations	1. Diet, perceived food quality 2. Food and eating practices 3. Breastfeeding practices 4. Beliefs about food, child feeding, and weight status	None	1. Quality and availability of food in native country promoted healthier diets, "pick fruit from the trees," fresh; in U.S., frozen and canned foods 2. Busy schedule and time pressures led to changes in meal routines 3. Little time to eat 3 meals a day; relied on leftovers and snacks

[a] Standard deviations not reported.
[b] In this study, type of income is not clear.
[c] Not reported.
Abbreviations: CA, Central American; DR, Dominican or Dominican Republic; F&V, fruit and vegetables; MA, Mexican American; PR, Puerto Rican or Puerto Rico; SA, South American.

nutrient-poor diet. This association was supported by four other studies.[37,40,42,45] Two of the studies reviewed show no association,[35,43] and one study demonstrates a healthier diet among less acculturated Hispanics.[44]

Monroe and colleagues[45] further observed significant difference in nutrient intake between first-, second-, and third-generation Mexican Americans. The largest degree of dietary change was observed among first- and second-generation Mexican Americans (with the exception of a 30% decrease in tortilla intake observed between second- and third-generation Mexican Americans). The caloric contribution from legumes, rice, and pasta was greatest for first-generation subjects, with Mexican-born individuals reporting slightly greater contributions from vegetables. Among U.S.-born males and females, an 18% and 14% decline, respectively, in calorie-adjusted mean intake of vegetables (including legumes) was seen. Concurrent with this decline in vegetables, there was a significant increase in intake of fats (such as mayonnaise, margarine, or butter) and an almost three times greater increase in salad dressing. These findings are similar to those of Batis et al.,[26] who reported that U.S.-born Mexican Americans had a higher intake of sugar, dessert, salty snacks, and saturated fats and a lower consumption of corn tortillas, high-fat milk, low-fiber bread, and Mexican fast foods in comparison with Mexican-born individuals. Alcohol intake also appears to differ with years of residence in the United States. When compared with Mexican immigrants, a 51% increase in beer consumption was observed for second-generation U.S.-born Mexican males.[45]

Several studies using language spoken as a proxy measure for acculturation show inconsistencies in relation to diet.[4,37,38,40,42,44] In some studies, gender also appears to play a role in the associations observed between acculturation and diet.[4] In the New Immigrant Survey[4] of 2,132 recent immigrants, participants were asked to score on a scale of 1–10 (where 10 means exactly the same and 1 means completely different) how much their diet had changed since immigrating. Respondents who reported speaking English at work reported the greatest degree of dietary change. Among women, being married to a U.S.-born spouse was associated with the greatest degrees of dietary change. This study also observed that eating more fruits was associated with an almost two-unit lower BMI in men and in women, while eating more meat and junk food was associated with an increase in BMI.[4]

Hubert, et al.[52] demonstrated a contrasting relationship between community residents and an agricultural labor camp population in Monterey County, California. Although the finding is not statistically significant, agricultural labor camp men who had lived in the United States for 15 years or more (most acculturated) had lower fat consumption than labor camp men residing in the United States for a shorter time (less acculturated). Among men in the labor camp, for every 10 years lived in the United States, a one-unit decrease in BMI was observed. In contrast, among men in the community, for every 10 years lived in the United States there was a one-unit increase (7–8 pounds) in BMI. Among men and women in the community sample, increasing BMI was positively associated with high-fat, fried, and fast foods.

In contrast to these studies,[26,37,40,42,45] others have shown a positive association between acculturation and healthy dietary habits. Lin et al.[44] studied dietary patterns in elderly Hispanics, primarily from Puerto Rico and the Dominican Republic. Five distinct dietary patterns were identified, including (1) fruits and breakfast cereal, (2) starchy vegetables, (3) rice, (4) whole milk, and (5) sweets. Hispanics in general had greater energy intake from the starchy vegetable or milk pattern; however, this differed according to acculturation. The most acculturated Hispanics adopted a nutrient-rich fruit and breakfast cereal diet, while the least acculturated consumed the fewest fruits and vegetables and the most fat (from cooking oils) and had the highest BMI and waist circumference.

Association between Acculturation and BMI

The relationship between acculturation and BMI is also complex and inconsistent,[35,40,52] and a direct association between acculturation and BMI has been observed that may be independent of diet. Ayala and colleagues[38] found that increased length of residence in the United States was positively associated with an increase in BMI and waist-to-hip ratio (WHR). Individuals who had lived in the United States for 13 years or less were less likely to be at risk for obesity based on WHR. Fitzgerald et al.[43] also reported a positive relationship between acculturation and BMI and found that less acculturated women were 54% less likely to be obese than highly acculturated women. In contrast to these findings, Gregory-Mercado et al.[40] observed that women with lower levels of acculturation had higher BMI. Hubert et al.[52] further documented generational differences among obese Mexican Americans. In their study, obese Mexican Americans were 1.6 times more likely than participants in the leanest groups to be second-generation Mexican Americans. The study also showed a strong positive association between BMI and generational status for community women and a positive relationship between fast-food consumption and BMI. In addition, obese men were more likely to speak English at home as their primary language.

Qualitative Studies

Qualitative studies attempt to explain the complex mechanisms by which Hispanic immigrants adopt unhealthy dietary behaviors. These studies present the major social barriers, perceptions, and beliefs that may explain why, with increased time in the United States, Hispanics show a decreased consumption of fruits and vegetables and a higher intake of fast foods and sodas.[48] While quantitative data allow us to observe associations between acculturation and diet, understanding why these associations occur is limited by these study designs. Hence, qualitative studies provide complementary insights and may provide a more in-depth explanation for food patterns and choices observed among the population of study. Qualitative studies can also yield insights about the potential barriers that influence an individual's food choices and other obesity-related health outcomes.

Table 4.2 presents a summary of five qualitative studies that explored the relationships between acculturation, diet, and BMI. The populations in these studies represent Mexican American, Puerto Rican, Dominican, South American, and Central American subgroups, among others. Three of the studies used an acculturation measure,[28,48,51] one did not measure acculturation,[50] and the fifth study asked an open-ended question about post-immigration eating habits.[49] As in the epidemiological studies, most participants were female. Overall, five salient themes emerged as barriers to healthy eating: (1) food cost, (2) food quality, (3) lack of time for food preparation, (4) lack of effort to prepare healthy meals, and (5) family and children's food preferences. In several studies, the higher price and lower quality or "freshness" of fruits and vegetables in the United States compared with the participant's native country were deterrents to purchasing these items.[28,49,50] For many participants, fruits and vegetables were perceived to be more "organic" or "fresher" in their native countries because one could pick them straight from the trees, while in the United States frozen and canned foods predominate.[28] In one study, Cason et al.[49] noted that the higher cost of fruits and vegetables also seemed to influence choices in the United States. Participants in eight focus groups reported a greater consumption of fast food and junk food mainly because of convenience. Additionally, six focus groups reported eating fewer fruits in the United States, and another four groups reported eating fewer vegetables. Focus groups that reported eating more fruits and vegetables in the United States also reported making more money in the United States than in their native countries.

Lack of time seemed to be a predominant barrier present in all five studies.[28,48–51] In a study involving 18 Hispanic adults living in the United States for 2.5 years or less, Himmelgreen et al.[51] found that 71.4% of participants reported having less time for food preparation and depended more on fast foods (76.5%). Further, 46% of participants reported an increased intake of healthy foods since arriving in the United States. However, 82.4% also reported an increase in weight and increased consumption of processed foods (66.7%), soda (61.1%), artificial juice (55.6%), and sweets (46.7%). Decreased time to prepare meals, increased work demands, reduced family interactions, and less control over children's food consumption have led to changes in meal preparation and dietary choices.[48–51] A study of 51 Hispanic mothers noted similar barriers to cooking traditional meals.[28] Time restrictions have led mothers to rely on leftovers and snacks, skipping meals or "eating on the go." Mothers also noted a decrease in length of breastfeeding due to work demands. In several studies,[28,49–51] mothers reported being concerned about their children's weight, as they seemed to have a growing preference for American foods, pizza, and hamburgers instead of *comida casera*, or traditional meals.

Stress, self-control, and social influences also appeared to be important factors in healthy eating, as noted by Hoke and colleagues[48] in a study of 15 overweight Mexican American women. Women reported overeating as a way to cope with stress as well as a lack of self-control with favorite foods. Cooking the family's favorite meals

Table 4.3. Intervention study of acculturation and BMI among Hispanics in the United States

Study	Study design	N	Sample characteristics	Acculturation measure	Dietary measure	BMI measure	Results
Barrera et al. (2012)[39]	¡Viva Bien! Intervention Care control, n = 138; culturally adapted intervention, n = 142 Colorado sample	280	100% female Mean age (yr)[a]: 57.11 Income[b] 79.6% U.S.-born; 15.8% Mexico-born	1. Acculturation Rating Scale for Mexican Americans-II (short form): Anglo orientation vs. Latina orientation[c]	Semi-quantitative FFQ assessed calories from saturated fat	Height and weight measured	Acculturation significantly associated with intervention outcomes: Anglo orientation positively associated with problem solving and social resources for dietary practices, and negatively associated with improvements in diet; Latina orientation negatively associated with improvements in dietary resources

[a] Standard deviations not reported.
[b] Not reported.
[c] Anglo orientation = closer to American culture; highly acculturated.
Abbreviations: BMI, body mass index; FFQ, food frequency questionnaire.

and the additional effort needed to cook a separate meal in order to maintain a healthy diet deterred women from eating healthfully. This study also asked participants about weight management practices. Many women reported being less active in the United States or trying diet pills or products such as green tea as weight management techniques.

Interventions

As our understanding of dietary acculturation expands and we learn more about the barriers that prevent Hispanics from maintaining a healthy weight and diet, it is important to translate these findings into culturally appropriate interventions that target obesity. Our literature search identified only one article that measured associations between acculturation and BMI in the context of a lifestyle intervention (table 4.3). Barrera et al.[39] used a tailored weight management and nutrition program for a Hispanic population at all levels of acculturation. In this intervention among 280 Hispanics, Barrera and colleagues measured acculturation using the Acculturation Rating Scale for Mexican Americans, which uses two subscales to measure Latina orientation versus Anglo orientation. The results showed that Latina orientation was associated with a lower intake of percentage of calories from saturated fat. U.S.-born women consumed more saturated fat at baseline than foreign-born women. At the six-month assessment, Anglo orientation was associated with improved problem solving and improvements in the use of dietary supportive resources such as sharing healthy low-fat recipes with friends and family members and walking or doing exercise activities with neighbors; Latina orientation was negatively associated with the use of dietary supportive resources.

Discussion

In this review of the literature on the relationship between dietary acculturation and risk of obesity among Hispanics in the United States, we specifically included those studies that inform the underlying mechanism by which the dietary transition that accompanies assimilation into an American lifestyle increases the obesity risk. Most of the studies reviewed, but not all, point toward the deleterious health effects for Hispanics of adopting a more energy-dense (calorie-dense) diet—in particular, an increase in BMI, which contributes to increased risk for obesity and cardiovascular disease. Interestingly, the influence of the acculturation process on dietary choices seems to vary by Hispanic subgroup.[41] Some possible reasons for these differences may lie in the social factors that contribute to the unhealthy disparities experienced by Hispanics, including neighborhood and individual SES,[43,53,54] food insecurity,[55] limited access to fresh fruits and vegetables,[56,57] the availability of traditional food items,[38] food taste preferences, limited time to prepare meals, influence of children in the home,[28] and a person's life story prior to immigration.[33,38]

Several studies show that living longer in the United States is associated with dietary choices and preferences consistent with the promotion of obesity. While not included in this review, Kaplan et al.[58] reported a highly significant difference in obesity rates for Hispanics living in the United States less than 5 years versus 15 years or more (5.1% vs. 63.8% for males; 7.9% vs. 58.2% for females). Individuals living in the United States for more than 15 years are 4.3 times more likely to be obese than those living in the United States less than 5 years. Other studies included in this review were able to determine a length-of-residence threshold for when these differences begin to appear; one qualitative study noted differences within 2.5 years of residence.[51] The duration of the dietary buffer that protects recent immigrants is shrinking, due in part to a nutrition transition taking place throughout Latin America.[34] As a result, immigrants may be arriving in the United States with higher BMIs. Therefore, it is important that public health professionals develop obesity and dietary interventions for Hispanic populations with low levels of acculturation that may be beneficial for new immigrants. Early dietary interventions coupled with programs that motivate active lifestyles can influence healthy behaviors early in the acculturation process.

Overall, trends predominantly point toward the adoption of unhealthy dietary choices with increased acculturation. Not all studies confirm this relationship, however, which may be partly due to differences in measurement (see table 4.1), socioeconomic and environmental context, and characteristics specific to Hispanic subgroups (such as geographic location and food selectivity and accessibility). Furthermore, some studies demonstrate selective dietary acculturation, where unhealthy traditional dietary behaviors may be replaced over time.[45] For example, a common finding in several studies is the consumption of whole milk instead of low-fat milk and the use of cooking oils and fats among recent, less-acculturated immigrants.[44,45,59] With increased length of residence in the United States, whole milk is replaced by nonfat or low-fat milk.[45]

Acculturation studies looking at dietary changes often overlook the strong and differential influence of individual-, family-, and community-level SES on the retention or adoption of healthy dietary behaviors.[23] Hispanics have lower SES than non-Hispanic Whites,[20] regardless of SES proxy, with more than 20.7% of Hispanics living below the federal poverty level, compared with 9.0% of non-Hispanic Whites.[24] Such financial constraints are likely to affect Hispanics' dietary acculturation. Hispanics living in predominantly low-income neighborhoods may experience limited access to healthy food options such as fresh fruits and vegetables.[57,60] As dietary acculturation research moves toward a better understanding of the process by which food selectivity takes places, it is essential to consider the relationship of SES and neighborhood context with acculturation in order to better understand the complex mechanisms that contribute to poor health outcomes and disparities.[15,20,23,24]

Acculturation research has several limitations—in particular, the inconsistent use of scales and proxies that result in positive, negative, and mixed associations.[15,18] Furthermore, the cross-sectional design of most studies precludes the ability to identify a temporal relationship between acculturation and dietary changes and/or risk for obesity, further limiting the conclusions that can be drawn regarding this relationship.

Much of the literature to date focuses on Mexican Americans and may not be appropriately applied to other ethnic groups such as Puerto Ricans, Cubans, Dominicans, and Central and South Americans (subgroups that are also expanding rapidly in the United States).[25,61] The differences in risk of obesity by Hispanic subgroup[57] warrant examination within these groups.

Language preference and/or proficiency, length of residence in the United States, age at time of immigration, country of birth, and immigration status are the most frequently assessed indicators of acculturation. Looking across all the quantitative studies reviewed in this chapter, we find that language use and proficiency as a proxy for acculturation (or as a scale measurement) appears to be the most consistent predictor for unhealthy dietary changes and risk for obesity among Hispanics. While these indicators show an association with health outcomes, they do not provide a mechanism for this relationship, nor are they able to capture fully the social and psychological context that predisposes Hispanic immigrants to making unhealthy choices.[16] Very few qualitative studies have explored the context of dietary choices, and these studies are often limited by the use of convenient ethnic subgroups, providing results that cannot be extrapolated to the entire Hispanic population. Another limitation of the current research is that studies looking at changes in dietary patterns may not examine the individual's diet, dietary behaviors, and/or dietary patterns in his or her place of origin. This limits dietary acculturation studies to a simple cross-sectional and static view of any changes that might have taken place in a person's dietary choices on exposure to the American diet.

Our review did not include data specific to physical activity, which is an integral factor in the development of obesity and cardiovascular disease. A contrasting relationship to that of acculturation and dietary choices is observed with physical activity and sedentary behaviors.[28,49] Individuals with lower levels of acculturation are less likely to be active than those who are more acculturated,[9,31] but the association is not as strong as with dietary habits.[31] A complete discussion of physical activity was outside the scope of this review, but physical activity is an important factor in weight control and obesity risk and can also be adversely affected by neighborhood and environmental context.

Lastly, few studies examine the elderly Hispanic population.[44] This lack of research on the elderly is important, given the current growth of both the Hispanic and elderly populations in the United States. Further studies are needed to inform the development of interventions for elderly Hispanics.

Conclusions

This review has highlighted the current literature and its limitations in understanding the dietary acculturation process that Hispanic immigrants experience in the United States. To address some of the limitations of acculturation research, there is a need for further study of theory-driven models of acculturation that may provide a model to understand the complex relationships between acculturation and diet.[15,36] A greater understanding of these relationships could promote the development of interventions that capitalize on both retaining healthier dietary habits from the native country and adopting healthy dietary habits in the United States, with the goal of reducing chronic disease risk.

LESSONS LEARNED
- The acculturation process seems to influence different Hispanic subgroups differently.
- Interventions tailored to recent immigrants may be beneficial in promoting a healthy and active lifestyle early in the acculturation process.
- There is a need for acculturation research to study further theory-driven models that can capture the effects of environmental, social, and cultural contexts and socioeconomic position in the complex mechanisms that lead to poor health choices and adverse health outcomes.

References

1. Flegal KM, Carroll MD, Kit BK, et al. Prevalence of obesity and trends in the distribution of body mass index among us adults, 1999–2010. JAMA. 2012 Feb 1;307(5):491–7.
2. Montoya JA, Salinas JJ, Barroso CS, et al. Nativity and nutritional behaviors in the Mexican origin population living in the US-Mexico border region. J Immigr Minor Health. Feb 2011;13(1):94–100.
3. Morales LS, Lara M, Kington RS, et al. Socioeconomic, cultural, and behavioral factors affecting Hispanic health outcomes. J Health Care Poor Underserved. 2002 Nov;13(4): 477–503.
4. Akresh IR. Dietary assimilation and health among Hispanic immigrants to the United States. J Health Soc Behav. Dec 2007;48(4):404–17.
5. Artinian NT, Schim SM, Vander Wal JS, et al. Eating patterns and cardiovascular disease risk in a Detroit Mexican American population. Public Health Nurs. 2004 Sep–Oct;21(5): 425–34.
6. Ayala GX, Baquer B, Klinger S. A systematic review of the relationship between acculturation and diet among Latinos in the United States: implications for future research. J Am Diet Assoc. Aug 2008;108(8):1330–44.
7. Benavides-Vaello S. Cultural influences on the dietary practices of Mexican Americans: a review of the literature. Hisp Health Care Int. 2005;3(1):27–35(9).
8. Bermudez OI, Tucker KL. Cultural aspects of food choices in various communities of elders. Generations. 2004 Fall;28(3):22–7.
9. Abraído-Lanza AF, Chao MT, Flóez KR. Do healthy behaviors decline with greater acculturation? Implications for the Latino mortality paradox. Soc Sci Med. 2005 Sep;61(6):1243–55.
10. Betancourt JR, Carrillo JE, Green AR, et al. Barriers to health promotion and disease prevention in the Latino population. Clin Cornerstone. 2004;6(3):16–26; discussion 27–9.
11. Koya DL, Egede LE. Association between length of residence and cardiovascular disease risk factors among an ethnically diverse group of United States immigrants. J Gen Intern Med. 2007 Jun;22(6):841–6.

12. Franzini L, Ribble JC, Keddie AM. Understanding the Hispanic paradox. Ethn Dis. 2001 Autumn;11(3):496–518.

13. Eamranond PP, Wee CC, Legedza AT, et al. Acculturation and cardiovascular risk factor control among Hispanic adults in the United States. Public Health Rep. 2009 Nov–Dec;124(6): 818–24.

14. Edelman D, Christian A, Mosca L. Association of acculturation status with beliefs, barriers, and perceptions related to cardiovascular disease prevention among racial and ethnic minorities. J Transcult Nurs. 2009 Jul;20(3):278–85.

15. Abraido-Lanza AF, Armbrister AN, Florez KR, et al. Toward a theory-driven model of acculturation in public health research. Am J Public Health. 2006 Aug;96(8):1342–6.

16. Perez-Escamilla R. Dietary quality among Latinos: is acculturation making us sick? J Am Diet Assoc. 2010 May;110(5 Suppl):S36–9.

17. Padilla R, Steiner JF, Havranek EP, et al. A comparison of different measures of acculturation with cardiovascular risk factors in Latinos with hypertension. J Immigr Minor Health. 2011 Apr;13(2):284–92.

18. Wallace PM, Pomery EA, Latimer AE, et al. A Review of acculturation measures and their utility in studies promoting Latino health. Hisp J Behav Sci. 2010 Feb;32(1):37–54.

19. Satia-Abouta J, Patterson RE, Neuhouser ML, et al. Dietary acculturation: applications to nutrition research and dietetics. J Am Diet Assoc. 2002 Aug;102(8):1105–18.

20. Carter-Pokras O, Zambrana RE, Yankelvich G, et al. Health status of Mexican-origin persons: do proxy measures of acculturation advance our understanding of health disparities? J Immigr Minor Health. 2008 Dec;10(6):475–88.

21. Corral I, Landrine H. Acculturation and ethnic-minority health behavior: a test of the operant model. Health Psychol. 2008 Nov;27(6):737–45.

22. Hunt LM, Schneider S, Comer B. Should "acculturation" be a variable in health research? A critical review of research on US Hispanics. Soc Sci Med. 2004 Sep;59(5):973–86.

23. Lopez-Class M, Castro FG, Ramirez AG. Conceptions of acculturation: a review and statement of critical issues. Soc Sci Med. 2011 May;72(9):1555–62.

24. Zambrana RE, Carter-Pokras O. Role of acculturation research in advancing science and practice in reducing health care disparities among Latinos. Am J Public Health. 2010 Jan;100(1): 18–23.

25. Van Wieren AJ, Roberts MB, Arellano N, et al. Acculturation and cardiovascular behaviors among Latinos in California by country/region of origin. J Immigr Minor Health. 2011 Dec;13(6):975–81.

26. Batis C, Hernandez-Barrera L, Barquera S, et al. Food acculturation drives dietary differences among Mexicans, Mexican Americans, and non-Hispanic whites. J Nutr. 2011 Oct; 141(10):1898–1906.

27. Mainous AG 3rd, Diaz VA, Geesey ME. Acculturation and healthy lifestyle among Latinos with diabetes. Ann Fam Med. 2008 Mar–Apr;6(2):131–7.

28. Sussner KM, Lindsay AC, Greaney ML, et al. The influence of immigrant status and acculturation on the development of overweight in Latino families: a qualitative study. J Immigr Minor Health. 2008 Dec;10(6):497–505.

29. Neuhouser ML, Thompson B, Coronado GD, et al. Higher fat intake and lower fruit and vegetables intakes are associated with greater acculturation among Mexicans living in Washington State. J Am Diet Assoc. 2004 Jan;104(1):51–7.

30. Guendelman S, Abrams B. Dietary intake among Mexican-American women: generational differences and a comparison with white non-Hispanic women. Am J Public Health. 1995 Jan;85(1):20–5.

31. Colby SE, Morrison S, Haldeman L. What changes when we move? A transnational exploration of dietary acculturation. Ecol Food Nutr. 2009 Jul–Aug;48(4):327–43.

32. Romero-Gwynn E, Gwynn D, De Lourdes Lopez M, et al. Dietary patterns and acculturation among immigrants from El Salvador. Nutr Today. 2000 Nov–Dec;35(6):8.

33. Pérez-Escamilla R, Putnik P. The role of acculturation in nutrition, lifestyle, and incidence of type 2 diabetes among Latinos. J Nutr. 2007 Apr;137(4):860–70.

34. Satia JA. Dietary acculturation and the nutrition transition: an overview. Appl Physiol Nutr Metab. 2010 Apr;35(2):219–23.

35. Hu DX, Taylor T, Blow J, et al. Multiple health behaviors: patterns and correlates of diet and exercise in a Hispanic college sample. Eat Behav. 2011 Dec;12(4):296–301.

36. Satia-Abouta J. Dietary acculturation: definition, process, assessment, and implications. Int J Hum Ecol. 2003;4(1):71–86.

37. Ghaddar S, Brown CJ, Pagan JA, et al. Acculturation and healthy lifestyle habits among Hispanics in United States–Mexico border communities. Rev Panam Salud Publica. 2010 Sep;28(3):190–7.

38. Ayala GX, Elder JP, Campbell NR, et al. Correlates of body mass index and waist-to-hip ratio among Mexican women in the United States: implications for intervention development. Women Health Iss. 2004 Sep–Oct;14(5):155–64.

39. Barrera M Jr, Toobert D, Strycker L, et al. Effects of acculturation on a culturally adapted diabetes intervention for Latinas. Health Psychol. 2012 Jan;31(1):51–4.

40. Gregory-Mercado KY, Staten LK, Ranger-Moore J, et al. Fruit and vegetable consumption of older Mexican-American women is associated with their acculturation level. Ethn Dis. 2006 Winter;16(1):89–95.

41. Derby CA, Wildman RP, McGinn AP, et al. Cardiovascular risk factor variation within a Hispanic cohort: SWAN, the Study of Women's Health Across the Nation. Ethn Dis. 2010 Autumn;20(4):396–402.

42. Fitzgerald N, Damio G, Segura-Perez S, et al. Nutrition knowledge, food label use, and food intake patterns among Latinas with and without type 2 diabetes. J Am Diet Assoc. 2008 Jun;108(6):960–7.

43. Fitzgerald N, Himmelgreen D, Damio G, et al. Acculturation, socioeconomic status, obesity and lifestyle factors among low-income Puerto Rican women in Connecticut, U.S., 1998–1999. Rev Panam Salud Publica. 2006 May;19(5):306–13.

44. Lin H, Bermudez OI, Tucker KL. Dietary patterns of Hispanic elders are associated with acculturation and obesity. J Nutr. 2003 Nov;133(11):3651–7.

45. Monroe KR, Hankin JH, Pike MC, et al. Correlation of dietary intake and colorectal cancer incidence among Mexican-American migrants: the multiethnic cohort study. Nutr Cancer. 2003;45(2):133–47.

46. Smith WE, Day RS, Brown LB. Heritage retention and bean intake correlates to dietary fiber intakes in Hispanic mothers—Qué Sabrosa Vida. J Am Diet Assoc. 2005 Mar;105(3):404–11.

47. Carrera PM, Gao XA, Tucker KL. A study of dietary patterns in the Mexican-American population and their association with obesity. J Am Diet Assoc. 2007 Oct;107(10):1735–42.

48. Hoke MM, Timmerman GM, Robbins LK. Explanatory models of eating, weight, and health in rural Mexican American women. Hisp Health Care Int. 2006;4(3):143–51(9).

49. Cason K, Nieto-Montenegro S, Chavez-Martinez A. Food choices, food sufficiency practices, and nutrition education needs of Hispanic migrant workers in Pennsylvania. Top Clin Nutr. 2006;21(2):145–58.

50. Gray VB, Cossman JS, Dodson WL, et al. Dietary acculturation of Hispanic immigrants in Mississippi. Salud Publica Mex. 2005 Sep–Oct;47(5):351–60.

51. Himmelgreen D, Daza NR, Cooper E, Martinez D. "I don't make the soups anymore": Pre- to post-migration dietary and lifestyle changes among Latinos living in West-Central Florida. Ecol Food Nutr. 2007;46(5–6):427–44.

52. Hubert HB, Snider J, Winkleby MA. Health status, health behaviors, and acculturation factors associated with overweight and obesity in Latinos from a community and agricultural labor camp survey. Prev Med. 2005 Jun;40(6):642–51.

53. Diez Roux AV. Investigating neighborhood and area effects on health. Am J Public Health. 2001 Nov;91(11):1783–9.

54. Dubowitz T, Subramanian SV, Acevedo-Garcia D, et al. Individual and neighborhood differences in diet among low-income foreign and U.S.-born women. Women Health Iss. 2008 May–Jun;18(3):181–90.

55. Dhokarh R, Himmelgreen DA, Peng YK, et al. Food insecurity is associated with acculturation and social networks in Puerto Rican households. J Nutr Educ Behav. 2011 Jul–Aug;43(4): 288–94.

56. Park Y, Quinn J, Florez K, et al. Hispanic immigrant women's perspective on healthy foods and the New York City retail food environment: a mixed-method study. Soc Sci Med. 2011 Jul;73(1):13–21.

57. Park Y, Neckerman KM, Quinn J, et al. Place of birth, duration of residence, neighborhood immigrant composition and body mass index in New York City. Int J Behav Nutr Phys Act. 2008 Apr 6;5:19.

58. Kaplan MS, Huguet N, Newsom JT, et al. The, association between length of residence and obesity among Hispanic immigrants. Am J Prev Med. 2004 Nov;27(4):323–6.

59. Romero-Gwynn E, Gwynn D. Dietary patterns and acculturation among Latinos of Mexican descent. East Lasing, MI: Julian Samora Research Institute, Michigan State University, 1997.

60. Grigsby-Toussaint DS, Zenk SN, Odoms-Young A, et al. Availability of commonly consumed and culturally specific fruits and vegetables in African-American and Latino neighborhoods. J Am Diet Assoc. 2010;110(5):746–52.

61. Goel MS, McCarthy EP, Philips RS, et al. Obesity among US immigrant subgroups by duration of residence. JAMA. 2004 Dec;292(23):2860–7.

CHAPTER 5

Obesity in Correctional Facilities
A Review of Epidemiology and Etiology

Kimberly Dong, MS, RD, and Alice Tang, PhD

Prevalence and incidence rates of chronic medical conditions such as obesity, hypertension, and diabetes have been steadily rising over the past few decades in the general, non-institutionalized U.S. adult population. Data from the 2009–10 National Health and Nutrition Examination Survey show that, based on body mass index (BMI), the prevalence of obesity was 35.5% among adult men and 35.8% among adult women; the prevalence of overweight (but not obesity) was 33.3%, more than double the rates of obesity in the early 1970s.[1] Over roughly the same period of time, rates of incarceration in the United States have risen dramatically, with a more than sevenfold increase between 1972 and 2009.[2] By the end of 2010, nearly 2.3 million adults were incarcerated in state and federal prisons or in local jails.[3] Although few data are currently available, it is expected that increases in rates of obesity and other chronic medical conditions in the correctional population will parallel those in the general population.

Health care costs, one of the top cost drivers for correctional facilities' budgets, are rising. In 2004, the Council of State Governments reported spending $3.7 billion annually on health care in state prisons, approximately 10% of correctional spending.[4] In 2007, the Federal Bureau of Prisons reported spending an estimated $736 million for inmate health care.[5] To our knowledge, health care costs for local jails have not been published. Obesity contributes to increased health care expenditures through (1) higher medical care and pharmacy costs to treat obesity-related illnesses (such as diabetes and cardiovascular disease), and (2) higher infrastructure costs, including larger beds, uniforms, restraints, and chairs, as well as size-appropriate medical equipment (e.g., longer hypodermic needles, larger MRI machines).[6] In this chapter we review the current literature on obesity rates in jail and prison populations as well as some of the etiology or potential factors that may contribute to this important issue. Since both obesity[1,6,7] and incarceration disproportionately affect members of minority groups,[4,7,8]

Kimberly Dong and Alice Tang are affiliated with the Department of Public Health and Community Medicine, Tufts University School of Medicine.

it is imperative to examine racial/ethnic, socioeconomic, and educational disparities in correctional facilities and how they relate to rates of obesity. In addition, we examine nutrition practices in prisons, as these may contribute to obesity among inmates over the long term. Where appropriate, distinctions will be made between jail and prison populations because the predisposing factors, as well as interventions to prevent or treat obesity, are likely to be different in these two settings.

Methods

The literature review in this chapter is divided into two parts. The first is a narrative review of peer-reviewed journal articles and reports or white papers published by the government or by nonprofit organizations. We used Medline/PubMed database resources to identify research articles focusing on obesity and nutrition in correctional populations up to June 2012. Search terms included a topic keyword and the words *prisons, correctional facilities, jails,* or *incarceration.* Topic keywords included *obesity, body mass index, heart disease, cardiovascular disease, nutrition, diet,* and *dietary intake.* Limits to the search strategy were English-language articles, human studies, and adult populations. The electronic search was followed by extensive manual searching of reference lists in the identified articles. We also searched the Internet for government reports and white papers, using the same search terms.

The second part of the review was based primarily on information obtained from mass media sources (newspaper and magazine articles) and informal interviews with food service experts within correctional facilities. Our initial source was the Rhode Island Department of Corrections, where the medical program director, physician, and dietitian described issues with weight gain in their facilities and provided sample menus and commissary lists from their institutions for evaluation. To obtain nutrition information from correctional facilities in other parts of the country, we contacted the Association of Correctional Food Service Affiliates' Chair Dietitians in Corrections, who then contacted nutrition professionals of the National Commission on Correctional Health Care (NCCHC) by email. Those interested in speaking with us and in providing sample menus and nutrition information from their facilities were asked to contact us directly. Respondents included the departmental food administrator at the California Department of Corrections and Rehabilitation and the state food service administrator, Food & Farm Services, at Georgia Correctional Industries. Interviews were conducted with these specialists (by Kimberly Dong, lead author of this chapter) by phone and email during May to June 2012.

Results

Narrative Literature Review

Disparities within the U.S. Incarcerated Population Large disparities exist in rates of incarceration in the United States: men, racial and ethnic minorities, and people of younger ages are much more likely to be incarcerated than their counterparts

Table 5.1. Estimated number of sentenced prisoners (per 100,000 U.S. residents) under state and federal jurisdiction, by sex, race, Hispanic origin, and age, 2010

Age	Male[a]				Female[a]			
	Total[b]	White[c]	Black[c]	Hispanic	Total[b]	White[c]	Black[c]	Hispanic
Total[d]	943	459	3,074	1,258	67	47	133	77
18–19	462	149	1,555	563	20	11	40	31
20–24	1,511	638	4,618	1,908	102	72	182	122
25–29	2,098	980	6,349	2,707	168	125	299	202
30–34	2,261	1,061	7,299	2,808	175	136	309	189
35–39	2,014	995	6,600	2,486	158	124	289	153
40–44	1,752	916	5,637	2,146	147	106	290	156
45–49	1,489	788	4,751	1,901	115	81	238	117
50–54	1,051	552	3,441	1,495	68	45	150	88
55–59	650	347	2,239	1,031	34	22	76	55
60–64	391	233	1,262	679	17	12	33	29
65+	143	95	418	294	4	3	7	8

Source: Guerino et al. (2011).[11]

[a] Counts based on prisoners with a sentence of more than 1 year.

[b] Includes American Indians, Alaska Natives, Asians, Native Hawaiians, other Pacific Islanders, and persons identifying two or more races.

[c] Excludes persons of Hispanic or Latino origin.

[d] Includes persons under age 18.

(table 5.1). Incarceration rates for some of these groups are particularly high, and disparities continue to increase. Blacks account for only 12% of the U.S. population but approximately 43% of the incarcerated population.[9,10] Across all racial groups, 1 in 44 males between the ages of 30 and 34 are incarcerated; for Black men in this age group, the rate is 1 in 13.[11] Men are approximately 14 times more likely than women to be incarcerated, but incarceration rates among women are increasing at a faster pace. For women, the highest rates are for Black women aged 30–34 years, for whom the incarceration rate is 1 in 324.[11]

As reported by Mauer and King,[12] the incarceration ratios by states show higher overall rates of imprisonment for Blacks than for all other races/ethnicities (6:1), but ratios differ widely by region, ranging from a high of 14:1 in Iowa to a low of 2:1 in Hawaii. As of 2007, seven states (Iowa, Vermont, New Jersey, Connecticut, Wisconsin, North Dakota, and South Dakota) had Black-to-White ratios of incarceration of greater than 10:1. These high ratios can be attributed to two types of sentencing practices: some states have above-average rates of incarceration among Blacks and average rates among Whites, while other states have average rates of incarceration among Blacks but lower-than-average rates among Whites. In addition, sentencing disparities exist: Whites are more likely to be incarcerated at local jails and to be released in a shorter time, while Blacks tend to be sentenced and held to longer prison terms for similar crimes. Consequently, Blacks are more likely than Whites to suffer negative consequences of prison terms, including separation from family and reduced employment prospects after release.

Rates of incarceration among Hispanics are nearly 3 times higher than those of Whites, but 2.4 times lower than those of Blacks.[11] In 2010, the highest rates of incarceration for Hispanics (approximately 1 in 37 U.S. residents) were those for males aged 25–39. The Hispanic-to-White ratio of incarceration is as high as 7:1 (in Connecticut).[12]

Prevalence of Obesity in U.S. Correctional Facilities To our knowledge, only two studies have reported on the prevalence of obesity in U.S. correctional facilities. Using data from the 2002 Survey of Inmates in Local Jails, the 2004 Survey of Inmates in State and Federal Correctional Facilities, and the 2002, 2003, and 2004 waves of the National Health Interview Survey–Sample Adult File (NHIS-SAF), Binswanger et al.[8] estimated and compared the prevalence of several chronic medical conditions (including obesity) among jail inmates, prison inmates, and the non-institutionalized U.S. population. Using the same data sources (except only the 2004 wave of the NHIS-SAF), Houle[7] reported the prevalence of obesity in adult males only and explored disparities by race/ethnicity and education. Body mass index, defined as weight (in kilograms) divided by height (in meters) squared, was used to define obesity ($BMI \geq 30 \, kg/m^2$) and was based on self-reported heights and weights in all of the surveys.

Binswanger et al.[8] found that both jail and prison inmates were significantly less likely to be obese than non-institutionalized adults, after accounting for differences in age, sex, race, education, U.S. birthplace, marital status, work, and alcohol consumption in the populations. Jail inmates were also significantly less likely to be overweight ($BMI = 25-30 \, kg/m^2$) than non-incarcerated adults. Prison inmates, however, were 22% more likely to be overweight than non-institutionalized adults, after adjusting for the same confounders (odds ratio $= 1.22$; 95% $CI = 1.12$ to 1.32). Houle[7] found similar results in that age-adjusted prevalence rates of obesity among adult male inmates in jails were significantly lower than those for non-institutionalized adult males (17.9% vs. 26.2%). Age-adjusted obesity rates for adult males in state and federal prison facilities (25% and 28.2%, respectively) were similar to those for non-institutionalized adult males. However, when pooled, the total male inmate population had a lower obesity prevalence than non-incarcerated adult males across all racial/ethnic and education subgroups. Houle's data did not include prevalence of overweight in any of the populations. Table 5.2 summarizes the prevalence of obesity in U.S. incarcerated vs. non-incarcerated populations reported by these two studies.*

---

* One major limitation of both studies discussed above is that BMI data are based on self-reports of height and weight. There may be systematic differences in self-reports of heights and weights between incarcerated and non-incarcerated populations, men and women, and jail and prison inmates. Surveys that include actual measured weights and heights would reveal a more accurate picture of rates of obesity and overweight in correctional facilities.

Table 5.2. Prevalence of overweight and obesity in the U.S. institutionalized and non-institutionalized populations, by age and race/ethnicity

| Characteristic[a] | Percent (95% CI) | | Prison inmates | |
	Non-institutionalized	Jail inmates	State	Federal
By age (yr)				
Overweight				
18–33	28.8 (25.5–32.1)	32.9 (29.9–35.9)	40.7 (37.8–43.6)	
34–49	35.8 (32.5–39.2)	39.4 (36.0–42.9)	46.7 (43.7–49.6)	
50–65	38.4 (35.2–41.7)	44.8 (41.7–47.9)	49.8 (47.1–52.5)	
Obese				
18–33	18.4 (18.0–18.9)	13.9 (13.5–14.2)	19.1 (19.0–19.3)	
34–49	25.4 (25.3–25.5)	19.1 (19.0–19.3)	24.7 (24.5–24.9)	
50–65	29.1 (28.9–29.3)	22.1 (22.0–22.1)	27.4 (27.0–27.8)	
By race/ethnicity				
Obese				
Non-Hispanic White	26.3 (25.0–27.6)	15.1 (12.8–17.4)	20.8 (19.4–22.4)	21.9 (18.2–25.6)
Non-Hispanic Black	30.9 (27.5–34.4)	20.0 (17.4–22.6)	27.9 (26.3–29.5)	31.8 (27.9–35.7)
Hispanic	27.4 (24.7–30.0)	17.8 (13.9–21.6)	27.3 (23.4–31.1)	26.1 (14.8–37.5)

Sources: For age: Binswanger et al. (2009)[8]; male and female adults aged 18–65; prevalences are sex-adjusted; state and federal prisons combined. For race/ethnicity: Houle (2011)[7]; adult males aged 25–59 years; prevalences are age-adjusted.

[a] Overweight = body mass index (BMI) 25.0–29.9 kg/m^2; obesity = BMI $\geq$ 30 kg/m^2.

While these data show that obesity prevalence is lower in the inmate populations as a whole than in the general population, the difference between jail inmates and prison inmates is interesting. Binswanger et al.'s finding[8] that overweight prevalence is significantly higher among prison inmates could be explained by inmates' weight gain during their prison terms. If such weight gain is a trend and that trend continues, increased rates of obesity in prisons could become more of an issue.

Potential Causes for Increased Obesity in Prisons The health status of inmates largely reflects their status prior to entry. Often, incarcerated individuals come from lower socioeconomic groups and may be more likely to smoke cigarettes, have lower-quality dietary intake, and have less physical activity[6,8]—all of which can increase the risk for obesity, cardiovascular disease, and other chronic diseases.[9] Female inmates often come from low socioeconomic groups and may have preexisting health conditions such as underweight, overweight, and/or nutrient deficiencies when entering jails and prisons, due to chaotic lifestyles prior to incarceration.[13] The stressful environment of correctional facilities can exacerbate the risk for obesity and heart disease, and the health of inmates can deteriorate during incarceration due to poor-quality dietary intake; physical inactivity; small, confined spaces; poor sleep; depression;

anxiety; and other mental health conditions.[8,14] It has been noted that, while incarcerated, women tend to gain weight, and this is attributed to high-starch meals, lack of exercise, boredom, and stress.[13] In addition, as the non-incarcerated and incarcerated population ages, chronic diseases become more prevalent, especially among obese people.

Two published studies report on weight gain among female prisoners. Plugge et al.[14] found that on entry into a U.K. prison, women were at high risk for cardiovascular disease; 85% smoked cigarettes, 87% were physically inactive, 86% did not eat at least five servings of fruits and vegetables per day, and 30% were overweight or obese. After one month in prison, none of these risk factors improved, except that the amount of tobacco smoked decreased (despite no change in the number of women smoking). Overall, these women gained an average of 1.5 kg of body weight during the first month in prison. An earlier study, conducted in 1979 among 56 nonpregnant female inmates in the Connecticut Correctional Institution at Niantic, found that 30.3% of the women were obese on admission and nearly half (48.5%) were obese after three months.[13] Ninety-one percent of those who stayed three months or longer had gained an average of 14 pounds, equivalent to 2 pounds per month. These data provide some insight into the issue of weight gain in longer-term correctional facilities.

Consequences of Obesity in Correctional Facilities Obesity increases the risk of many diseases, such as diabetes, hypertension, heart disease, arthritis, asthma, fatty liver, and cancer. Heart disease is the leading cause of death in men and women in the U.S. general population, accounting for 25% of deaths.[15] This is not surprising, given that, currently, about one-third of U.S. adults are obese (35.7%) and that obesity is a major risk factor for heart disease.[16] Mortality statistics published by the U.S. Department of Justice demonstrate a robust connection between mortality and chronic diseases in those who are incarcerated (table 5.3). Between 2001 and 2009, heart disease and cancer were the top causes of illness-related deaths by far.[17] In 2009 alone, nearly 60% of all illness-related deaths were caused by heart disease (29%) and cancer (30%). Not surprisingly, inmates aged 55 years and older had the highest mortality rates among all age groups due to heart disease and cancer over the nine-year period.[17]

Health care costs have consistently been found to be significantly higher for overweight and obese individuals than for normal-weight individuals.[18] In a review of the literature, Bachman[19] found that health care costs increase with higher BMI, with increases ranging from 21% to 54% in class I obesity (BMI = 30–34.9 kg/m^2), 43% to 57% in class II obesity (BMI = 35–40 kg/m^2), and 78% to 111% in class III obesity (BMI > 40 kg/m^2) compared with normal-weight patients. Increases were in the range of 2%–23% for those who were overweight (BMI = 25–29.9 kg/m^2) compared with those of normal weight. Increased costs were primarily due to increased needs for medications for diabetes and cardiovascular disease. In correctional facilities, an increase in proportion of overweight and obese inmates can place additional strains

Table 5.3. Number of state prisoners' deaths, by cause of death, 2001–9

Cause of death	2001	2002	2003	2004	2005	2006	2007[a]	2008	2009
All causes	2,877	2,942	3,165	3,129	3,172	3,239	3,392	3,452	3,408
Illness	2,573	2,621	2,843	2,787	2,819	2,833	2,981	3,030	3,014
Heart disease	749	804	821	838	851	866	710	859	870
Cancer	628	650	776	710	763	765	600	858	911
Liver disease	225	201	248	219	237	244	190	234	258
AIDS-related	272	242	210	146	154	132	120	98	94
All other illnesses[b]	699	724	788	874	814	826	1,361	981	881
Suicide	169	168	199	200	213	220	216	197	201
Homicide	39	48	49	49	56	55	57	40	55
Drug/alcohol intoxication	35	37	23	22	37	57	41	58	50
Accident	23	31	26	34	30	33	29	26	31
Other/unknown	38	37	25	37	17	41	68	101	57

Source: Noonan et al. (2011).[17]

  [a] In 2007, a high number of cases were missing cause-of-death information. These cases were classified as "all other illnesses."

  [b] Includes other specified illnesses (such as cerebrovascular disease, influenza, cirrhosis, and other nonleading natural causes of death) as well as unspecified illnesses.

on the prison health care system, including (as previously noted) additional infrastructure needs (larger uniforms, beds, restraints, and chairs), size-appropriate medical equipment (e.g., longer hypodermic needles), more frequent transportation to hospitals, and increases in medical care and pharmacy costs.[6]

Nutrition and Lifestyle Interventions in Correctional Facilities To our knowledge, there are no recently published studies of controlled trials focusing on nutrition and physical activity interventions within correctional facilities. However, one study from the WISEWOMAN national program funded by the Centers for Disease Control and Prevention (CDC) suggests the feasibility of incorporating effective interventions within a correctional facility. The WISEWOMAN program offers heart disease screening and lifestyle education interventions (including developing healthier diets, increasing physical activity levels, and stopping smoking) to underinsured and uninsured women who participate in the National Breast and Cervical Cancer Early Detection Program. The WISEWOMAN program in South Dakota included one site at the Women's Prison in Pierre.[20] Although the authors found no differences in baseline rates of several risk factors for heart disease (hypertension, overweight, obesity, low-HDL cholesterol, and high total cholesterol) after adjusting for demographic differences between the incarcerated and non-incarcerated participants, they reported significantly higher rates of attendance in the lifestyle intervention sessions among the incarcerated women (53%) than among the non-incarcerated women (23%). In addition, 42.5% of the incarcerated women completed all of the intervention sessions, compared with only 3.6% of the non-incarcerated women (adjusted odds ratio = 21.4; 95% CI = 14.0 to 32.8; $p < .01$). These results demonstrate that prisons may offer an ideal environment and opportunity to conduct lifestyle interventions, as inmates may have more time to dedicate to programs. However, more work needs to be done to improve and maximize participation rates within this setting.

Other results from the South Dakota study[20] suggest several other potential benefits of conducting nutrition/lifestyle interventions in a prison setting. First, the authors found that both total cholesterol levels and smoking rates were significantly lower at baseline among incarcerated women than among non-incarcerated women, even after adjusting for demographic differences between the two groups. These findings were attributed to the diet and the smoke-free environment imposed by the prison. Further analysis of the menus at the prison corroborated the authors' hypothesis that the meals followed the American Heart Association's recommendations for cardiovascular risk reduction. Second, incarcerated women with high cholesterol levels were more likely to be unaware of their condition than non-incarcerated women. This suggests the need not only for screening to identify those at risk on entry into the correctional facility but also for creating effective educational strategies to properly inform inmates of their health conditions. To our knowledge, the effects of the lifestyle intervention on the health status of the incarcerated women have not yet been published. The prison setting offers the opportunity for health screenings and interventions, and the environment is conducive to high levels of participation. Proper scientific testing of nutrition and lifestyle interventions is critically needed.

Mass Media Sources and Informal Interviews

Current Nutrition Practices in Correctional Facilities Menu planning for correctional facilities varies according to regulations and standards set by the governing agency, accreditation status, food service contracts, and court mandates.[21] Both the NCCHC and the American Correctional Association (ACA) offer nutrition standards and best practices based on the Dietary Reference Intakes (DRIs) established by the Institute of Medicine.[22] However, few correctional facilities implement these practices on a full scale unless they are accredited by the NCCHC or ACA. Many facilities may use current, nationally accepted guidelines to plan menus, such as the U.S. Department of Agriculture's My Plate, the USDA and Department of Health and Human Services' Dietary Guidelines for Americans, and the American Heart Association's dietary recommendations.[22] Some juvenile correctional facilities may adhere to the USDA's National School Lunch and Breakfast Program nutrition requirements. Most facilities, however, focus only on fulfilling caloric and food safety needs,[22,23] unless otherwise required. Some facilities aim to provide certain amounts of specific food groups or specific nutrients, such as dietary fat and calcium.

There are many challenges to planning nutritious, affordable, palatable, and low–security risk foods for inmates, including few incentives for facilities to implement standards that are not mandatory. Major challenges to menu planning include budget limitations and contract requirements, which may influence the availability of healthy food. Due to state budget limitations, many correctional facilities are challenged with keeping meal costs to 60–90 cents per meal, or less than $3 per inmate per day[24] (B. Wakeen, personal communication). Milk replacements (mixtures of soy-based products), artificial sweeteners, and fortified foods and beverages are often used because they are less costly than the original products (B. Wakeen, personal communication). As in other food service environments, there are challenges in meeting food preferences based on differences in ethnicity, culture, and region of the country. In addition, correctional facilities face unique nutrition challenges such as security issues limiting access to specific foods and eating utensils. Common contraband items include certain fruits, sugar, yeast, select spices, and glass, plastic, or metal containers, utensils, and knives.[22] For example, some correctional facilities serve chicken only as chicken patties (to prevent the use of chicken bones as a weapon) or limit pepper (so that it cannot be thrown in someone's face).[22] Fresh fruits may be categorized as contraband because inmates may take fruit back to their cell to make "hooch," or alcohol, by fermenting the fruit in hidden spaces. Limited kitchen space and staffing can affect cooking methods. Finally, careful attention must be paid to meeting the food preferences of a large majority of prisoners in order to prevent unrest and rioting.

Provision of therapeutic diets in correctional facilities varies. Some may have diabetic/carbohydrate-controlled, low-fat/low-cholesterol, low-sodium, lactose-free, gluten-free, high-calorie/high-protein, vegetarian, and allergen-free diets.[22] Due to the increased rates of hypertension, heart disease, and diabetes, some facilities offer a general heart-healthy menu. To accommodate dietary preferences due to religious practices, such as for Muslim or Jewish inmates, a general vegetarian-style menu may be offered that adheres to relevant dietary restrictions. However, most institutions offer therapeutic or other special diets that are as similar as possible to the diet served to the main population, for financial and logistical reasons and to avoid showing favoritism or creating possibilities for trading food.[22]

Sample Prison Menus According to a recent survey of U.S. correctional facilities, most institutions served, on average, 2,000–4,000 calories/day.[23] Table 5.4 shows a sampling of menu offerings in male correctional facilities in three states (California, Rhode Island, and South Carolina), and table 5.5 shows caloric and macronutrient (carbohydrates, proteins, and fats) ranges for these menus compared with recommendations for adults in the general population to maintain a healthy BMI. All three menus are at higher caloric levels than most adults need to maintain a healthy BMI with a sedentary lifestyle. In addition to the quantity of food, dietary quality must be assessed, since this can be compromised due to budget constraints. In general, the macronutrients are at levels appropriate for the calorie ranges, but the quality of these foods often needs improvement. Some of the foods may be highly processed

Table 5.4. Sample menus from California Department of Corrections and Rehabilitation, Rhode Island Department of Corrections, and South Carolina Department of Corrections

Meal	California	Rhode Island	South Carolina
Breakfast	Stewed prunes	Fresh fruit	Orange drink
	Oatmeal	Bran flakes	Hard boiled eggs
	Danish	Hard cooked eggs	Grits
	Eggs	Bread	Cereal
	Wheat toast	Margarine	Biscuits
	Nonfat milk	Salt/pepper/sugar	Coffee
	Coffee		Milk
Lunch	Lunchmeat sandwich	Turkey salad	Bologna
	Chips	Torpedo roll	Cheese
	Cookies	Lettuce/tomato	Bun
	Fresh fruit	Mayo	Mayo
	Sugar-free beverage	Pasta salad with broccoli, carrots, celery	Mustard
		Beverage	Macaroni salad
			Salad bar
			Iced tea
			Orange drink
Dinner	Salad/dressing	Braised stew beef	Grilled chicken
	Breaded fish	Salad/dressing	Onion gravy
	Scalloped potatoes	Mashed potatoes	Steamed rice
	Pinto beans	Carrots	Steamed cabbage
	Green peas	Fruit	Cornbread
	Catsup	Bread	Cake
	Wheat bread	Margarine	Iced tea
	Applesauce cake	1% milk	Milk
	Sugar-free beverage	Salt/pepper	

Sources: For California: printed with permission from Laurie Maurino, RD, Departmental Food Administrator, California Department of Corrections and Rehabilitation. For Rhode Island: printed with permission from Fred Vohr, MD, Medical Program Director, Rhode Island Department of Corrections. For South Carolina: Collins and Thompson (2012).[24]

(such as refined grains and lunch meats), high in sodium, and high in starch. Additionally, some of the vegetables and fruits offer minimal nutrition, with salads made predominantly from iceberg lettuce and fruits canned in heavy syrups. Most often, meats and fish are breaded and fried, and heart-healthy dietary fats are rarely, if ever, offered. An issue that is often overlooked is the potential physiological effect of poor-quality diets on behavior and violence.[25]

Even though calorie levels may be high, correctional facility menus may still be at risk of specific micronutrient deficiencies, which must be monitored. All dietary analyses of menus assume inmates eat and drink all of the food and beverages provided during meals, making it challenging to assess inmates' actual dietary quality and adequacy. In addition, given the limited information on nutrition facts panels,

Table 5.5. Comparison of nutritional requirements for meals at correctional facilities in California, Rhode Island, and South Carolina

Calories/ macronutrients	Recommended levels (for reference)		California (weekly average)[c]	Rhode Island (weekly average)[d]	South Carolina (42-day average)[e]
	Male[a]	Female[b]			
Total calories	2,400	1,800	2,800	2,900	2,600
Carbohydrates	45%–65%	45%–65%	—	52%	53%
	1,080–1,560 Cal	810–1,170 Cal		1,508 Cal	1,379 Cal
Proteins	10%–35%	10%–35%	—	14%	14%
	240–840 Cal	180–630 Cal		406 Cal	376 Cal
Fats	20%–35%	20%–35%	30%	34%	33%
	480–840 Cal	360–630 Cal	840 Cal	986 Cal	845 Cal

Sources: For California: California Department of Corrections and Rehabilitation, courtesy of Laurie Maurino, RD. For Rhode Island: Rhode Island Department of Corrections, courtesy of Michael Fine, MD, Fred Vohr, MD, and Debbie Mathieu, RD. Nutritional content was analyzed using Nutrition Data System for Research (v2010, Nutrition Coordinating Center, University of Minnesota, Minneapolis, MN) based on standard recipes that may not be representative of actual nutrient content of items. For South Carolina: Collins and Thompson (2012).[24]

[a] Male characteristics are: 35 years of age, 5′ 10″, 154 pounds, sedentary, body mass index (BMI) of 22 kg/m², and a nonsmoker.

[b] Female characteristics are: 35 years of age, 5′ 4″, 128 pounds, sedentary, BMI of 22 kg/m2, and a nonsmoker.

many micronutrients may fall below 100% of the DRI, depending on the nutrition information provided by food companies and the limitations in the software used to conduct nutritional analysis.

Inmates have other options for food consumption besides the meals served. Depending on the facility and their own financial resources, inmates are usually able to purchase food and beverages from on-site commissaries/canteens. The food and beverage choices available from canteens and commissaries include dairy products (cheese and ice cream), meat (beef jerky, sausage, canned fish), pastries and cookies, candies, soda and fruit drinks, ramen noodles, and potato chips. Generally, the products offered from the commissaries are not monitored by dietitians, are not held to regulations or standards, and are often high in calories, fat, sugar, and sodium. These commissary options offer inmates more selection than the meals served, are affordable alternatives to supplement their food intake, and may significantly increase caloric intake, which may well contribute to weight gain. This, in addition to the lack of transparency of nutrient content data, poses a challenge for correctional food service affiliates in lobbying for healthier food options.

Current Efforts to Improve Nutrition in Correctional Facilities The NCCHC recommends that all inmates have a heart-healthy diet, but this is not required for accreditation.[20] Providing menus that are consistent with heart-healthy guidelines can correct for nutritional deficiencies acquired prior to incarceration and continue health promotion during incarceration. Prison meals, if in keeping with heart-healthy guidelines, could provide dietary intake that is healthier for inmates than what they might be eating in the community.[20]

Current American Medical Association (AMA) policy focuses on getting correctional facilities to provide medical care that meets community standards, leaving nutrition standards unaddressed.[21] During the 2010 AMA annual meeting, the American Association of Public Health Physicians presented the report *Dietary Intake of Incarcerated Populations*, in which they suggested that "our AMA Council on Science and Public Health be instructed to collaborate with the United States Department of Agriculture (USDA) to establish and publicize appropriate standards for institutional menus for incarcerated adult and adolescent populations as recommended by the NCCHC and such other organizations advocating for optimal health care in correctional facilities."[21 [p. 1]] The AMA is presently advocating for states to mandate adherence to the current DRIs and Dietary Guidelines for Americans as a criterion for accreditation and/or standards compliance, until national dietary guidelines specific to adolescent and adult populations become available, and to urge the Food and Nutrition Board of the Institute of Medicine to examine the nutrient status and dietary requirements of incarcerated populations and issue guidelines on menu planning.[26]

As briefly mentioned earlier, inmates' food preferences are also an important factor to consider. Some institutions may administer brief food preference surveys to inmates. If this practice were adopted more widely, institutions might take favorite food options and adopt healthier versions and preparation methods for serving them. For example, offering low-fat or skim milk rather than whole milk or offering a higher-fiber bread rather than white bread would promote inmates' health. Although whole-grain bread often costs more than refined bread, depending on vendors and contracts, inmates could be trained to bake whole-grain breads, which would introduce a cheaper alternative and an additional skill set that might be useful to inmates when seeking employment after discharge.[13]

Food vendors must work closely with correctional facilities to develop healthier, cost-effective foods and beverages to assist with meeting healthier nutrition guidelines. Finding lower-sodium options for lunch meats and breads and switching from fruits canned in heavy syrup to unsweetened fruit or fruit canned in natural juices would also improve the nutrient content of foods offered. Cooking techniques could be improved so that foods such as vegetables are not overcooked, which can lead to loss of key water-soluble nutrients, decreasing the nutrient value of these vegetables. As mentioned earlier, other healthy snack options should be offered in commissaries.

Sample Vocational Programs for Inmates As we have noted, time spent in correctional facilities may offer inmates the best opportunity for health education and screening since they are more likely to be a participatory audience. Vocational programs may also offer opportunities to provide additional health education and empower inmates to gain skills that may be useful while incarcerated and during the transition to civilian life. Some correctional facilities, such as the Ashley County Jail in Arkansas and Georgia Correctional Industries, have seasonal gardens and farms on site. These gardens can be beneficial in decreasing food costs, increasing fruit and vegetable intake, and providing nonviolent inmates with an opportunity to volunteer in the garden, giving them a positive outlet and additional skills that are useful for procuring employment after release.[26] For the Ashley County Jail, the only costs associated with the gardens are for seeds, fertilizer, and water, making it affordable, especially with the help of volunteer inmates to work the gardens. In addition, the Ashley County Jail gardens do not use chemicals, so the produce is 100% natural. Some of the items grown in the Ashley County Jail include cucumbers, squash, potatoes, black-eyed peas, watermelons, corn, cantaloupe, tomatoes, and okra. Excess produce is frozen and stored, and some that cannot be stored is given to local senior centers across the county.

Georgia currently has two facilities with gardens on site that are worked with inmate labor as part of an on-the-job training program. They also have a farming operation that raises cattle for beef, hogs and chickens for meat and eggs, and dairy cows for the dairy operation. In addition, the farm is responsible for canning farm-grown vegetables that are used statewide, and another benefit is that sodium is not used in any of the canning processes for these products. For Georgia, the gardens reduce the cost of fresh produce and allow a greater variety of fresh vegetables on the menu. Approximately 42% of the items on the Georgia menu use fresh and canned vegetables, grits, and cornmeal from the garden and meats, dairy, eggs, and milk from the farms (A. Pataluna, personal communication).

When considering the benefits of a garden in a correctional facility, some issues such as having adequate space and climate must be taken into account, as well as which types of crops thrive in the particular climate and environment. Initial capital for land, equipment, plants, seeds, fertilizer, and soil must be considered, and the maintenance costs must be budgeted (A. Pataluna, personal communication). Some of the benefits of farming include the cultivation of fresh, readily available vegetables that provides an enjoyable vocational opportunity for inmates (A. Pataluna, personal communication). However, sometimes vocational opportunities such as prison gardens are not as beneficial as anticipated. California Department of Corrections and Rehabilitation no longer uses gardens because such a food supply can be unreliable; in the past, the gardens sometimes produced insufficient quantities to serve all the inmates at one prison (L. Maurino, personal communication). Some other issues to consider with vocational programs are finding creative solutions for budgeting, especially during periods of economic downturn; security issues, with inmates using gardening tools as weapons; and some negative backlash from vendors who oppose competition (L. Maurino, personal communication).

Other vocational programs may assist inmates with the development of culinary skills, which provides additional nutrition education that can be useful to inmates inside the prison or to people returning from incarceration to the community. In Massachusetts, the Department of Correction Food Service policy states that the department is committed to "provide all inmates assigned to food service with the opportunity through training and education to acquire skills and abilities that may assist in obtaining gainful employment after release."[27 [p. 760]] Massachusetts has implemented a culinary arts program located at its Milford Headquarters to teach inmates skills in food preparation, food service, and health/sanitation.[27] All revenue generated from the Milford Café is used for expenses related to the operation of the cafeteria program, inmate programs, employee benefits, and other expenses approved by the commissioner. The goal of the program is to be self-sufficient for all operating expenses, except for the salaries of the staff.

Also in Massachusetts, there is the Fife and Drum Restaurant, which is located inside the Northeastern Correctional Center, a minimum-security prison outside Concord. This restaurant offers daily hot lunches to the public, prepared from scratch for $3.21 per meal, cooked and served by inmates. The inmates learn many skills beyond basic chopping and serving, including customer service and business management. The culinary program spends about $500 per week on food, a cost completely offset by what customers pay.[28] Inmates have a sense of pride in what they cook and are generally grateful for this opportunity, not only because they learn useful skills but because it helps to make time pass more quickly. Evaluations addressing the efficacy of vocational programs need to be conducted to assess the impact of these opportunities.

Conclusions

Prisoners often are seen as deviant and therefore not important as recipients of health care or subjects of health policy. This view is short-sighted, however, if only because many inmates will return to society, in the best cases as functioning citizens. As rates of obesity and cardiovascular disease increase in the United States, the number of unhealthy individuals entering correctional facilities will also increase. Young men and women from lower-socioeconomic communities, who may already be struggling with health and psychosocial disadvantages that accumulate over the lifetime, are more likely than others to become incarcerated.[8,12] These additional stressors from race/ethnicity-related and economic factors, compounded with the stress of prison life, can increase the risk of physiological changes that may lead to multiple cardiovascular risk factors such as obesity, hypertension, diabetes, and heart disease. The current evidence base is weak but thus far shows that the prevalence of some chronic medical conditions is higher among prison populations than in the general U.S. population. More rigorous studies of obesity are needed, using standardized measurements of heights and weights, to obtain better estimates of the rates of obesity in jails and prisons. We and others postulate that imprisonment is an opportune time to improve the health of inmates by implementing strategies, such as providing healthier diets, to address the rising rates of overweight, obesity, and chronic diseases. This is important not only to the health of individual inmates but also to the health of correctional facilities and of society as a whole, by controlling medical costs during incarceration and after release.

- More research is needed on differences between prisons and jails in obesity risk, as well as on interventions to reduce cardiovascular disease risk among inmates.
- Correctional institutions should integrate interventions on weight gain and obesity, as well as educational efforts to teach weight management, into existing programs.
- Oversight agencies should establish clearly defined guidelines for adequate nutritional intake in correctional facilities, regulated by nutrition and other health care professionals. Many inmates are at increased risk for chronic diseases, inadequate nutritional intake, and physical inactivity, so the national dietary guidelines may not be suitable.
- More research must be conducted to assess nutrient needs for incarcerated individuals. Like schools, universities, and long-term care facilities, correctional facilities must have consistent standards.
- Additional research is needed on differences in nutritional requirements for juvenile and adult inmates, as well as the cost-effectiveness of healthy menus.

Acknowledgments

The authors thank Debbie Mathieu, RD, Dietitian, Rhode Island Department of Corrections; Fred Vohr, MD, Medical Program Director, Rhode Island Department of Corrections; and Laurie Maurino, RD, Departmental Food Administrator, California Department of Corrections and Rehabilitation, for providing sample menus and commissary lists from their correctional institutions. They thank Barbara Wakeen, MA, RD, LD, CCFP, CCHP, Association of Correctional Food Service Affiliates, Chair Dietitians in Corrections; Laurie Maurino; and Amy Pataluna, RD, LD, State Food Service Administrator, Food & Farm Services, Georgia Correctional Industries, for their willingness to share their insights based on their experiences and expertise working in correctional facilities. Special thanks to Josiah Rich, MD, MPH, Professor of Medicine and Community Health, Brown University Medical School, the Miriam Hospital; Michael Fine, MD, former Medical Program Director, Rhode Island Department of Corrections; and Barbara Wakeen, for contributing their expertise and advocacy efforts to draw attention to these issues.

References

1. Flegal KM, Carroll MD, Kit BK, Ogden CL. Prevalence of obesity and trends in the distribution of body mass index among US adults, 1999–2010. JAMA. 2012 Feb 1;307(5):491–7.
2. Pew Charitable Trusts. Prison count 2010: state population declines for the first time in 38 years. Washington, DC: Pew Charitable Trusts, 2010. Available at: http://www.pewtrusts.org

/uploadedFiles/wwwpewtrustsorg/Reports/sentencing_and_corrections/Prison_Count _2010.pdf.

3. Glaze L. Correctional population in the United States, 2010. Washington, DC: U.S. Deparment of Justice, Office of Justice Programs, Bureau of Justice Statistics, 2011. Available at: http://bjs.ojp.usdoj.gov/content/pub/pdf/cpus10.pdf.

4. Pew Center on the States. One in 100: behind bars in America 2008. Washington, DC: Pew Charitable Trusts, 2008. Available at: http://www.pewstates.org/uploadedFiles/PCS_Assets /2008/one%20in%20100.pdf.

5. Office of the Inspector General, Audit Division, Federal Bureau of Prisons. The Federal Bureau of Prison's efforts to manage inmate health care. Washington, DC: U.S. Department of Justice, 2008. Available at: http://www.justice.gov/oig/reports/BOP/a0808/final.pdf.

6. Leddy MA, Schulkin J, Power ML. Consequences of high incarceration rate and high obesity prevalence on the prison system. J Correct Health Care. 2009 Oct;15(4):318–27.

7. Houle B. Obesity disparities among disadvantaged men: national adult male inmate prevalence pooled with non-incarcerated estimates, United States, 2002–2004. Soc Sci Med. 2011 May;72(10):1667–73.

8. Binswanger IA, Krueger PM, Steiner JF. Prevalence of chronic medical conditions among jail and prison inmates in the USA compared with the general population. J Epidemiol Community Health. 2009 Nov;63(11):912–9.

9. Cyrus N. Prison food law. Boston, MA: Legal Electronic Document Archive at Harvard Law School, 2005. Available at: http://leda.law.harvard.edu/leda/data/733/Naim05.html.

10. Garland BE, Spohn C, Wodahl E. Racial disproportionality in the American prison population: using the Blumstein method to address the critical race and justice issue of the 21st century. Justice Policy J. 2008:5(2):1–42.

11. Guerino P, Harrison PM, Sabol WS. Prisoners in 2010. Washington, DC: U.S. Department of Justice, Office of Justice Programs, Bureau of Justice Statistics, 2011. Available at: http:// bjs.ojp.usdoj.gov/content/pub/pdf/p10.pdf.

12. Mauer M, King RS. Uneven justice: state rates of incarceration by race and ethnicity. Washington, DC: Sentencing Project, 2007. Available at: http://www.sentencingproject.org/doc /publications/rd_stateratesofincbyraceandethnicity.pdf.

13. Shaw NS, Rutherdale M, Kenny J. Eating more and enjoying it less: U.S. prison diets for women. Women Health.1985 Spring;10(1):39–57.

14. Plugge EH, Foster CE, Yudkin PL, et al. Cardiovascular disease risk factors and women prisoners in the UK: the impact of imprisonment. Health Promot Int. 2009 Dec;24(4):334–43.

15. Centers for Disease Control and Prevention. Heart disease facts. Atlanta, GA: Centers for Disease Control and Prevention. Available at: http://www.cdc.gov/heartdisease/facts.htm.

16. Centers for Disease Control and Prevention. Adult obesity facts. Atlanta, GA: Centers for Disease Control and Prevention. Available at: http://www.cdc.gov/obesity/data/trends .html.

17. Noonan ME, Carson EA. Prison and jail deaths in custody, 2000–2009—statistical tables (NCJ236219). Washington, DC: U.S. Department of Justice, Office of Justice Programs, Bureau of Justice Statistics, 2011. Available at: http://bjs.ojp.usdoj.gov/content/pub/pdf /pjdc0009st.pdf.

18. Wolf AM, Finer N, Allshouse AA, et al. PROCEED: Prospective Obesity Cohort of Economic Evaluation and Determinants: baseline health and healthcare utilization of the US sample. Diabetes Obes Metab. 2008 Dec;10(12):1248–60.

19. Bachman KH. Obesity, weight management, and health care costs: a primer. Dis Manag. 2007 Jun;10(3):129–37.
20. Khavjou OA, Clarke J, Hofeldt RM, et al. A captive audience: bringing the WISEWOMAN Program to South Dakota Prisoners. Women Health Iss. 2007 Jul–Aug;17(4):193–201.
21. Council on Science and Public Health. Dietary intake of incarcerated populations: Report 4 of the Council on Science and Public Health. Chicago, IL: American Medical Association, 2011. Available at: http://www.ama-assn.org/resources/doc/csaph/a11csaph4-summary.pdf.
22. Wakeen BA, ed. Nutrition and foodservice management in correctional facilities. Chicago, IL: Academy of Nutrition and Dietetics, 2008.
23. Wakeen B. Dietitian's corner-conferenc luncheon wrap-op. In: Insider. Burbank, CA: Association of Correctional Food Service Affiliates, 2011. Available at: http://www.acfsa.org/Insider/insider2011Winter.pdf.
24. Collins SA, Thompson SH. What are we feeding our inmates? J Correct Health Care. 2012 Jul;18(3):210–8.
25. Bohannon J. Psychology:The theory? Diet causes violence. The lab? Prison. Science 2009 Sep 25;325(5948):1614–6.
26. Thielan T. Jail garden: cuts food costs, provides variety. In: Insider. Burbank, CA: Association of Correctional Food Service Affiliates, 2011. Available at: http://www.acfsa.org/Insider/insider2010Fall.pdf.
27. Massachusetts Department of Correction. Food service policy (No: 103 Doc 760). Milford, MA: Massachusetts Department of Correction, 2012. Available at: http://www.mass.gov/eopss/docs/doc/policies/760.pdf.
28. Mullen S. Prison meal deal: where the staff serves lunch . . . and time. Boston, MA: 90.9 WBUR, Boston's National Public Radio News Station, 2012. Available at: http://www.wbur.org/npr/146110728/prison-meal-deal-where-the-staff-serves-lunch-and-time.

CHAPTER 6

Weight Loss Interventions in the Mexican American Community

Natalie A. Ceballos, PhD

As pointed out in previous chapters, according to the National Health and Nutrition Examination Survey, between 2009 and 2010 more than one-third of adults and almost 17% of youths in the United States were obese.[1] Although recent reports suggest that the rise in obesity rates in the United States may be slowing or reaching a plateau,[1-3] obesity rates among Hispanic/Latino adults have continued to rise, with estimates of 39.3% for Mexican Americans and 37.9% for all Hispanics/Latinos combined (compared with 44.1% for non-Hispanic Blacks and 32.6% for non-Hispanic Whites; see chapter 3 on trends in African American rates, particularly among adolescents).[4] The health consequences of obesity may include coronary heart disease, type 2 diabetes, cancers, hypertension, and stroke, among others.[4]* These are conditions that tend to have a disproportionate effect on Hispanics/Latinos, and hence the development of effective weight loss interventions is especially crucial for this population.[5] Although the variety of existing nutrition, fitness, and weight loss tools has expanded in recent years (e.g., web-based programs, affordable pedometers, diet-meal delivery),[6] the continued rise in prevalence of obesity among Hispanics/Latinos suggests that barriers to weight loss have not been overcome in this population.

According to Mier et al.,[7] persistent health disparities require the adoption of more culturally sensitive approaches to behavioral prevention/intervention efforts. Cultural factors surrounding weight loss may present a challenge for Hispanics/Latinos.[8] For instance, qualitative work by Diaz et al.[9] indicates that Hispanics/Latinos may find health professionals' advice to lose weight to be in conflict with the culturally constructed notion that overweight people are robust and healthy. At the same time, participants in Diaz and colleagues' study also reported losing many of their healthy traditional habits as they adapted to mainstream U.S. culture. These

---

Natalie A. Ceballos is in the Department of Psychology at Texas State University, San Marcos.

* See other chapters in this volume for more on the health consequences of obesity. Among others, chapters 2, 11, and 19 provide helpful inventories of health risks associated with obesity.

participants expressed positive feelings about weight loss interventions involving group education and stressed the importance of peer interaction in the weight loss process. Previous studies have suggested that socially and culturally sensitive health interventions increase the external validity of behavioral programs.[7,10] Thus, tailored weight loss interventions with a culturally relevant focus are promising approaches to combat obesity among Hispanics/Latinos.

The validity of culturally sensitive behavioral interventions for weight loss among Hispanics/Latinos is not a trivial issue, as this group now constitutes the largest minority group in the United States, representing 16% of the total population.[11] It is similarly important to recognize the heterogeneity within this group, as important differences are obscured when Hispanic/Latino subgroups are combined into a single population for research studies. The majority of Hispanics/Latinos in the United States are of Mexican descent (63%), followed by Puerto Ricans (9.2%), Central Americans (7.9%), South Americans (5.5%), Cubans (3.5%), Dominicans (2.8%), Spaniards (1.3%), and "other Hispanics/Latinos" (6.8%).[11] Members of each subgroup may have preferences for specific ethnic cuisines, distinct notions of what constitutes desirable body types for each gender, and different needs depending on the socioeconomic status (SES) of the community in which they live. The issue of SES is particularly important in the context of nutritional transition theory,[12] as recent research suggests that the burden of obesity is increasingly being shifted to the less well-off members of society. Consideration of acculturation level and generational issues is also needed, as various studies have noted that a higher level of acculturation to the mainstream U.S. culture is associated with females' preference for a thinner body type[13,14] and males' preference for a lean, muscular, athletic appearance.[15] At the same time, studies suggest that Mexican American immigrants are shifting both toward a more Americanized diet that includes unhealthy fast food and toward a heavier reliance on automobiles, which may lead to obesity.[12,15]

Statement of the Problem

Culturally sensitive intervention efforts for obesity and overweight are growing in popularity, and a review of published weight loss interventions focusing on Hispanics/Latinos is needed to examine their efficacy overall. This mission is particularly important and timely given the continued rise in obesity and obesity-related illnesses (coronary heart disease, type 2 diabetes, cancers, hypertension, stroke) among Hispanics/Latinos, despite the plateau in weight gain among other racial and ethnic groups in the United States.[1-4]

To this end, the current review examines articles on interventions for adolescents and adults, with a primary focus on the Mexican American subgroup of Hispanic/Latinos in the United States. Studies of interventions in Hispanic/Latino populations without Mexican American participants were not included in the review. The range of interventions examined includes programs designed to address reduction of weight, body mass index (BMI), and/or adiposity and programs that sought to change levels of physical activity, sedentary behaviors, and motivations or perceptions of barriers to weight loss. The review concludes with a discussion of the state of interventions focusing on Mexican Americans and some recommendations for future behavioral interventions in this population.

Methods
Procedure

Articles were retrieved by searching the indexing databases PubMed, Google Scholar, and PsycINFO. Search terms included combinations of *weight loss*, *Hispanics*, *Mexican Americans*, *Latinos*, *promotoras*, *culturally sensitive*, *intervention*, *diet*, *physical activity*, and *obesity*. Studies published between 1992 and 2012 were considered for review. Only behavioral interventions were included. Although studies focusing on participants in poor health were not excluded per se, articles with a primary focus on clinical populations (e.g., weight loss among patients with type 2 diabetes, cancer, or lupus) were excluded, as these topics involve comorbid health issues that are beyond the scope of the current review.

The articles selected for review either were exclusively designed for Hispanic/Latino participants or included a large proportion of Hispanic/Latino participants. Articles were required to contain culturally sensitive *surface structure* components and/or *deep structure* components for Hispanic/Latino populations, as defined by Resnicow et al.[16] and Mier et al.[7] According to this framework, cultural sensitivity is a bidimensional concept that includes surface structure components (e.g., intervention materials, messages, channels, settings, and recruitment strategies) that match the characteristics of a priority population, as well as deep structure components (e.g., cultural, social, historical, environmental, and psychological factors) that influence health behaviors in the population.

Study Population

To be included in the review, articles must describe studies in which the participants were exclusively Hispanic/Latino or in which 30% or more of the participants endorsed Hispanic/Latino ancestry. This review focuses primarily on Mexican Americans; however, the common research practice of combining Hispanic/Latino subgroups into one common group prevented this level of interpretation for many studies. Thus, as an indirect measure for studies that did not specify the distribution of participants across Hispanic/Latino subgroups, the demographic characteristics of the recruitment area were retrieved from the 2010 U.S. Census, along with descriptions of the dominant Hispanic/Latino subgroup(s) in the recruitment area. Studies for which such population characteristics could not be ascertained were excluded from this review. All data on age, gender, acculturation level, and SES were included, and the potential influence of these factors was considered where applicable.

Results

The studies selected for review are summarized in tables 6.1 (interventions for adults) and 6.2 (interventions for adolescents), listed in chronological order of publication.

Interventions for Adults

Programs designed to combat obesity in adults are typically focused on interventions among groups of individuals who are already overweight or obese and/or those who are interested in reducing weight. Studies reviewed in this section include approaches that involve only the individual or the individual and the family, with a focus on nutritional education (including culturally appropriate recipes) and physical activity. The inclusion of *promotoras de salud* appears to be a useful approach in many communities.*

Cousins et al.[17] examined the potentially differential effectiveness of three programs for weight loss among obese Mexican American women (average age = 33 years): (1) a family-based approach (family group, n = 27), (2) an individual-based program (individual group, n = 32), and (3) a "manual-only" comparison (comparison group, n = 27), in which participants received only a culturally tailored manual (*Cuidando el Corazon*, detailed below) with no additional intervention. Participants were recruited through a combination of media promotion and personal contacts at community churches and health agencies. Assessments occurred at baseline and at 3, 6, and 12 months. Acculturation was measured using the methods of Cuellar et al.[18]

The bilingual manual, *Cuidando el Corazon*, included a low-fat, low-calorie diet (1,200 calories/day for women), nutritional information, culturally specific recipes, an exercise plan, and behavioral modification strategies. The comparison group, as noted above, received only this manual. The individual group both received the *Cuidando el Corazon* and attended classes taught by bilingual registered dietitians. For the first six months of the program, the individual group attended one class per week (24 classes in total). Classes included nutritional information, feedback on food diaries, behavioral modification for weight loss, group exercise, food tasting, and cooking demonstrations. For the next six months, the individual group attended monthly maintenance classes (6 classes in total), which focused on active problem-solving strategies for preventing relapse. The family group also attended 24 weekly and 6 monthly classes taught by bilingual registered dieticians, and this group received a tailored *Cuidando el Corazon*. They also received information on partner support and parenting skills to encourage healthy lifestyles. For this group, spouses were also encouraged to attend sessions, and separate, age-appropriate sessions were held for preschool-aged children.

The attrition rate was 51%. The average acculturation score was 2.88 (where exclusively Mexican orientation = 1.0 and exclusively Anglo orientation = 5.0).[18] Average

---

* For more on the importance of *promotoras* in effective interventions in Hispanic/Latino communities, see chapters 2 and 15–17.

Table 6.1. Summary of studies on weight loss interventions for Hispanic/Latino adults in the United States

Authors	Intervention/approach	Population	Outcome and significance[a]
Cousins et al. (1992)[17]	1-year RCT; family-based, individual, and comparison groups	Obese Mexican-American women	Weight reduction in family and individual groups was greater than in comparison group ($ps < .001$ and $p < .003$, respectively).
Domel et al. (1992)[22]	11-week nutrition and health intervention vs. comparison group	Hispanic/Latina women; BMIs $\sim 36 \, \text{kg/m}^2$ at baseline	Covariate-adjusted final weight and BMI in intervention group was less than in comparison group ($p < .001$).
Avila and Hovell (1994)[24]	10-week RCT; exercise, nutrition, and behavioral modification	Low-income Mexican-American women, overweight by > 20%	Intervention group had significant reductions in BMI, hip and waist circumference, and total serum cholesterol ($ps < .05$). Changes in comparison group n.s.
Clarke et al. (2007)[25]	8-week physical activity and dietary program vs. normal weight comparison group	Overweight/obese Hispanic/Latina mothers of young children	Pre- vs. post-program scores showed increases in pedometer activity ($p < .05$) and decreases in body weight, body fat %, and waist circumference ($ps < .05$).
Faucher and Mobley (2010)[27]	20-week RCT; education on portion control; used *promotoras de salud*[a]	Low-income, obese Mexican-American women	Intervention n.s.; however, a main effect of self-weighing was noted ($p = .02$).
Bopp et al. (2011)[29]	6-month RCT; faith-based approach to exercise and health education	Hispanic/Latino adults (81% Mexican American); 62% female; BMIs $\sim 28 \, \text{kg/m}^2$ at baseline	Intervention group: 66% identified health reasons for physical activity (vs. 36% in comparison group); 47% accurately described physical activity recommendations (vs. 16% in comparison group).
Mier et al. (2011)[30]	12-week walking program; used community health workers	Mexican-American women from *colonias*; 63% obese at baseline	Intervention significantly increased the number of hours walked per week ($p = .002$) and decreased stress levels ($p = .02$).
Ashida et al. (2012)[33]	3-month personalized health message intervention	Mexican American adults, 44% male; average BMI $\sim 30 \, \text{kg/m}^2$ at baseline	Having at least one family network member who encouraged fruit/vegetable consumption and regular physical activity increased motivation to change ($p = .01$ and $p = .05$, respectively). Forty percent of participants did not have encouragers for these behaviors.

[a] p values of less than .05 (e.g., $p < .05$ for single result; $ps < .05$ for multiple results) denote statistically significant outcomes.
Abbreviations: BMI, body mass index; n.s., did not reach statistical significance; RCT, randomized controlled trial.

Table 6.2. Summary of studies on weight loss interventions for Hispanic/Latino adolescents in the United States

Study	Intervention/approach	Population	Outcome and significance[a]
Flores (1995)[36]	12-week RCT; aerobic dance + health education intervention	Seventh-grade students, 54% female, 43% Hispanic/Latino, BMIs ~23 kg/m²	Males: differences n.s. Females: intervention group had greater reduction of BMI ($p < .05$) and resting heart rate ($p < .01$).
Goran and Reynolds (2005)[39]	8-week RCT; IMPACT CD-ROM + classroom lessons and family homework assignments	Fourth-grade students, 60% female, 58% Hispanic/Latino, BMIs ~20 kg/m²	Treatment × sex interaction for BMI z-score ($p = .02$), intervention led to lower BMI for girls but higher BMI for boys; similar pattern occurred for reduction of % body fat ($p = .009$).
Shaibi et al. (2006)[41]	16-week RCT; resistance training intervention	Overweight Hispanic/Latino adolescent males	Intervention group increased lean mass ($p < .05$), decreased % body fat ($p < .05$), and improved insulin sensitivity ($p < .05$). Relative to comparison group, changes in lean mass and insulin sensitivity were greater in the intervention group ($ps < .05$).
Spruijt-Metz et al. (2008)[44]	1-week, school-based intervention to increase physical activity and decrease sedentary behaviors	Middle school females, 73% Hispanic/Latina, 60% normal weight, 74% physically active	Intervention reduced time spent on sedentary behavior ($p < .05$) and increased intrinsic motivation for physical activity ($p < .05$).
Davis et al. (2009)[47]	16-week RCT; nutrition (N) vs. nutrition + strength training (N+ST) vs. nutrition + strength/aerobic combination (N+CAST) vs. controls (C)	Hispanic/Latina females, 83% Mexican-American, BMI ≥ 85th percentile	N+CAST decreased added sugar consumption relative to controls ($p = .02$), and N decreased sugar consumption relative to both N+CAST and controls ($p = .005$). N+CAST decreased weight vs. increase in weight of N+ST group ($p = .01$). N+CAST and C decreased BMI vs. increase in N+ST group ($p = .01$). N+CAST decreased total fat mass vs. increase in N+ST group ($p = .045$).
Barkin et al. (2011)[48]	6-month prospective RCT; behavioral modification + physical activity sessions vs. standard counseling	Hispanic/Latino parent-child dyads; children had BMIs ≥ 85th percentile, majority of parents were obese	Intervention did not outperform standard of care. Comparison group was more likely to decrease BMI ($p = .03$). Children were more likely to increase BMI over time if their parents did as well ($p = .008$).
Romero (2012)[50]	5-week hip-hop dance intervention + health education	Low-income adolescents, 54% male, 75% Mexican-American	Females had a significant increase in physical activity ($p = .01$); males had a decrease in neighborhood barriers to exercise ($p < .05$).

[a] p values of less than .05 (e.g., $p < .05$ for single result; $ps < .05$ for multiple results) denote statistically significant outcomes.
Abbreviations: BMI, body mass index; n.s. = did not reach statistical significance; RCT, randomized controlled trial.

education level was 10 years, and 24% of participants reported yearly incomes under $10,000. Participants had an average baseline weight of 168 lbs with a BMI of 31 kg/m^2. After one year in the study, average weight changes in the comparison, individual, and family groups were −1.5, −4.6, and −8.3 lbs, respectively. Corresponding BMI reductions were −0.3, −0.8, and −1.6 kg/m^2.

A statistically significant difference was noted between the time course of weight loss (baseline, 3-, 6- and 12-month weight loss) in the comparison group versus the individual group ($p < .003$) and in the comparison group versus the family group ($p < .001$); however, the individual and family groups were not statistically different from one another. Although post hoc tests were not reported, the largest differences seem to have occurred at the 6-month time point. Despite their statistical similarity, it is important to consider that the overall weight loss of the family group was twice that of the individual group, and only the family group was able to sustain a weight loss that shifted them from the obese to the overweight/pre-obese BMI category.[19] Cousins et al.[17] note that, although weight losses were relatively small, a loss of 10 pounds may have beneficial effects on health.[20,21]

Domel et al.[22] examined a weight loss program for Spanish-speaking, Hispanic/Latina women living in low-income areas of Dallas, Texas. Distribution across Hispanic/Latino subgroups was not specified; however, 38% of the Dallas population is Hispanic/Latino, and the majority of these residents report Mexican heritage (32% of total population).[11] Thirty-four women completed the study (average age = 41 years). Average education level was 8.9 years, and average baseline BMI was 36 kg/m^2.

The intervention group was recruited from churches through handouts and announcements in English and Spanish. Promotional events, newspaper articles, and public service announcements on Spanish-language radio stations were also used. The comparison group was recruited from a neighborhood recreational center in another part of the same city, using flyers and word of mouth; these participants were paid $25 for their participation.

Spanish-language program materials were delivered by one of four people: the principal investigator, a Hispanic/Latino bilingual dietitian, a health educator, or a social worker. Program materials focused on health for the entire family and included ethnically appropriate recipes, pamphlets in comic book format, and audiocassettes in radio show format.

The attrition rate was 55%. The intervention group reduced BMIs by −1.6 kg/m^2 and decreased their weight by −8.7 lbs, whereas the comparison group increased their BMI by 0.1 kg/m^2 and gained 0.8 lb. Covariate-adjusted final weight and final BMI were smaller in the intervention group than in the comparison group ($p < .001$); however, in their original research article, Domel et al.[22] did not report the specific covariates used in the statistical analyses. At a three-week follow-up session, the intervention group had maintained its weight loss and had, on average, lost an additional pound. A previous review of this study discussed several limitations, including a lack of detail regarding randomization, session duration, and content.[23]

Avila and Hovell[24] conducted a 10-week physical activity intervention for weight loss among Mexican American women. Participants were recruited from a low-income area of San Diego, California, using flyers at clinics, churches, supermarkets, and a local English-as-a-second-language class. Participants had a mean age of 42 years; 74% were married, and 69% were homemakers. Participants had minimal levels of acculturation to the U.S. mainstream. Ninety percent had completed the sixth grade, but only 35% had completed high school.

Participants were randomly assigned to an intervention group (n = 22) or a control group (comparison group, n = 22). The intervention group attended eight one-hour sessions focusing on exercise, nutrition, and behavioral modification. Participants were encouraged to pair with another participating Latina (i.e., to use the "buddy" system) to provide motivation and assistance with weight loss. The comparison group attended the same number of weekly sessions with an alternative topic (the importance of cancer screening).

By the end of the study, the intervention group had reduced its BMIs by an average of $-1.4 \, \text{kg/m}^2$ ($p < .05$). The comparison group increased its BMIs by $0.3 \, \text{kg/m}^2$. The intervention group also decreased hip and waist circumference by -1.2 and -2.05 inches, respectively ($p < .01$), and decreased total serum cholesterol by $-67 \, \text{mg/dl}$ ($p < .01$). Such changes were not noted in the comparison group. Three months post-treatment, the intervention group had an additional BMI reduction of $-1.3 \, \text{kg/m}^2$. Lindberg and Stevens[23] noted that this study had high attrition rates: three-month follow-up data were available for 8 participants in the comparison group and 10 participants in the intervention group.

Clarke et al.[25] conducted an eight-week diet and physical activity program, which included 93 overweight and obese mothers of young children, plus a comparison group of 31 SES- and ethnicity-matched mothers with BMIs less than 25. Average age of participants was 27 years, and 56% of participants were Hispanics/Latinos from Austin, Texas. Distribution across Hispanic/Latino subgroups was not reported, but the population of Austin is 23% Hispanic/Latino, and a majority of individuals report Mexican heritage (21% of total population).[11] The majority of participants were employed and cohabitating with a romantic partner. Participants were recruited through fliers posted at community centers and public health clinics. The use of inexpensive pedometers is one of the most innovative components of this program, as the perceived financial expense of exercise activities is an oft-cited reason for avoiding exercise in low-income populations.[26]

The intervention consisted of eight weekly classes at community centers and clinics, including a lecture/discussion plus 30 minutes of exercise. Dietary education included cooking demonstrations and menu planning with ethnic foods. Information was provided on recipe modifications, portion control, food budgeting, and caloric density of fast foods. Social support, self-monitoring, role modeling, and stress management were also covered. Participants were instructed to exercise at home at least five days per week for 45 minutes per session with moderate intensity; compliance was measured using pedometers. Retention rates were 75% for the intervention group and 82% for the comparison group. The attendance rate was 74% for the women who completed the study; participants were allowed to bring their children with them to the intervention.

Average baseline BMI for participants in the intervention group was $35 \, kg/m^2$, versus $21 \, kg/m^2$ for the comparison group. Seventy-four percent of the intervention group was obese, and the rest were overweight. By the end of the program, the intervention group had increased activity ($p < .05$) and decreased weight ($p < .05$), with an average loss of −6.6 lbs. Body fat percentage and waist circumference also decreased ($p < .05$; −1.4% and −1.4 inches, respectively). At the week 24 follow-up, the intervention group exhibited a modest additional weight loss, bringing the average total weight loss for the intervention group to −6.9 lbs.

Faucher and Mobley[27] conducted a 20-week randomized controlled trial (RCT) focusing on portion control. Nineteen low-income Mexican American women were recruited from a community center, all of whom were interested in losing weight. Participants were assigned to either an intervention group or a standard care group. All educational materials were in Spanish, and intervention sessions were provided by a *promotora de salud*.

In the comparison group, participants had a physical examination and one dietary education session with a primary care provider and the *promotora*. Educational materials included a food pyramid, portion control counseling, and tools for logging dietary intake and daily activity. This session was more extensive than what is provided in typical health visits, which tend to last around three to five minutes.[27]

The intervention group attended four two-hour group meetings during study weeks 1, 3, 7, and 13. Meetings focused on portion control and were conducted by researchers and a *promotora*. The curriculum was financially sensitive, culturally appropriate, and focused on the participants and their families. Lessons included meal preparation, recipe sharing, and portion control aids (i.e., one serving of meat = the size of a deck of playing cards).

Participants in the intervention group were "on average" 35 years of age. All reported Mexico as their country of origin and had lived "on average" 9.4 years in the United States. Ninety percent of this group reported Spanish as their primary language. The majority of the intervention group (91%) were married or cohabitating; 93% were homemakers. Ninety percent of the intervention group had children living at home. Average baseline weight of the intervention group was 183.3 lbs, with a BMI of $34 \, kg/m^2$. After the intervention, this group had an average weight loss of −6.5 lbs, with a BMI reduction of $-1 \, kg/m^2$. The comparison group had an average baseline weight of 193.3 lbs with a BMI of $34 \, kg/m^2$. At the end of the study, the comparison group had an average weight loss of −2.8 lbs with a BMI reduction of less than $1 \, kg/m^2$.

Although the extent of weight loss in the intervention group versus the comparison group was not statistically significant, the intervention group lost twice as much weight. An additional finding was a statistically significant main effect of self-weighing across groups ($p = .02$). Participants who weighed themselves regularly (e.g., daily, weekly, or monthly) lost 10 times more weight than those who did not (10.3 lbs vs. 0.3 lbs). Sixty-seven percent of participants who weighed themselves regularly had been randomly assigned to the intervention group.

Although previous research has shown a relationship between self-weighing and weight loss,[28] this study by Faucher and Mobley is perhaps the first to replicate this finding among low-income Mexican American women, despite low statistical power and an attrition rate of 34%.

Bopp et al.[29] described a six-month RCT entitled Faithful Footsteps, which was designed to influence knowledge and attitudes about physical activity in 50 Hispanic/ Latino adults (average age = 43 years). Sixty-two percent were female; 81% were of Mexican descent; 77% were married; 73% were employed; and 68% reported an education level of less than a high school diploma. The average BMI was 27.9 kg/m².

Intervention and comparison programs were conducted in the church setting, and both recruitment and intervention activities were facilitated by priests and priest-appointed congregation members. Study materials were available in Spanish and English, were culturally relevant to Hispanics/Latinos, and incorporated Roman Catholicism. The intervention included a six-week period in which health education displays were posted in public areas around the church and viewed by a large number of congregation members, an eight-week team-based walking contest, and a health fiesta featuring children's activities. The comparison group received a six-week educational unit of unrelated information (on job safety).

Forty-two percent of participants completed both baseline and six-month follow-up assessments. Data analyses were limited to descriptive statistics and focused only on knowledge and attitudes about physical activity. In the intervention group, 66% of participants identified health reasons for participating in physical activity (vs. 36% in the comparison group), and 47% were able to describe physical activity recommendations accurately (vs. 16% in comparison group).

Bopp and colleagues acknowledged that their outcomes assessment was not rigorous but stated that the intervention group's enhanced awareness of healthy behaviors may represent a preliminary step in the contemplation of change. Further, the authors found their data to be supportive of a faith-based setting as an appropriate place for delivering physical activity interventions to some groups of Hispanics/Latinos.

Mier et al.[30] described a walking program for Mexican American women living in *colonias* in Hidalgo County, Texas. *Colonias* are unincorporated, impoverished settlements lacking basic services, and their inhabitants represent one of the most underserved populations in the United States.[30] Sixteen women (average age = 32 years) participated; 62% were married and 94% percent were born in Mexico. Fifty-six percent reported less than a high school education, and 56% were unemployed. At baseline, 63% were obese, 18.8% were overweight, and 18.8% had a BMI in the normal range.

The intervention was a 12-week, non-experimental, one-group, pre-test (baseline) and post-test (three-month follow-up) assessment, which focused on enhancing physical activity by increasing participants' walking time in hours per week. The intervention group was given a Spanish handbook (*Vamos a Caminar* [Let's Walk]) based on the AARP's *Physical Activities Workbook*[31] and modified for cultural sensitivity.

Community health workers presented the intervention and considered participants' schedules and childcare needs when planning program sessions. One session was conducted each week for 12 weeks, and participants were encouraged to walk at a moderate pace for 30 minutes per day. Sessions focused on barriers to walking, injury prevention, benefits of physical activity, establishing and following a walking plan, and the use of social support from other *colonia* residents who were participating in the program.[32] Participants who completed the study received a free pedometer.

Attendance rate was 92%; all participants attended at least 7 of the 12 sessions; however, in their original article, Mier et al.[30] did not report the attrition rate of the study. The study's high attendance rate is possibly attributable to the use of community health workers.[30] At the three-month follow-up, participants had increased their walking time from 297 to 1,212.75 minutes per week ($p = .002$). Participants also reported a decrease in stress ($p = .02$). Based on these data, the researchers found the home-based walking program to be an effective means of increasing physical activity among women from *colonias*.

Ashida et al.[33] conducted a study in which participants' baseline health information was used to create tailored health interventions. Participants included 475 Mexican American adults (average age = 41 years) from 161 families. Forty-four percent of participants were male, and average baseline BMI was approximately 30 kg/m². Recruitment and initial data collection were accomplished by telephone contact (random dialing of numbers obtained from phone books of targeted neighborhoods), door-to-door recruitment in selected neighborhoods, in-person recruitment of individuals from community centers and health clinics, and networking through already enrolled participants. At the time of initial recruitment, information was obtained in English or Spanish regarding age, gender, level of education, country of birth, and family health history.[34]

Two weeks after a baseline assessment of personal and family health history, participants were mailed personalized health intervention messages that were tailored to their specific needs. Materials included one or more of the following from the Centers for Disease Control and Prevention's Family Healthware[35] tool: a pedigree depicting participant's family history of health issues; health risk assessments for heart disease, diabetes, and cancer; and personalized behavioral risk-reduction recommendations. A three-month telephone follow-up interview assessed (through structured questionnaires) participants' motivation to adopt a healthier lifestyle, including motivation to change diet and physical activity behaviors, social network characteristics, and current diet and physical activity behaviors. The extent of each participant's overall social network was determined based on responses to a question about friends and family who had played a significant role in the respondent's life over the past year. A second question asked how many social network members had also encouraged the respondent to eat more fruits and vegetables and/or obtain regular exercise. For each healthy behavior, a dichotomous variable was created to indicate whether or not the respondents had at least one supporter of that behavior. Ashida and colleagues did not report any qualitative data collection or analyses.

Ninety-six percent of participants completed the three-month follow-up. At baseline, participants consumed about 1.5 servings of fruits and vegetables per day and engaged in 100.44 minutes of physical activity per week. At the three-month follow-up, 53% of participants indicated a desire to increase their fruit and vegetable consumption, and 51% were motivated to increase physical activity. Sixty-one percent of participants had more than one family member who encouraged fruit and vegetable consumption. Fifty-eight percent had more than one family member who encouraged physical activity. Logistic regression models were used to predict motivation to improve diet and increase physical activity. Results indicated that having at least one family member who encouraged fruit and vegetable consumption and regular physical activity significantly increased motivation to change ($p = .01$ and $p < .05$, respectively). Unfortunately, 40% of participants did not have any family members who encouraged these behaviors.

This study not only reveals the importance of building social support for the success of diet/exercise-themed lifestyle interventions but also suggests that personalized intervention approaches with clear visual aids and minimal participation requirements are a feasible means of motivating behavioral change in this underserved population.

Interventions for Adolescents

Obesity prevention and intervention efforts among adolescents are particularly timely, as recent estimates indicate that 18.6% of boys and 15.0% of girls in the United States are obese.[1] Further, research suggests that overweight children are more likely to become overweight adults.[36,37] Studies reviewed in this section focus on preventing obesity among Hispanic/Latino adolescents through nutritional education and enhancement of physical activity; in addition, adolescents who are already overweight or obese are encouraged to adopt healthier lifestyles. Innovative approaches such as dance interventions and computer games may help to hold the interest of adolescent populations.

Flores[36] reported an RCT to assess the effectiveness of the Dance for Health program to reduce BMIs and improve health among minority adolescents. Participants were 81 seventh-graders (average age = 12.6 years) recruited from physical education classes at a middle school in East Palo Alto, California. Approximately 40% were Hispanic/Latino, and 54% were female. Distribution of participants across Hispanic/Latino subgroups was not specified; however, the population of East Palo Alto is 65% Hispanic/Latino with a majority of individuals reporting Mexican heritage (54% of total population).[11] Forty-one percent of participants spoke Spanish at home, and 74% were born in the United States.

The intervention group participated in three 50-minute aerobic dance sessions per week for 12 weeks. Sessions included 10 minutes of warm-up/cool-down with 40 minutes of moderate- to high-intensity dancing. Dance routines were choreographed by the instructors, using hip-hop songs suggested by the students. A culturally sensitive health curriculum was presented to the intervention group in two sessions each week. Flores states that English was a second language for many of the Hispanic/Latino students; thus, the health education materials, while in English, were adapted so that they would be very simple to read and understand. The health education sessions were composed of 10 minutes of didactic activity and 20 minutes of other activities. There were 25 lessons: 6 on nutrition, 5 on exercise, 3 on obesity and unhealthy weight practices, and 11 on other issues (e.g., coping with peer pressure). The comparison group spent an equivalent amount of time participating in standard playground activities.

Statistical significance was noted, for females only, in changes in BMI ($p < .05$) and resting heart rate ($p < .01$) relative to the comparison group. Among girls in the intervention group, BMI was decreased by $-0.8 \, kg/m^2$ and heart rate was decreased by -10.9 beats per minute (bpm) at the end of the program. Among girls in the comparison group, BMI increased ($0.3 \, kg/m^2$) and resting heart rate decreased slightly (-0.2 bpm). With average pre-intervention BMI values of 22.9 and $22.2 \, kg/m^2$, respectively, girls in the intervention and comparison groups were in the overweight range.[38] Reduction of BMI in the intervention group moved these participants to the median range for their age,[38] a clinically meaningful change. Although the finding was not statistically significant, Flores[36] also noted an intervention-related trend toward BMI reduction and improvement of health parameters among male participants.

Several reasons were given for why males may not have benefited as thoroughly from the intervention. Flores suggests that the attitude toward physical activity was somewhat worse among boys in the intervention group than those in the comparison group. Flores states that "although the boys seemed to enjoy the dance, they might need more unstructured free play time for the class to work very well for them."[36] [p. 192] Earlier in the article, "other activities" (vs. dance activities) were defined as typical, unstructured playground activities. Alternatively, the relatively poor attitude of boys toward the dance intervention might be explained in part by the notion (prevalent among adolescent males in many cultures, including the Latino culture) that dancing is an activity for females. Tailoring exercise interventions to target adolescent males is an important issue for future trials, as some studies suggest that male adolescents may be at greater risk of obesity than females.[37]

Goran and Reynolds[39] explored the computer-based curriculum entitled Interactive Multimedia for Promoting Physical Activity (IMPACT). Participants were 122 fourth-graders (average age = 9.4 years) from Los Angeles County, California. Sixty percent were female, and 58% were Hispanic/Latino. Distribution across Hispanic/Latino subgroups was not specified; however, the population of Los Angeles County is approximately 48% Hispanic/Latino, with the majority of individuals reporting

Mexican heritage (36% of total population).[12] Average baseline BMI was 19.5 kg/m^2, which is overweight for boys and borderline overweight for girls in this age group.[11] The study initially recruited 209 participants, but data from only 122 participants were retained for main outcome analyses. This study was reviewed earlier by Norman et al.[40]

The IMPACT intervention was eight weeks in length and consisted of eight CD-ROM interactive lessons of 45 minutes each, four classroom lessons of 45 minutes each, and four family-based homework assignments of 45 minutes each. IMPACT is an interactive educational learning game designed to increase physical activity, decrease sedentary behavior, and alter related psychosocial variables. The intervention was designed to be compelling and fun and involves adventure scenarios such as "a group of children traveling around the globe in search of magic ingredients to concoct an antidote to the elixir generated by the evil Snidwitt, who wants everyone to hate being physically active."[39 [p. 764]] The IMPACT intervention was subjected to focus groups to ensure gender and cultural sensitivity.[39] The comparison group received non-health-related educational CD-ROMs.

The authors noted a treatment-by-sex interaction for BMI z-score ($p = .02$). The intervention led to lower BMI values among girls but higher values among boys; a similar effect was noted for percent body fat ($p = .009$). These sex differences were present despite modifications to enhance the gender sensitivity of the intervention. Comparisons based on ethnicity were not feasible, and so it is unclear whether modifications to the program to increase cultural sensitivity were successful.[39]

Shaibi et al.[41] conducted a 16-week resistance training intervention (two sessions per week), which included a non-exercising comparison group. Participants were 22 overweight Hispanic/Latino adolescent males from Los Angeles County, recruited through medical clinics, advertisements, and local schools. Distribution across Hispanic/Latino subgroups was not reported. The population of Los Angeles County is 48% Hispanic/Latino, with the majority of individuals reporting Mexican heritage (36% of total population).[11] The authors did not explicitly tailor the intervention for Hispanics/Latinos; however, the study addresses a culturally relevant issue—that is, the drive for muscularity among Hispanic/Latino males and the need to develop healthy interventions to bring about such changes.[42]

Attendance rate for the study was 96%. The intervention group benefited significantly from resistance training, largely through changes in body composition, as overall weight did not change. The intervention group increased total lean mass by 7.4% and decreased percentage body fat by −6.7% ($p < .05$). For lean body mass, the extent of improvement in the intervention group was significantly greater than that in the comparison group ($p < .05$). The intervention group also significantly improved their insulin levels ($p < .05$), a result not seen in the comparison group. Finally, unlike the intervention group, the comparison group had an overall weight gain during the study ($p < .05$).

Only 4% of participants in the study failed to attend sessions. Delivering the intervention through a community center and employing personal trainers to whom the adolescents could relate may have contributed to the program's success. Because overweight youths frequently exhibit better performance in activities requiring explosive muscular strength, these individuals may be more enthusiastic and compliant in resistance training programs.[41] This study was also reviewed by Davis et al.[43]

Spruijt-Metz et al.[44] assessed an intervention entitled Get Moving!, a culturally sensitive program to increase physical activity and decrease sedentary behavior. There were 459 female participants (average age = 12.5 years), 73% of whom were Hispanic/Latino. Distribution of Hispanic/Latino subgroups was not specified. The statewide Hispanic/Latino population in California is 37.6%, with a majority of residents reporting Mexican heritage (30.7% of total state population).[11] At baseline, 60% of participants were of normal weight and 74% were physically active.

The program duration was nine months. Baseline and follow-up measures were employed at the beginning of the fall semester and end of the spring semester, respectively. The intervention group took part in a media-based physical activity program delivered during five to seven in-class sessions for five to seven consecutive school days in the spring semester. The program included information about the benefits of physical activity and the deleterious effects of sedentary behavior. It also included interactive learning activities (referred to as *teachable moments*), the end products of which were student-designed public service announcements aimed at increasing physical activity and decreasing sedentary behaviors among girls.[44]

Physical activity and sedentary behavior were assessed using a modified previous-day physical activity recall instrument, which measured behavior in blocks of 30-minute bouts throughout the day.[44] At baseline, the intervention group had an average sedentary activity rating of 3.82 and an intrinsic motivation-to-exercise rating of 1.11. After completing the intervention, their sedentary activity ratings decreased by −3.44 and intrinsic motivation-to-exercise ratings increased by 1.16 ($p < .05$). In the comparison group, sedentary activity ratings increased by 0.50 and intrinsic motivation-to-exercise ratings decreased by −0.06. The intervention failed to significantly increase physical activity. However, because a majority of participants (60%) were of normal weight and were physically active (74%) at baseline, outcomes of this study were at risk for ceiling effects. At a minimum, this study demonstrates that involving the target population in developing lifestyle interventions (e.g., public service announcements) improves program outcomes.[44–46]

Davis et al.[47] reported a 16-week culturally tailored RCT focusing on improving health parameters in 41 Hispanic/Latina girls (average age = 15 years, attending grades 9–12) with BMIs ≥ 85th percentile. Eighty-three percent of the participants were Mexican American. Most were from low-income or lower-middle-income families. Participants were randomized to either the control group, receiving no treatment (C), or one of three intervention groups: (1) nutrition intervention only (N), (2) nutrition + strength training (N+ST), or (3) nutrition + combination of strength and aerobic training (N+CAST). The N group received one laboratory-based, 90-minute, culturally tailored dietary intervention per week to decrease sugar consumption and increase dietary fiber. Trained research staff also used motivational interviewing techniques to enhance participants' motivation for healthy eating. The N+ST group received the dietary intervention and motivational interviewing plus two 60-minute progressive strength training sessions each week. The N+CAST group received the dietary intervention and motivational interviewing plus two 60-minute strength/aerobic exercise sessions per week. Combined exercise sessions consisted of 30 minutes of progressive strength training plus 30 minutes of progressive cardiovascular activity (i.e., elliptical machines or aerobics classes).

Of the 50 original participants, 41 completed the study. Intervention-related changes included but were not limited to the following. Decreases in the consumption of added dietary sugar were most pronounced in the group receiving only the dietary intervention (the N group). The N+CAST group decreased total sugar consumption relative to the control group ($p = .02$), but the N group decreased sugar consumption significantly relative to both the N+CAST and the control groups ($p = .04$). Reductions in weight, BMI, and total fat mass were most consistent in the N+CAST group; the N+ST group actually gained weight, BMI, and total fat mass. Specifically, the N+CAST group decreased in weight (−1.1%) compared with the increase in weight in the N+ST group (2.6%; $p = .01$). The N+CAST (−1.6%) and C (−1.6%) groups decreased in BMI compared with an increase in the N+ST group (3.0%; $p = .01$). The N+CAST group (−4.3%) decreased in total fat mass compared with an increase in the N+ST group (1.8%; $p < .05$).

This study was unique in that it was the first to comprehensively compare combinations of nutritional, aerobic, and strength training interventions in the form of an RCT among adolescent, overweight, Hispanic/Latino females. These data suggest that combined aerobic and strength training may be a beneficial addition to dietary interventions for this population. The study was one of a series of interventions described by this team of investigators, who have published a comprehensive review of their research program,[43] including an overview of the study by Shaibi et al.,[41] discussed above.

Barkin et al.[48] reported a six-month prospective RCT focusing on weight loss among Hispanic/Latino parent-child dyads. Distribution of participants across Hispanic/Latino subgroups was not specified. The study was conducted in Forsyth County, North Carolina, an area that is approximately 12% Hispanic/Latino, with the majority of individuals reporting Mexican heritage (8.1% of total population).[11] Most participants reported low levels of acculturation, and most spoke Spanish at home and with their friends. Children were aged 8–11 years and had an average BMI ≥ the 8th percentile. Fifty-four percent of adolescent participants were female. The average parental age was 34 years, and the majority of parents were obese. The report presented demographic information for 106 parent-child dyads; however, only 72 of these completed all assessments. Thus, 72 participants were included in the main outcome analyses.

The researchers conducted focus groups to ensure the cultural sensitivity of the study materials. Both Spanish- and English-language versions of the study documents were available, and participants were free to choose documents in the language they preferred. All reading materials, for both parents and children, were written at the third-grade level. Bilingual researchers and educators presented the program.

The intervention group participated in six sessions over the six-month study period. An initial behavioral modification session was conducted at a community primary care clinic, and this was followed by five physical activity sessions (one per month) at the local YMCA, led by a bilingual program manager of Hispanic/Latino descent. Inexpensive, accessible activities included soccer, dance, volleyball, and outdoor games. YMCA sessions were one hour in duration and included a 20-minute educational session using materials from the American Heart Association, a 30-minute group physical activity session, and 10 minutes of parent-child goal setting (setting concrete goals for the next month's physical activity). The comparison group had only two "enhanced, office-based, standard of care" sessions (baseline + six-month follow-up) at the community primary care clinic.[48] Sessions featured general information about improving nutrition and increasing physical activity.

The retention rate was 68%. Barkin and colleagues noted that most participants were transient inhabitants of Forsyth County, and their transience may have contributed to retention difficulties. Across groups, children decreased BMI by $-0.4 \, \text{kg/m}^2$ by the end of the study; for parents the decrease was $-0.9 \, \text{kg/m}^2$. A mixed effects linear regression model indicated that the intervention did not outperform the enhanced office-based standard of care. The comparison group was more likely (vs. the intervention group) to decrease BMI over the six-month study ($p = .03$). Children were more likely to increase BMI over time if their corresponding parent increased BMI as well ($p = .008$).

Based on these data, Barkin and colleagues suggest that among Hispanic/Latino families from Mexico with limited acculturation, more credibility may be conferred when information is provided in a clinical setting rather than a YMCA. The authors cited the Hispanic/Latino cultural notion of *respeto*[49] as an explanation of this finding and suggested that formal, clinic-based interventions involving the entire family may be particularly efficacious for this population.[48]

Finally, Romero[50] reported a five-week pilot test of the Latin Active hip-hop dance intervention, designed to increase physical activity among low-income Mexican American adolescents. Participants were 73 adolescents, 54% of whom were male. Seventy-five percent self-identified as Mexican or Mexican American, and another 6% reported mixed ethnic heritage of Mexican descent; 51% were second-generation Americans. Eighty percent were from low-income households.

The program content was largely based on feedback from focus groups composed of parents and teens from the same school from which participants were recruited for the intervention study.[50] The focus groups indicated that 85% of students were interested in hip-hop music and in learning to break-dance as a form of physical activity. The authors stated that lessons were created in collaboration with key stake-holders (middle school students and teachers, health educators, and local break-dancers) providing culturally similar social role models.

The study had a pre- and post-test survey design. In the intervening period, participants received 10 Latin Active lessons of 50 minutes each, delivered twice per week for five weeks. Classes were delivered in English, but when necessary, the instructor would also deliver instructions in Spanish. At the beginning of class, the instructor spent 20 minutes discussing various neighborhood barriers to exercise and the benefits of physical activity. This was followed by 30 minutes of break-dancing (5-minute group warm-up, 10-minute group practice of dance moves, 10 minutes of individual practice and one-on-one assistance, and 5–10 minutes of group freestyle or "battle circle"). Ninety percent of the instructors were female.

Ninety percent of the students targeted for recruitment ultimately joined the Latin Active program. Seventy-seven percent of them completed both pre- and post-test surveys based on the California Healthy Kids Survey and the ambient hazards scale.[51] Data for boys and girls were analyzed separately. At baseline, girls had a physical activity rating of 1.97, which had increased to 2.97 by the second testing session, reflecting a facilitation of exercise habits ($p = .01$). Initially, boys reported many neighborhood barriers to exercise (baseline rating = 2.11). At the post-intervention assessment, this score had decreased to 1.47, reflecting a decrease in boys' perception of barriers ($p < .05$), which was due largely to their enhanced awareness of neighborhood parks.

Increases in activity were seen only among the girls, a finding that may be attributed to the fact that 90% of the instructors were female. It is unclear whether Hispanic boys were reluctant to accept female dance teachers or male teachers would provide better role models. It is also possible that boys may have been reluctant to participate actively in dance activities, which they may have perceived as "female" activities. Perhaps tailoring the intervention for better gender and culture matching of instructors and students would improve the success of this program.[50] The boys in the study seemed to respond most favorably to the education/discussion portion of the program, as reflected in a decreased perception of neighborhood barriers to exercise. This, in itself, is an important accomplishment, as high crime rates and lack of green space are often cited as barriers to exercise among low-income participants.[52] At a minimum, the significant changes from pre-to post-intervention suggest that hip-hop–based dance programs deserve further study in randomized controlled trials.[50]

Discussion

Table 6.3 summarizes some important factors to consider for weight loss interventions in Hispanic/Latino populations, along with representative publications discussing these issues. Across the studies reviewed in this chapter, several trends emerge. Although weight loss intervention studies in general tend to suffer from high attrition rates,[53] studies focusing on Hispanics/Latinos, particularly those who live in low-

Table 6.3. Summary of factors to consider for interventions in Hispanic/Latino populations

Factor	Representative publications
Use of lay health advisors, or *promotoras de salud*	Rhodes et al. (2007)[56]
Participant demographics (e.g., gender, socioeconomic status, Hispanic/Latino subgroup)	Kaplan and Bennett (2003)[57]; Shaibi et al. (2006)[41]; Clarke et al. (2007)[25]; Davis et al. (2010)[43]
Participants' acculturation levels	Diaz et al. (2007)[9]; Barkin et al. (2011)[48]
Suitability of individual- vs. group/family-based approaches	Faucher and Monley (2010)[27]; Barkin et al. (2011)[48]
Culturally sensitive recruitment and retention of participants	Mier et al. (2010)[30]; Resnicow et al. (1999)[16]; Yancey et al. (2006)[55]
Clinical vs. statistical significance of weight loss outcomes	Jacobson and Truax (1991)[59]

income areas, tend to have higher than usual rates of attrition.[54] Qualitative studies suggest that flexibility may be the key to increasing retention rates in this population. Yancey et al.[55] suggested several "best practice" strategies for recruitment and retention of low-income Hispanic/Latino participants. Convenience is a major concern and may be addressed by providing evening/weekend study hours to accommodate participants' work schedules. Providing childcare may also be an important issue for some participants, particularly women. Some low-income participants may also benefit from study-provided transportation, especially in areas where public transportation is not efficient or readily available. Other strategies suggested by Yancey and colleagues include formalizing communication of appreciation for participants' investment of time and effort (e.g., by verbal recognition, certificates of participation, letters of gratitude), providing incentives or compensation for time spent on study activities (e.g., monetary honoraria, food, raffle tickets), and maintaining contact with participants through the use of birthday cards and reminder communications. Minimal field staff turnover and documentation of multiple friend and family contacts in order to avoid mobility-related loss to follow-up are also recommended.[55] Further, qualitative data suggest that social support (e.g., use of the "buddy system") may help women to complete a weight loss program successfully.[24,55] Addressing nutritional issues within the family and enlisting social support for behavioral interventions may also be necessary, as some participants reported attempts by peers and family members to subvert the participant's weight loss goals.[14] Sabotage by peers or family could be a defense reaction to the threat of change and/or could reflect the cultural notion that overweight bodies are healthy and attractive.[9,14]

The acculturation level of the study population is another important consideration. As mentioned above, Diaz et al.[9] found that, although new immigrants from Mexico reported a reduction in healthy eating and exercise habits on arrival in the United States, they also tended to believe that overweight bodies reflect robust health, while thin bodies are unhealthy. Diaz and colleagues also noted that participants preferred weight loss programs conducted in a group setting with the opportunity for peer interaction. Related work suggests that the employment of bilingual lay health advisors, community health workers, or *promotoras*, is an effective means of delivering health-related interventions among Hispanic/Latino communities, particularly when recent immigrants are the target population.[56] *Promotoras* are typically part of the communities in which they work, and as such, these lay health advisors are more likely to understand the needs of the community and to effectively deliver culturally relevant health promotion messages.[56] Lay health advisors who are of the same gender and ethnicity as the target population may be most effective.[27,56]

The socioeconomic status of the target population is an important consideration for any type of health intervention. From a methodological standpoint, studies that fail to examine or control for the potential impact of SES on health outcomes may run the risk of falsely identifying gender and/or ethnicity effects that are instead due largely to SES differences between groups.[57] It is of particular importance to the current review to note that SES correlates differentially with obesity among Mexican American males and females: obesity is more prevalent among high-income males and less prevalent among high-income/high-education females.[4] Further, women from some low-income areas have concerns about the safety of exercising outdoors.[26]

Integration of innovative, cutting-edge approaches may enhance interventions to improve health parameters and to prevent the development of obesity among adolescents.[37] Computerized educational games, dance interventions (particularly for females), and resistance training (for males) are promising approaches to facilitate weight loss and increase physical activity among adolescents. However, interventions for children must be sensitive to the importance of peer acceptance and adolescents' desire to conform to cultural notions of ideal appearance. In particular, previous studies suggest that Hispanic/Latino adolescent girls may feel pressure to conform to the appearance ideals of their heritage and thus may be concerned about losing too much weight.[14,58]

Finally, in all studies of health interventions and outcomes, it is important to note that results may be clinically significant without necessarily reaching the level of statistical significance, typically defined as having a probability threshold of not more than $p < .05$. For instance, as noted by Jacobsen and Truax,[59] conventional statistical comparisons between groups tell us very little about the true efficacy of a treatment. Further, these authors suggest that the size of an effect is largely independent of its clinical significance. In terms of clinical significance, the standards of efficacy tend to be set by consumers—that is, the recipients of the intervention, their peers and significant others, and the larger community. In this review, a behavioral change was considered clinically significant if the intervention succeeded in moving a patient/participant closer to the range of the healthy population.[59,60]

One trend noted in this review is that comparatively few behavioral intervention studies have included male participants; most have focused on women. Among those studies that did include Hispanic/Latino males, even culturally sensitive interventions seemed to be less effective among males than among females. This trend was noted in several studies across both adolescent and adult participant samples. For example, in the family-based subgroup of the study by Cousins et al.,[17] male partners attended educational sessions with their mates only 50% of the time and attributed their lack of compliance to the cultural notion that diet and meal planning are "women's activities." In the adolescent intervention studies by Flores,[36] females underwent meaningful changes relative to the comparison group, but such effects were typically absent or nonsignificant trends among males. Flores attributed this gender difference to males' preference for more unstructured exercise rather than structured aerobic dance classes. Similarly, gender differences were noted by Goran et al.[39] in their computerized intervention, despite their attempts to present gender-sensitive content and the mainstream notion that video games are more popular among males than among females.

In a notable exception to the trend for conducting behavioral intervention studies among women only, the resistance training intervention reported by Shaibi et al.[41] targeted adolescent Hispanic/Latino males and focused on a more traditionally male activity (weight lifting). The study took place in a community center and employed personal trainers to whom the participants might relate. Successful changes in body composition and improvements in insulin sensitivity were noted, and the program had a 96% attendance rate. Reaching out to the underserved population of adolescent Hispanic/Latino males is particularly important because, although overweight/obese adolescents of both genders are more likely than their peers to become overweight/obese adults, males are at higher risk than females.[37] Further, a study by Neumark-Sztainer et al.[42] found that Hispanic/Latino and "other/multiethnic" males (compared with non-Hispanic Whites, African Americans, and Asian Americans) were most likely to self-report dangerous strategies such as steroid use to enhance muscularity. Thus, tailored weight loss interventions must be sensitive to the interactive influences of gender and culture on participants' ideal body image and should encourage healthy methods to improve fitness, taking into consideration not only fat loss but also participants' potential desire for enhanced muscularity. Future studies should also focus on interventions targeting the underserved population of low-income, Hispanic/Latino men.

Another key limitation of the existing weight loss literature for Hispanic/Latino populations is that, to date, the vast majority of published studies of culturally sensitive interventions have not included participants who are truly representative of the heterogeneous population of Hispanics/Latinos in the United States. Frequently, participants are classified as *Hispanic/Latino* without attention to membership in ethnic subgroups (e.g., Mexican American, Puerto Rican, Cuban, South American, Central American). Whenever possible, future studies should endeavor to enroll participants across a variety of Hispanic/Latino subgroups so that the efficacy of interventions can be measured with Hispanic/Latino subgroup as a between-subjects factor. At a minimum, studies featuring a combined Hispanic/Latino group should specify whether their participant population is truly representative of the distribution of Hispanic/ Latino subgroups in the United States or in the specific area being studied.

Assessment of acculturation level, including some consideration of generational issues, is also needed. For instance, a body image study by Olvera et al.[13] found that compared with their less acculturated peers, Hispanic/Latino boys and girls who were more acculturated to the U.S. mainstream were more likely to rate thinner body figures as more attractive than larger body figures. Qualitative studies have found that females tend to desire weight loss to achieve the thin ideal portrayed by celebrities in the United States, whereas males typically indicate a drive for muscularity and less body mass in order to facilitate performance in sports and other physical activities.[14] In either case, dissatisfaction with one's body can lead to unhealthy means of weight loss and/or enhancement of muscularity.[42,61] Less acculturated individuals' belief that a larger body type is healthier and more attractive may also present a challenge to weight loss interventions and may be particularly influential in terms of recruitment.[9]

Finally, as noted earlier, SES may differentially predict obesity among Hispanic/ Latino men and women,[4] with higher obesity prevalence among high-income males and lower obesity prevalence among high-income/high-education females. Further, low-income populations frequently live in neighborhoods where safe and affordable opportunities for physical activity are not readily available.[26] This challenge to weight loss interventions contributes to study attrition and potentially inhibits participants' success in reaching their weight loss goals. Unfortunately, the influence of SES has not been examined consistently across studies. Finding innovative ways to address roadblocks to successful weight loss in low-income populations should be a major focus of future intervention efforts.

Conclusions

Obesity is a significant problem in the United States, particularly among Hispanics/ Latinos. Culturally sensitive interventions seem to provide clinically meaningful, if not statistically significant, improvements in BMI, body composition, and motivation for healthy behaviors. *Promotora*-mediated and family-based interventions appear to be particularly effective for adult women, and flexibility may improve retention rates in such programs. Computerized educational games and dance programs are cutting-edge approaches to obesity intervention and prevention among adolescents. New, tailored approaches are needed to address obesity and overweight among Hispanic /Latino males of all ages; this group should be a major focus for future interventions.

LESSONS LEARNED
  • Culturally sensitive interventions, such as the use of *promotoras de salud*, or community health advisors, provide clinically meaningful improvements in motivation, BMI, and body composition.

- Adult women tend to prefer interventions that involve family and peer support in establishing healthier lifestyles.
- Flexible and easily accessible interventions, with provision of incentives, may improve program retention.
- Adolescents tend to prefer interventions that include educational games, dance training (for females), and resistance training (for males).
- To date, the majority of successful studies have focused on Latinas. Additional work is needed to determine how best to recruit and treat Latinos who are in need of weight loss intervention.

References

1. Ogden CL, Carroll MD, Kit BK, et al. Prevalence of obesity in the United States, 2009–2010 (NCHS Data Brief, No. 82). Hyattsville, MD: National Center for Health Statistics, 2012. Available at: http://www.cdc.gov/nchs/data/databriefs/db82.pdf.
2. Ogden CL, Carroll MD, Curtin LR, et al. Prevalence of high body mass index in U.S. children and adolescents, 2007–2008. JAMA. 2010 Jan 20;303(3):242–9.
3. Flegal KM, Carroll MD, Ogden CL, et al. Prevalence and trends in obesity among U.S. adults, 1999–2008. JAMA. 2010 Jan 20;303(3):235–41.
4. Centers for Disease Control and Prevention. Adult obesity facts. Atlanta, GA: Centers for Disease Control and Prevention, 2012. Available at: http://www.cdc.gov/obesity/data/adult.html.
5. Cossrow N, Falkner B. Race/ethnic issues in obesity and obesity-related comorbidities. J lin Endocrinol Metab. 2004 Jun;89(6):2590–4.
6. Arem H, Irwin M. A review of web-based weight loss interventions in adults. Obes Rev. 2011 May;12(5):e236–43.
7. Mier N, Ory MG, Medina AA. Anatomy of culturally-sensitive interventions promoting nutrition and exercise in Hispanics: a critical examination of existing literature. Health Promot Pract. 2010 Jul;11(4):541–54.
8. Lindberg NM, Stevens VJ. Immigration and weight gain: Mexican American women's perspectives. J Immigr Minor Health. 2011 Feb;13(1):155–60.
9. Diaz VA, Mainous AG, Pope C. Cultural conflicts in the weight loss experience of overweight Latinos. Int J Obes (Lond). 2007 Feb;31(2):328–33.
10. Bernal G, Bonilla J, Bellido C. Ecological validity and cultural sensitivity for outcome research: issues for the cultural adaptation and development of psychosocial treatments with Hispanics. J Abnorm Child Psychol. 1995 Feb;23(1):67–82.
11. U.S. Census Bureau. The Hispanic population: 2010. Washington, DC: U.S. Census Bureau, 2010.
12. Popkin BM, Gordon-Larsen P. The nutrition transition: worldwide obesity dynamics and their determinants. Int J Obes Relat Metab Disord. 2004 Nov;28 Suppl 3:S2–9.
13. Olvera N, Suminski R, Power TG. Intergenerational perceptions of body image in Hispanics: role of BMI, gender, and acculturation. Obes Res. 2005 Nov;13(11):1970–9.
14. Alm MA, Soroudi N, Wylie-Rosett J. A qualitative assessment of barriers and facilitators to achieving behavior goals among obese inner-city adolescents in a weight management program. Diabetes Educ. 2008 Mar–Apr;34(2):277–84.

15. Ryabov I. The impact of community health workers on behavioral outcomes and glycemic control of diabetes patients on the U.S.-Mexico Border. Int Q Community Health Educ. 2010;31(4):387–99.

16. Resnicow K, Baranowski T, Ahluwalia JS, et al. Cultural sensitivity in public health: defined and demystified. Ethn Dis. 1999 Winter;9(1):10–21.

17. Cousins JH, Rubovits DS, Dun JK, et al. Family versus individually oriented intervention for weight loss in Mexican American women. Public Health Rep. 1992 Sep–Oct;107(5):549–55.

18. Cuellar I, Harris L, Jasso R. An acculturation scale for Mexican American normal and clinical populations. Hisp J Behav Sci. 1980 Sep;2(3):199–217.

19. World Health Organization. Global database on body mass index, BMI classification. Geneva, Switzerland: World Health Organization, 2012. Available at: http://apps.who.int/bmi /index.jsp?introPage=intro_3.html.

20. Langford HG, Davis BR, Blaufox D, et al. Effect of drug and diet treatment of mild hypertension on diastolic blood pressure. The TAIM research group. Hypertension. 1991 Feb;17(2): 210–7.

21. Watts NB, Spanheimer RG, DiGirolamo M, et al. Prediction of glucose response to weight loss in patients with non-insulin-dependent diabetes mellitus. Arch Intern Med. 1990 Apr;150(4):803–6.

22. Domel SB, Alford BB, Cattlett HN, et al. A pilot weight control program for Hispanic women. J Am Diet Assoc. 1992 Oct;92(10):1270–1.

23. Lindberg NM, Stevens VJ. Review: weight loss interventions with Hispanic populations. Ethn Dis. 2007 Spring;17(2):397–402.

24. Avila P, Hovell MF. Physical activity training for weight loss in Latinas: a controlled trial. Int J Obes Relat Metab Disord. 1994 Jul;18(7):476–82.

25. Clarke KK, Freeland-Graves J, Klohe-Lehman DM, et al. Promotion of physical activity in low-income mothers using pedometers. J Am Diet Assoc. 2007 Jun;107(6):962–7.

26. Mier N, Medina AA, Ory MG. Mexican Americans with type 2 diabetes: perspectives on definitions, motivators and programs of physical activity. Prev Chronic Dis. 2007 Apr;4(2): A24.

27. Faucher MA, Mobley J. A community intervention on portion control aimed at weight loss in low-income Mexican American women. J Midwifery Women Health. 2010 Jan–Feb;55(1): 60–4.

28. O'Neil PM, Brown JD. Weighing the evidence: benefits of regular weight monitoring for weight control. J Nutr Educ Behav. 2005 Nov–Dec;37(6):319–22.

29. Bopp M, Fallon EA, Marquez DX. A faith-based physical activity intervention for Latinos: outcomes and lessons. Am J Health Promot. 2011 Jan–Feb;25(3):168–71.

30. Mier N, Tanguma J, Millard AV, et al. A pilot walking program for Mexican American women living in colonias at the border. Am J Health Promot. 2011 Jan–Feb;25(3):172–5.

31. AARP. Physical activities workbook. Washington, DC: AARP, 2002. Available at: http:// www.aarp.org/health/conditions-treatments/info-05-2010/health_publications_order _form.html.

32. Mier N, Millard AV, Flores I, et al. Community-based participatory research: lessons learned from practice in South Texas colonias. TPHA J. 2007;59(1):16–8.

33. Ashida S, Wilkinson AV, Koehly LM. Social influence and motivation to change health behaviors among Mexican-origin adults: implications for diet and physical activity. Am J Health Promot. 2012 Jan–Feb;26(3):176–9.

34. Wilkinson AV, Spitz MR, Strom SS, et al. Effects of nativity, age at migration, and accultura- tion on smoking among adult Houston residents of Mexican descent. Am J Public Health. 2005 Jun;95(6):1043–9.

35. Yoon PW, Scheuner MT, Jorgensen C, et al. Developing Family Healthware, a family history screening tool to prevent common chronic diseases. Prev Chronic Dis. 2009 Jan;6(1):A33.

36. Flores R. Dance for health: Improving fitness in African American and Hispanic adoles- cents. Public Health Rep. 1995 Mar–Apr;110(2):189–93.

37. Rowland K, Coffey J, Stephens MB. Clinical inquiries: are overweight children more likely to be overweight adults? J Fam Pract. 2009 Aug;58(8):431–2.

38. Centers for Disease Control and Prevention. Data table of BMI-for-age charts. Atlanta, GA: Centers for Disease Control and Prevention, 2011. Available at: http://www.cdc.gov/growth charts/html_charts/bmiagerev.htm.

39. Goran MI, Reynolds K. Interactive Multimedia for Promoting Physical Activity (IMPACT) in children. Obes Res. 2005 Apr;13(4):762–71.

40. Norman GJ, Zabinski MF, Adams MA, et al. A review of eHealth interventions for physical activity and dietary behavior change. Am J Prev Med. 2007 Oct;33(4):336–45.

41. Shaibi GQ, Cruz ML, Ball GD, et al. Effects of resistance training on insulin sensitivity in overweight Latino adolescent males. Med Sci Sports Exerc. 2006 Jul;38(7):1208–15.

42. Neumark-Sztainer D, Story M, Falkner NH, et al. Sociodemographic and personal charac- teristics of adolescents engaged in weight loss and weight/muscle gain behaviors: who is doing what? Prev Med. 1999 Jan;28(1):40–50.

43. Davis JN, Ventura EE, Shaibi G. Interventions for improving metabolic risk in overweight Latino youth. Int J Pediatr Obes. 2010 Oct;5(5):451–5.

44. Spruijt-Metz D, Nguyen-Michel ST, Goran MI, et al. Reducing sedentary behavior in minority girls via a theory-based tailored classroom media intervention. Int J Pediatr Obes. 2008;3(4): 240–8.

45. Naylor PJ, Macdonald HM, McKay KE. Action Schools! BC: a socioecological approach to modifying chronic disease risk factors in elementary school children. Prev Chronic Dis. 2006 Apr;3(2):A60.

46. Kim S, Flaskerud JH, Koniak-Griffin D, et al. Using community-partnered participatory re- search to address health disparities in the Latino community. J Prof Nurs. 2005 Jul–Aug;2(4): 199–209.

47. Davis JN, Tung A, Chak SS, et al. Aerobic and strength training reduces adiposity in over- weight Latina adolescents. Med Sci Sports Exerc. 2009 Jul;41(7):1494–503.

48. Barkin SL, Gesell SB, Poe EK, et al. Changing overweight Latino preadolescent body mass index: the effect of the parent-child dyad. Clin Pediatr (Phila). 2011 Jan;50(1):29–36.

49. Hirsch JS. En el norte la mujer manda—gender, generation, and geography in a Mexican transnational community. Am Behav Sci. 1999 Jun;42(9):1332–49.

50. Romero AJ. A pilot test of the Latin Active hip hop intervention to increase physical activity among low-income Mexican American adolescents. Am J Health Promot. 2012 Mar;26(4): 208–11.

51. Heath GW, Pate RR, Pratt M. Measuring physical activity among adolescents. Public Health Rep. 1993;108 Suppl 1:42–6.

52. Huang SY, Hogg J, Zandieh S, et al. A ballroom dance classroom program promotes moder- ate to vigorous physical activity in elementary school children. Am J Health Promot. 2012 Jan–Feb;26(3):160–5.

53. Pratt CA. A conceptual model for studying attrition in weight-reduction programs. J Nutr Educ. 1990;22(4):177–82.

54. Osei-Assibey G, Kyrou I, Adi Y, et al. Dietary and lifestyle interventions for weight management in adults from minority ethnic/non-white groups: a systematic review. Obes Rev. 2010 Nov;11(11):769–76.

55. Yancey AK, Ortega AN, Kumanyika SK. Effective recruitment and retention of minority research participants. Annu Rev Public Health. 2006;27:1–28.

56. Rhodes SD, Foley KL, Zometa CS, et al. Lay health advisor interventions among Hispanics/Latinos: a qualitative systematic review. Am J Prev Med. 2007 Nov;33(5):418–27.

57. Kaplan JB, Bennett T. Use of race and ethnicity in biomedical publication. JAMA. 2003 May 28;289(20):2709–16.

58. Cachelin FM, Rebeck RM, Chung GH, et al. Does ethnicity influence body-size preference? A comparison of body image and body size. Obes Res. 2002 Mar;10(3):158–66.

59. Jacobson NS, Truax P. Clinical significance: a statistical approach to defining meaningful change in psychotherapy research. J Consult Clin Psychol. 1991 Feb;59(1):12–9.

60. Jacobson NS, Follette WC, Revenstorf D, et al. Variability in outcome and clinical significance of behavioral marital therapy: a reanalysis of outcome data. J Consult Clin Psychol. 1984 Aug;52(4):497–504.

61. Ackard DM, Peterson CB. Association between puberty and disordered eating, body image and other psychological variables. Int J Eat Disord. 2001 Mar;29(2):187–94.

PART II   **COMMENTARIES**

CHAPTER 7

In the Way or On the Way?
Asking Ourselves about the Role of Contextual Factors in Community-Based Obesity Research

Shiriki K. Kumanyika, PhD, MPH, T. Elaine Prewitt, DrPH, JoAnne Banks, PhD, RN, and Carmen Samuel-Hodge, PhD

> We've got to remember that it's not easy and people need the kind of support that's relevant to them in order to make it sustainable. Science is important and research is important, but this is really about people's lives, and the science should be a by-product of that. The science should inform and help us to really make the differences in people's lives we are trying to make.   —*Presenter at the 2006 National Invited Workshop of the African American Collaborative Obesity Research Network, Philadelphia*

O besity is one of many critical health issues in African American communities,[1] but health may take a back seat to more immediate concerns such as inadequate housing, high unemployment, family stresses, or high levels of violence.[2] These more immediate concerns are themselves determinants of health and may be affected by health,[3] although they are not often seen that way or considered in the domain of traditional health research or practice, either by the public or by professionals. Notwithstanding the high levels of obesity within African American communities,[4,5] there is more to daily functioning and survival than deciding how many calories to eat or whether to exercise. Indeed, the stresses of daily functioning under conditions of structural violence may contribute to overeating and obesity.[6-8] The issue of where initiatives to address obesity fit with community priorities has come up repeatedly within the African American Collaborative Obesity Research Network (AACORN), a

Shiriki Kumanyika is affiliated with the Department of Biostatistics and Epidemiology, University of Pennsylvania Perelman School of Medicine, in Philadelphia; T. Elaine Prewitt, with the Department of Health Policy and Management at the University of Arkansas for Medical Sciences, in Little Rock; JoAnne Banks, with the Department of Nursing, Winston Salem State University, in Winston-Salem, North Carolina; and Carmen Samuel-Hodge, with the Nutrition Department of the Schools of Public Health and Medicine, University of North Carolina at Chapel Hill.

national research network that seeks to improve the quality, quantity, and effective translation of obesity research in African American communities.[9] The issue of community priorities has influenced our thinking as we plan and conduct workshops, set research agendas, and reflect generally on how to achieve our goals.

One question that arises is how forcefully one should push the topic of obesity when there are more pressing problems.[2] A related and especially challenging question is how researchers who focus on obesity should view these other problems. Does one ignore or try to work around these other issues because they seem to be "in the way"? Or, by expanding the horizons of obesity researchers, could considering these other community priorities be "on the way" to realistic, sustainable solutions that also fit with the prevailing perceptions and needs in the communities? These questions are broadly and highly relevant to most types of research with communities— particularly so when the objective is to address health disparities affecting socially or politically disadvantaged communities in which low social capital and limited financial resources lead to constant challenges and a chronic negative influence on quality of life.[10]

AACORN has found these questions worthy of serious consideration because we are oriented to community-centered research conducted in partnership with communities. We submit that the fundamental survival problems posed by the contexts in which people live cannot be considered as being in the way while we pursue narrowly framed, single-focus solutions; nor can the potentially overwhelming nature of the many problems faced by communities be used as an excuse to focus, ineffectively, on everything while accomplishing nothing. Rather, we must struggle with ways to understand and consider contextual factors as being on the way to the solution. Our interventions would then not only keep the context in view but also ultimately enhance and be enhanced by the larger picture. In this chapter we share some highlights of the evolution of our thinking to get to this point.

Expanding the Paradigm: Shifting Thinking toward People and Communities

Frameworks that allow academic researchers and communities to consider the multiple contextual factors that influence individual behaviors are critical in developing and implementing sustainable health promotion interventions. Figure 7.1 provides one such framework. This expanded paradigm represents a synthesis of deliberations that occurred before, during, and after AACORN's 2004 interdisciplinary workshop, "Toward Achieving Healthy Weight in African American Communities."[11] The need to shift our perspective, when designing obesity prevention and treatment interventions, from a disease-oriented toward a more people- and community-oriented view became clear to us early in our organizational life and was directly addressed when planning the 2004 workshop. Fearing a rehash of well-known problems and ineffective solutions, we sought to expand our perspective by inviting scholars from disci-

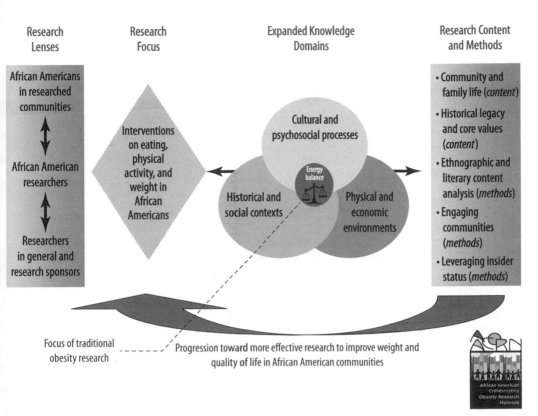

Research
Focus

Expanded Knowledge
Domains

Research Content
and Methods

African Americans
in researched
communities

African American
researchers

Researchers
in general and
research sponsors

Interventions
on eating,
physical
activity, and
weight in
African
Americans

Cultural and
psychosocial processes

Energy
balance

Historical and
social contexts

Physical and
economic
environments

• Community and
family life (*content*)

• Historical legacy
and core values
(*content*)

• Ethnographic and
literary content
analysis (*methods*)

• Engaging
communities
(*methods*)

• Leveraging insider
status (*methods*)

Focus of traditional
obesity research

Progression toward more effective research to improve weight and
quality of life in African American communities

FIGURE 7.1. AACORN's expanded obesity research paradigm. Source: Copyright African American Collaborative Obesity Research Network.

plines or fields of study not commonly included in discussions about the development of obesity interventions, such as family sociology, literature, philosophy, economics, marketing, and transcultural psychology. At that workshop we also saw the situation from the perspectives of community members who had been involved as partners in research projects.

Starting in the center (see fig. 7.1), the energy-balance focus (that is, the balance between calories in and calories out) that is core to weight control is shown to be influenced by many contextual variables. The behavioral determinants of weight status are embedded in historical and social contexts (e.g., historical legacy of slavery; social processes in families and communities), cultural and psychosocial processes (e.g., aesthetic, moral, religious, and social values; individual and collective responses to historical and current social conditions), and physical and economic environments (e.g., neighborhood characteristics, resources, media, and food marketing—including food availability, food promotion, and food costs). There are liabilities and assets to be considered within each of these domains. Understanding assets to avoid a deficit view of communities is a key premise. The overall message is that efforts to design interventions on eating, physical activity, and weight can be enhanced by considering these contextual influences.

At the left of the diagram, the research lenses identify different stakeholder groups. What is seen, asked, and heard about communities depends on who is looking or listening and their perceptual lenses. Valuable information can be gained from the perspectives of (1) members of the community of interest, (2) researchers in relevant fields whose expertise incorporates insights based on lived experiences in or shared identity with the community of interest, and (3) researchers and research sponsors who see themselves as outside the community but who have relevant interests and expertise. Taking advantage of these different perspectives makes working with communities essential, as in community-based participatory research (CBPR).[12]

The right side of figure 7.1 addresses content and methods. Important content areas are family and community interactions related to food and activity; historical legacies of sociopolitical inequality and how these legacies may influence interactions with the health care system; and how foods are marketed to African Americans.[11,13] The potential value of ethnographic and other types of qualitative investigations that yield potentially richer insights than those obtained from quantitative approaches is emphasized; content analysis of literary works was identified as a novel approach. Involving researchers who are also community insiders and see issues through dual lenses, where possible, is identified as a specific methodological recommendation.

Our expanded paradigm underscores the need to involve multiple, interacting parts of behavioral contexts. For example, factors that lead people to consume too many calories may include (1) historical factors emanating from slavery; (2) cultural and psychosocial meanings of food based on history, traditions, and family and life experiences specific to the circumstances of African Americans; and (3) other factors that affect the population in general but may be generally less favorable in African American communities: limited personal income; food prices; food availability in neighborhoods, workplaces, schools, and homes; transportation, as it affects the ability to obtain food outside the neighborhood; and the frequency and content of food advertising on television and through other channels.[13–16] Factors associated with relatively low physical activity levels in African Americans may include (1) cultural attitudes and behaviors that emanate from exposure to forced labor during slavery or low-paying manual work; (2) the limited availability or high cost of indoor recreational facilities, lack of safe parks, and/or street crime that deter outdoor activity; (3) poorly equipped physical activity facilities in schools; (4) reliance on television for engaging children after school hours; and (5) the promotion of cars and sedentary entertainment as symbols of social status.[14,16,17]*

---

* See chapter 8 on the relationship of safety and obesity prevention among African Americans. See the chapters in part III for numerous examples of creative programs targeting obesity and overweight in underserved U.S. communities that face all or some of the challenges to healthy weight elucidated here.

Community-Based Participatory Research

How to design and implement obesity research that is appropriately contextualized and conducted in partnership with the community was the main theme of AACORN's 2006 national workshop, "Participatory Research on African American Community Weight Issues: Defining the State of the Art."[18] This second workshop aimed to clarify concepts, principles, and issues in CBPR approaches and their implications for obesity research. A specific session featured colleagues in other areas of community or public health research or activism who reviewed and reflected on community needs and priorities. They addressed topics such as housing quality and related effects on community life, strategies for addressing gang violence, and the effects of high levels of incarceration on community life, and reflected on how these issues and circumstances might interact with efforts to address obesity.

Both the 2004 and the 2006 AACORN workshops fostered discussion that would break new ground in conceptual and methodological approaches to addressing obesity. A major conclusion from the 2006 CBPR-oriented workshop was that a better understanding of community context would be a critical foundation for developing and implementing effective research approaches for African Americans. The potential drawbacks of opening the door to competing priorities were recognized. However, cooperation and mutual awareness among those working on different problems were deemed to be more helpful for researchers and communities than trying to prioritize one focus over the other. We recognized that community members have diverse interests and also that obesity-related health problems are often prominent among the top concerns raised by community members. Several presentations at the 2006 workshop underscored that physical activity and food issues could be approached under the banner of environmental justice, benefiting from collective action. Mobilizing communities to take action (while providing sustained support) can also benefit communities' capacity for taking on other challenges, particularly where the community efficacy is currently low or resources are very limited.

Challenges

Community-based participatory research has particular relevance for obesity research in that it considers social, structural, and contextual factors in the causal chain of disease and blends academic with community perspectives.[12] The targeted behaviors and their multifaceted influences are highly socially and structurally embedded in community contexts. Academic (biomedical, biochemical, and physiological) and community (economic, ecological and sociocultural) views of food and physical activity may differ sharply, requiring adjudication through a collaborative, iterative process. Such adjudication through the building of trust and mutual respect is difficult— CBPR is challenging.[12] Tensions may arise from the academic side upon the suggestion that factors that are far removed from or only indirectly related to food or physical activity should be taken into account (e.g., poverty, housing, crime). This is especially so when one considers that academic professionals must function and survive in a research and funding culture that usually requires a single-minded focus on a specified problem. Additionally, academics may resist taking context into account, especially those academics who trained in disciplines where traditional research is grounded in an assumed position of objectivity and neutrality and tends to be deliberately decontextualized.[12,19] Traditionally, decisions about a research question, research design, implementation, and dissemination of findings are an outgrowth of the critical and impartial synthesis of the literature and delineation of gaps in knowledge. Challenges to this traditional view become clear, however, when conducting CBPR, which argues for approaches in which communities and university-based researchers co-create knowledge. The endogenous knowledge and skills of community partners and the expertise of university-based researchers are viewed equitably in a preferably long-term research partnership conducted according to the principles of CBPR.[19,20]

One example of the decontextualized view of much health research is the high value placed on randomized trials, which are oriented to establishing causality with priority assigned to the ability to make unbiased comparisons between or among the groups being studied (internal validity). In this scenario, relevant daily life and historical contextual factors, both measured and unmeasured, are thought to be balanced across the groups being compared. This approach, however, may sacrifice assessment of the impact of these contextual factors (external validity). Contextual factors cannot be factored out of consideration in the real world and may determine the ultimate policy and program relevance of the intervention.[21]* Failure to take into account the impact of social and environmental forces on individual behavior can be a major hindrance to the ecological validity of much research that is otherwise considered to be well-designed. This need for relevance to context holds for non-experimental studies as well. For example, Finkelstein et al.[22] concluded that controlling for individual characteristics (i.e., taking them out of consideration through statistical techniques) was not sufficient for understanding disparities in coronary heart disease risk factors among participants in the multisite WISEWOMAN project. They noted "our findings suggest that the differences in community characteristics account for many racial/ethnic disparities in cardiovascular disease risk factors. Efforts to eliminate the disparities are likely to require communitywide interventions that seek to even the playing field."[22] [p. 515]

---

* In this volume, the editors have sought to achieve a balance. We have included systematic literature reviews when the volume of work allowed for it and more inclusive reviews when much of the work lay outside the framework of randomized controlled trials published in the restricted world of peer-reviewed academic publications. We have also intentionally included a large number of reports from the field (part III), as well as the four commentaries in part II (beginning with this chapter), which enabled us to represent a wide array of communities in which obesity and overweight are important concerns but for which there is no abundance of scientific, academic research. Doing so has the added benefit of ensuring that we do not lose sight of the many structural factors that seem to be relevant to the phenomenon of high rates of obesity and overweight but might be factored out in a randomized controlled trial.

Where there is a single-minded focus on obesity as the main issue, there will be a reluctance to yield to other community concerns. These concerns may stand in the way from an academic perspective. By the same token, such single-minded research may be considered to be in the way as far as the community is concerned. Perceptions of what is in the way may depend on how vivid the other issues are (i.e., their perceived magnitude and severity and the apparent immediacy of addressing them). The inclination to consider concerns other than obesity may also depend on the available resources. If resources are tight and earmarked for obesity, paying attention to issues other than obesity may seem impractical.

What is viewed as in the way versus on the way may differ depending on the knowledge, understanding, and self-interests of the research partners—community versus academic. Community members' perspectives may be influenced, at least initially, by limited knowledge of or concern about the research process, including potential barriers and facilitators within the academic environment, why a control group is necessary, or why people are assigned at random rather than being able to choose their intervention group. Procedures that may seem indispensable to researchers may be "in the way" for community partners. In addition, certain types of research may be acceptable to community partners only when a clear benefit is involved and when the intervention fits well with their setting. As reported by Yanek et al.[23] for Project Joy, a faith-based cardiovascular disease risk-reduction study in Black churches, many pastors refused to decide on participation without first knowing their randomization assignment; some then decided to opt out once learning their assignment. In the same study, the standard (non-spiritual) intervention condition was impossible to implement because a spiritual component was added as a natural adaptation of the program.*

Similarly, university researchers may be unaware of the contexts within which communities are operating—historical, cultural, psychosocial, economic, and other—and how these contexts directly or indirectly influence intervention delivery or outcomes. Additionally, researchers may not have the time, funds, or interest to address issues that they perceive as unlikely to have a direct, positive influence on the main outcomes of a study or on their careers. The extent to which such differences in research partners' perceptions are recognized and the way they are addressed determines whether CBPR can be undertaken effectively.

Opportunities

It is critical to recognize that in some communities, weight and weight-related food and physical activity issues may be lower on the list of priorities and less immediate than issues such as employment, safety, academic advancement of schoolchildren, residential/neighborhood issues, substance abuse, and incarceration. Community ranking of these priorities may be driven by the pressing and immediate requirements

---

* See chapters 12 and 18 for accounts of two faith-based obesity/overweight interventions.

for survival. It may be necessary to cross a threshold of progress on these issues in order to optimize attention and motivation to focus on issues such as obesity. Through partnerships, obesity researchers might be better able to identify communities or groups within communities where weight-related issues are at the forefront or identify how actions related to food and physical activity can be undertaken to complement other types of initiatives.

Thoughtful consideration of CBPR principles and the "on the way" perspective in obesity research allows for in-depth insight that is not afforded by research models grounded in the traditional biomedical paradigm. Through CBPR, obesity researchers can work with communities in ways that allow attention to competing or multiple priorities and potentially expand research partnerships to include colleagues who address other issues. For example, effective interventions to reduce or prevent violence would lead naturally to more opportunities for children to engage safely in outdoor activity. Dialogue between obesity researchers and researchers who focus on these and other community priorities would promote a better understanding of ways to approach and work with communities with the potential for simultaneously addressing a variety of concerns.

Implications

Many researchers, community members, and research funders have probably asked themselves some version of the question "In the way? Or On the way?" The question will be more salient for some than others. Researchers who consider themselves members of the ethnic group or community in question may have a greater interest in or sense of obligation toward addressing broader community issues or may be more likely than other researchers to encounter expectations of offering the community more than their research expertise.[11] As the number of researchers tackling obesity-related issues in African American communities continues to expand and more research is conducted, communities may become increasingly attuned to noticing which researchers are complicit in ignoring the broader issues of context, compared with those who are able to frame research based on knowledge of the ambient, contextual layers in which weight-related issues are embedded. AACORN's expanded obesity research paradigm (fig. 7.1) articulates the importance of combining insights from academic and community perspectives. A simplified version, developed as a tool to facilitate discussions in communities (fig. 7.2),[24] can help with identifying specific social, cultural, physical, and economic determinants of obesity that are contextual determinants of individual eating and physical activity behaviors. This approach is consistent with the increasing recognition that "upstream" interventions to change environmental contexts are fundamental to addressing a broad array of health disparities.[3,10]

Successful and sustainable research projects conducted by academic and community partnerships must find ways to facilitate discussions that allow consensus building, clarity of perceptions about what is in the pathway to the solution, and ground

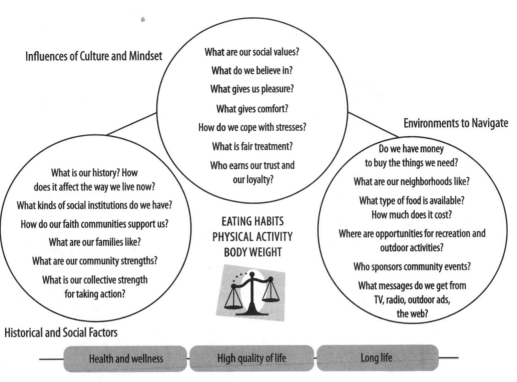

Influences of Culture and Mindset

What are our social values?

What do we believe in?

What gives us pleasure?

What gives comfort?

How do we cope with stresses?

What is fair treatment?

Who earns our trust and our loyalty?

Environments to Navigate

What is our history? How does it affect the way we live now?

What kinds of social institutions do we have?

How do our faith communities support us?

What are our families like?

What are our community strengths?

What is our collective strength for taking action?

EATING HABITS
PHYSICAL ACTIVITY
BODY WEIGHT

Do we have money to buy the things we need?

What are our neighborhoods like?

What type of food is available? How much does it cost?

Where are opportunities for recreation and outdoor activities?

Who sponsors community events?

What messages do we get from TV, radio, outdoor ads, the web?

Historical and Social Factors

Health and wellness · High quality of life · Long life

FIGURE 7.2. AACORN's community-centered view of influences on eating, physical activity, and body weight. Source: Copyright African American Collaborative Obesity Research Network.

rules about how to negotiate and successfully proceed. Ultimately, all partners must understand contexts and value diverse perspectives.[9]

Acknowledgments

The authors are charter members of the African American Collaborative Obesity Research Network (AACORN; www.aacorn.org). The development of this commentary was supported by a Robert Wood Johnson Foundation research and infrastructure grant to AACORN. The opinions expressed in this chapter do not necessarily reflect those of the Robert Wood Johnson Foundation.

References

1. Braithwaite RL, Taylor SE, Treadwell HM, eds. Health issues in the black community. Hoboken, NJ: Jossey-Bass, 2009.
2. Kumanyika S. Obesity, health disparities, and prevention paradigms: hard questions and hard choices. Prev Chronic Dis. 2005 Oct;2(4):A02.

3. Williams DR, Costa MV, Odunlami AO, et al. Moving upstream: how interventions that address the social determinants of health can improve health and reduce disparities. J Public Health Manag Pract. 2008 Nov;14 Suppl:S8–17.

4. Ogden CL, Carroll MD, Kit BK, et al. Prevalence of obesity and trends in body mass index among US children and adolescents, 1999–2010. JAMA. 2012 Feb 1;307(5):483–90.

5. Flegal KM, Carroll MD, Kit BK, et al. Prevalence of obesity and trends in the distribution of body mass index among US adults, 1999–2010. JAMA. 2012 Feb 1;307(5):491–7.

6. Gutierrez G. A theology of liberation: history, politics, and salvation. Maryknoll, NY: Orbis Books, 1988.

7. Farmer P. Pathologies of power: health, human rights, and the new war on the poor. Berkeley, CA: University of California Press, 2003.

8. Hooks B. Sisters of the yam: black women and self-recovery. Cambridge, MA: South End Press, 1993.

9. Kumanyika SK, Gary TL, Lancaster KJ, et al. Achieving healthy weight in African-American communities: research perspectives and priorities. Obes Res. 2005 Dec;13(12):2037–47.

10. Kumanyika SK, Morssink CB. Bridging domains in efforts to reduce disparities in health and health care. Health Educ Behav. 2006 Aug;33(4):440–58.

11. Kumanyika SK, Whitt-Glover MC, Gary TL, et al. Expanding the obesity research paradigm to reach African American communities. Prev Chronic Dis. 2007 Oct;4(4):A112.

12. Leung MW, Yen IH, Minkler M. Community based participatory research: a promising approach for increasing epidemiology's relevance in the 21st century. Int J Epidemiol. 2004 Jun;33(3):499–506.

13. Grier SA, Kumanyika SK. The context for choice: health implications of targeted food and beverage marketing to African Americans. Am J Public Health. 2008 Sep;98(9):1616–29.

14. Lovasi GS, Hutson MA, Guerra M, et al. Built environments and obesity in disadvantaged populations. Epidemiol Rev. 2009;31:7–20.

15. Baskin ML, Odoms-Young AM, Kumanyika SK, et al. Nutrition and obesity issues for African Americans. In: Braithwaite RL, Taylor SE, Treadwell HM, eds. Health issues in the black community. Hoboken, NJ: Jossey-Bass, 2009.

16. Taylor WC, Carlos Poston WS, Jones L, et al. Environmental justice: obesity, physical activity, and healthy eating. J Phys Act Health. 2006;3(Suppl 1):S30–54.

17. Casagrande SS, Whitt-Glover MC, Lancaster KJ, et al. Built environment and health behaviors among African Americans: a systematic review. Am J Prev Med. 2009 Feb;36(2):174–81.

18. African American Collaborative Obesity Research Network (AACORN). Participatory research on African American community weight issues: defining the state of the art. Compendium of speaker presentation summaries. AACORN 2nd Invited Workshop, Philadelphia, PA, Aug 14–15, 2006. Available at: http://www.aacorn.org/uploads/files/AACORN2ndInvited WorkshopCompendium2006FINAL102.pdf

19. Wuest J. Professionalism and the evolution of nursing as a discipline: a feminist perspective. J Prof Nurs. 1994 Nov–Dec;10(6):357–67.

20. Wallerstein NB, Duran B. Using community-based participatory research to address health disparities. Health Promot Pract. 2006 Jul;7(3):312–23.

21. Green LW, Glasgow RE. Evaluating the relevance, generalization, and applicability of research: issues in external validation and translation methodology. Eval Health Prof. 2006 Mar;29(1):126–53.

22. Finkelstein EA, Khavjou OA, Mobley LR, et al. Racial/ethnic disparities in coronary heart disease risk factors among WISEWOMAN enrollees. J Women Health (Larchmt). 2004 Jun;13(5):503–18.

23. Yanek LR, Becker DM, Moy TF, et al. Project Joy: faith based cardiovascular health promotion for African American women. Public Health Rep. 2001;116 Suppl 1:68–81.

24. African American Collaborative Obesity Research Network (AACORN). A community-centered view of influences on eating, physical activity, and body weight. Philadelphia, PA: AACORN, 2007. Available at: http://www.aacorn.org/AbouComm-2517.html.

CHAPTER 8

The Importance of Public Safety in Promoting Physical Activity and Curbing Obesity within African American Communities

Keshia M. Pollack, PhD, MPH, Lauren M. Rossen, PhD, MS, Caterina Roman, PhD, Melicia C. Whitt-Glover, PhD, and Laura C. Leviton, PhD

With the continuing efforts to implement policy and environmental strategies to promote physical activity as a way of curbing the obesity epidemic, some scholars are thinking about the nexus of obesity reduction through exercise and public safety. Public safety encompasses traffic, crime and violence, and perceptions of safety. While important, safety concerns related to interpersonal violence (including sexual abuse and intimate-partner violence)—or interpersonal violence's possible connections with obesity—are not included in this commentary.*

Fears related to public safety have ramifications for individual and community health and are particularly relevant to obesity-related health behaviors such as physical activity. There is growing evidence that communities characterized by high levels of violence often lack safe and usable parks and playgrounds and score low on walkability measures, thus limiting community members' access to safe opportunities for outdoor physical activity.[1-7] These potential barriers to participating in physical activ-

---

Keshia M. Pollack is an associate professor in the Department of Health Policy and Management at the Johns Hopkins Bloomberg School of Public Health and is affiliated with the Johns Hopkins Center for Injury Research and Policy and the Hopkins Center for Health Disparities Solutions. Lauren M. Rossen is a postdoctoral research fellow with the Infant, Children and Women's Health Statistics Branch in the Office of Analysis and Epidemiology at the National Center for Health Statistics, Centers for Disease Control and Prevention. Caterina Roman joined the Department of Criminal Justice at Temple University in 2008 after 18 years at the Urban Institute in Washington, DC. Melicia C. Whitt-Glover is president and CEO of Gramercy Research Group in Winston-Salem, North Carolina. Laura C. Leviton is a special advisor for evaluation at the Robert Wood Johnson Foundation, having overseen evaluation of more than 80 of the foundation's programs, including several with a focus on preventing childhood obesity.

* The arguments developed in this chapter synchronize well with the overarching point of view on the interaction of immediate and distal factors influencing rates of obesity and overweight presented in the introduction and chapter 7.

ity may increase the risk of obesity, especially for individuals who live in low-income urban settings where safety concerns are common.[4-9] Moreover, these environmental characteristics are particularly relevant for African American communities because inequities in environments conducive to physical activity have been hypothesized to contribute to disparities in weight and physical activity behaviors.[1,10,11] A recent analysis estimated that differences in neighborhood access to physical activity facilities and food outlets explained between 13% and 28% of the Black-White gap in adolescent body mass index (BMI).[12] While there is a large literature that investigates physical and financial access to community resources for physical activity, relatively few studies have examined specific factors related to public safety in association with physical activity behaviors and weight. Additionally, there are other potential pathways by which safety may influence weight that remain underexamined in the literature, such as how safety affects dietary behavior.*

The purpose of this chapter is to reflect on the extant literature, to discuss public safety as it pertains to obesity, specifically in African American communities, and to propose a theoretical model illustrating the ways in which public safety and obesity are connected in African American communities. This commentary emphasizes the role of physical activity, given a growing theoretical and empirical focus on the links between safety and physical activity. In addition, we describe some emerging hypotheses about how safety relates to physiological responses to stress, as well as dietary behavior. We also provide suggestions for how improved safety can help in addressing obesity, and we conclude with some comments on how alliances can be forged across academic fields to develop a common agenda of both research and practice that supports environments conducive to safe physical activity and healthy eating.

Although we recognize that public safety is an important consideration for curbing obesity among all populations, we focus on African Americans because of the high prevalence of obesity and low levels of physical activity in this population,[13-17] the large concentration of African American adults and children who live in low-income urban settings where safety concerns are common,[5-9] and the limited attention to the intersection between obesity, active living, and public safety, which is particularly relevant for this population.[6,7] Moreover, obesity and violence generally have been considered separate epidemics in African American communities,[18,19] and thus we begin to explore relationships between these two public health problems. The discussion of public safety and related health risks could certainly be extended to other racial and ethnic subpopulations that predominantly reside in disadvantaged urban environments. Our review of the literature on these issues in Hispanic populations was limited, however, so we focus mainly on studies that were conducted with African Americans or that highlight disparities.

---

* Several other chapters in this volume also work with the observation that inequities in the built environment—including inequities in the safety of different neighborhoods—have a strong bearing on the distribution of obesity and overweight. See, for example, chapters 2, 6, 7, 10, 12–14, 18, 22, 29, and 31.

African Americans, Obesity, and Physical Activity

The burden of obesity disproportionately affects African Americans of all ages. While approximately 35% of non-Hispanic White adults (≥ 20 years) are obese (BMI ≥ 30 kg/m^2), the prevalence among non-Hispanic Black adults is nearly 50% overall, and it is 59% among African American women.[13] Nearly one in four African American children (2–19 years; 24.3%) are obese (age- and sex-specific BMI percentile ≥ 95), compared with only 14% of non-Hispanic White children.[14] African American children are twice as likely as non-Hispanic White children to have a BMI higher than the 97th percentile for age and sex.[14] The high prevalence of obesity is a concern because of known correlations between obesity and mortality, comorbidities, and disability.[20]*

Physical activity is a critical determinant of energy balance and health and is often described as a necessary component of any multifaceted intervention to address obesity.[21] Individuals who regularly engage in physical activity tend to weigh less, have lower rates of several chronic diseases (e.g., cardiovascular disease, diabetes, cancer, hypertension), and report better health outcomes than those who are not regularly active.[22] Disparities in physical activity among subpopulations have been reported, though they are complex.[23] A full exploration of the current state of knowledge on physical activity in African Americans is beyond the scope of this chapter. What is important and clear from the research is that physical activity levels for all racial and ethnic subpopulations require improvement.[21] Moreover, research is just beginning to disentangle the influences of perceived and objective environmental hazards on physical activity, influences that probably vary across socioeconomic groups and racial and ethnic subpopulations.[10,24]

How Does Safety Correlate with Obesity?

We did not identify any conceptual models in the existing literature that illustrate how safety may influence obesity. However, one highly relevant framework for us to build upon was proposed by Loukaitou-Sideris and Eck[25] and connects crime and physical activity. The intent of their framework was to highlight how settings may influence physical activity and, in particular, the situational characteristics (factors immediately surrounding a location) that create the opportunities for crime and incivilities. We adapted their model, and in figure 8.1 we depict a hypothetical set of relationships that consider how aspects of public safety may be linked to obesity. These pathways may be direct or indirect and may contain feedback loops that create a complex web of intertwined relationships. We use the framework not as a definitive theoretical model but to provide a backdrop for drawing on the extant literature.

Safety as a Barrier to Participating in Outdoor Physical Activity

The influence of unsafe neighborhoods has been suggested as one mechanism for reduced physical activity,[26] as time spent outdoors is positively associated with physical

---

* See also chapters 2, 3, 6, and 7 for overviews of rates of obesity across races and ethnicities.

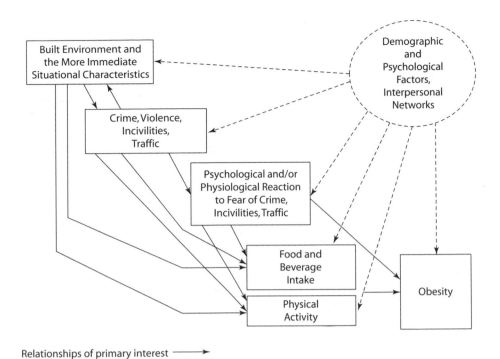

Relationships of primary interest ———➤

Other relationships some of which - - - ➤
may interact with primary interest
relationships

FIGURE 8.1. How safety may influence obesity. Source: Adapted from Loukaitou-Sideris and Eck (2007).[25]

activity and has declined significantly in recent decades.[26,27] Based on the existing literature, safety is hypothesized to correlate with obesity through both direct biophysical pathways and indirect pathways mediated by physical activity (fig. 8. 1). The dominant hypothesis is that safety concerns related to the built environment are barriers to participation in outdoor physical activity and thereby indirectly affect obesity. High levels of crime and violence and other safety issues also may influence decisions about where physical activity facilities (e.g., gyms) are located, which could result in a scarcity of such facilities in areas where safety is a large concern. Since there is evidence that African Americans are less likely than others to have access to dedicated places to exercise,[2] the potential effects of fears related to traffic hazards or crime associated with more informal places to exercise (e.g., parks, active transportation— such as getting places by walking and cycling—opportunities) may be particularly relevant for this population. Specifically, these fears and perceptions related to safety may prohibit both adults and children from walking or playing outside.[27–29]

Parents often cite concern about traffic safety and crime as a barrier to outdoor physical activity and active transportation for children.[30] A qualitative study of youths in Baltimore described several safety-related barriers to physical activity among low-income African American adolescents, including risk of injury from unsafe and poorly maintained equipment/facilities, the presence of incivilities such as syringes or broken glass, fear of crime and gang or drug violence, and inadequate monitoring or security in outside areas.[31] Adolescents reported that perceived crime or incivilities are a barrier to using parks or playgrounds, even if these facilities are nearby.[31]

Perceived and objective measures of neighborhood safety have been associated with reduced levels of objectively assessed or self-reported physical activity[8,9,27-29] and with higher BMI among youths.[5] Associations between traffic safety and physical activity have also been reported: adolescents living in neighborhoods with better traffic safety are more likely to engage in active transportation (e.g., walking, biking).[32] Additionally, neighborhood crime and hazards related to traffic have been associated with higher BMI.[26] Despite children's higher levels of physical activity, routine exposure to high volumes of traffic or other environmental hazards such as crime remains a safety concern (as evidenced by the term "captive walkers"—that is, urban, low-income children who lack alternative transportation to school and are therefore forced to walk).[33]

African American parents cite many safety concerns associated with physical activity for girls,[34] which may exacerbate gender-related disparities in physical activity. Specifically, evidence shows that African American parents are more concerned about safety for girls than for boys and are more likely to let boys play outside and keep girls inside.[34] These perceptions may be a barrier to outdoor physical activity for girls, which could contribute to gender disparities in activity and obesity and to poor health outcomes. Among adults, studies cite more environmental/safety-related barriers to physical activity among women than among men; however, this does not necessarily hold true for African American women compared with women in other racial/ethnic groups.[35-39]

Children without access to safe activity spaces (e.g., recreation centers, parks, playgrounds) will often use alternative play spaces such as vacant lots and streets,[31] placing them at risk of injury from traffic and pedestrian accidents. This risk is compounded by the greater degree of hazardous traffic conditions in poor, urban settings. In general, African Americans have disproportionately high exposures to these hazardous conditions, placing them at greater risk than Whites for injury and mortality due to traffic and pedestrian accidents.[40] These traffic-related safety concerns pose a barrier to outdoor physical activity or active living and transportation for all ages.[40]

Public Safety, Fear, and the Physiological Response

Public safety could also connect with obesity through stress response pathways, which we also illustrate in figure 8.1. Cortisol levels have been shown to be associated with levels of perceived chronic stress and with abdominal fat deposition.[41] The association between obesity and cortisol is attributed to the hypothalamic-pituitary-adrenal (HPA) axis, one of two major neuroendocrine systems associated with the stress response, which leads to deregulation of cortisol.[42] Chronic exposure to environmental stresses, such as those resulting from the exigencies of inner-city living, may play a role in the development of visceral obesity through hyperactivation of the HPA axis.[43] External stressors such as high levels of community crime or violence may contribute to higher cortisol levels.[44] The Institute of Medicine report *From Neurons to Neighborhoods*[45] highlights the cascade of negative health consequences associated with chronic stress in childhood. Exposures to stressors or adverse childhood experiences can alter brain physiology in a way that affects the salience of rewards and punishments, as well as control of decision making and mood. These pathways have been implicated in the development of obesity, high blood pressure, cardiovascular disease, and inflammation.

Another potential pathway by which stress may influence obesity is through dietary behaviors. In a 2001 review article, Björntorp[46] hypothesized that elevated cortisol levels could induce *stress eating*, one negative coping strategy, which may also contribute to obesity beyond the direct effects on visceral fat deposition. In support of this hypothesis, a number of studies have examined the phenomenon of *comfort eating*, a similar term used to designate the need for certain individuals in a state of negative affect to consume sweet, fatty, energy-dense foods, thereby increasing the risk of weight gain.[47] These associations are complex and variable; eating behaviors due to stress vary by sociodemographic factors.[48]

We also identified research that recognizes racism and poverty as important perceived stressors and barriers to maintaining a healthy weight for African Americans living in the Deep South.[49] Another study showed that both African American and European American children who are exposed to negative socioenvironmental climates over time were more likely to have altered serum cortisol levels when compared with children in nonnegative socioenvironmental climates; the effect was magnified for African American children.[50] The possible connections between public safety and obesity via pathways that incorporate physiological responses are plausible, and it is likely that exposure to chronic social and environmental stresses could also affect obesity, especially through food intake dysregulation. These connections are important and warrant further investigation as we continue to learn more in the effort to quell the epidemic of obesity among African Americans and other vulnerable populations.

Relationship between Safety and Diet

Despite very little empirical evidence to date that links public safety to dietary intake and, subsequently, to obesity, there is some information to suggest that more research is needed to examine this potential pathway. For example, in many low-income urban areas, residents rely on small corner stores for day-to-day food purchases.[51] Many of these stores, as a response to or as a preventive measure against crime, have a Plexiglas window or door separating the consumer from the store staff, and often the consumer must request certain items that the staff will retrieve and exchange through the window.[52] This barricade makes it difficult for consumers to read nutrition information, compare food products and prices, or inspect the quality of produce—if it is even available. Although storeowners recognize that this window restricts consumers' choice and purchasing behavior, the predominant concern among owners is safety, and many report fears of robbery, theft, or assault.[52] Moreover, one study reported that an increase in criminal activities deterred retail development (this study also found that an increase in density of retail employment led to an increase in crime, which raises concerns about endogeneity).[53] There is also some evidence that fears related to neighborhood crime may influence which stores residents are willing to travel to, though safety issues remain underexamined in this context.[54,55] These connections are important, and studies are needed on the possible effect of safety on healthy eating.

Can Improved Public Safety Affect Obesity Rates?

There is some evidence to suggest that improving public safety can affect obesity rates by increasing opportunities for safe physical activity. For instance, the direct benefits of traffic safety for increased physical activity are becoming clear as the literature begins to frame traffic safety as an obesity prevention issue. A 2006 review by the Centers for Disease Control and Prevention Task Force on Community Preventive Services concluded that physical activity is affected by community-scale urban design and land use policies that create pedestrian-friendly environments, such as communitywide zoning and building codes.[56] Certain types of street-scale urban design and land use policies were also found to increase physical activity. These policies improve street lighting and introduce traffic-calming features such as raised crosswalks. The benefits of crime prevention are also straightforward: if residents are less active outside because they fear violence and crime, then preventing crime and violence may have the added benefit of preventing obesity.

The hypothesized connections also pertain to school settings. Evidence suggests that characteristics of school safety and climate are important to consider when developing school-based interventions aimed at instilling healthy practices to reduce overweight and obesity among children. For example, active commuting to school has declined rapidly over the past four decades. Data from the National Household Transportation Survey indicate that between 1969 and 2009, the proportion of K–8 students who regularly walked or biked to school dropped from 47.7% to 12.7%.[57] Factors associated with decreased likelihood of active transportation to school are related to safety concerns, including parental concerns,[58] real or perceived high crime rates, [30] and school policies prohibiting walking.[30]

Support for how reductions in crime and violence could affect obesity is lacking in the literature, but drawing on the model we presented earlier (fig. 8.1), it seems plausible that if fear of crime or violence is associated with obesity, then reducing the occurrence of crime and changing the perception of fear may affect obesity. Future studies should explore specific pathways by which objective and perceived safety influences physical activity and obesity in order to identify key leverage points that could be targeted for intervention. Approaches to preventing crime (such as problem-oriented policing or crime prevention through environmental design) have an evidence base supporting their effectiveness.[59]

More research is needed to determine whether improving safety through these kinds of evidence-based interventions leads to concomitant improvements in exercise and weight. These are important areas that warrant future exploration and may help to elucidate the connection between safety and obesity in African American communities that are disproportionately burdened by both public health problems.

Future Directions

Public health practitioners may find it difficult to bring attention to issues such as chronic disease when communities are experiencing pressing societal issues such as unemployment and violence. By linking obesity to public safety, it may be possible to garner public support for obesity prevention activities. Work must be done on the part of researchers to unite multidisciplinary areas of expertise that will allow these links to be embedded within the framework of research examining links between features of the environment and obesity. Too often, studies are framed with a narrow theoretical lens, resulting in a focus on one outcome of interest with a constrained set of predictors. This tendency to focus narrowly can limit the overall import of the studies, as well as the breadth of implications that could emerge for obesity prevention policy and practice.

The health outcomes related to obesity and lack of safety tend to cluster in urban communities. This does not mean that residents of rural neighborhoods are immune from these health concerns; rather, research indicates that some urban populations are particularly vulnerable to myriad health conditions.[60] The framework of syndemics would seem to apply to this pattern. The term *syndemic* is applied to two or more epidemics that interact synergistically and contribute to an excess burden of disease in a population.[61] As we have noted, both obesity and violence have been considered epidemic in some communities, so this framework is useful for our discussion here. The Syndemics Prevention Network suggests that syndemics occur when health problems cluster by person, place, or time and that "to prevent a syndemic, one must not only prevent or control each affliction, but also the forces that tie those afflictions together."[61 [p. 2]] In other words, issue-specific solutions are unlikely to be as effective as those that focus on upstream forces—in this case, public safety.

Public health solutions to syndemics should be developed in an integrated, comprehensive way that addresses the common underlying determinants. Developing comprehensive ecological frameworks that integrate threads of safety, victimization, and fear with behaviors tied to obesity that can be tested (and retested) could help advance the body of evidence needed to mount effective obesity prevention programs and interventions. For example, policies to improve community clean-up efforts may not only remove barriers to outdoor physical activity but also reduce exposure to neighborhood hazards that increase the risk of injury and victimization. Such complex systems approaches are well suited to address the complex web of public health problems and epidemics that disproportionately burden African American, Hispanic, and disadvantaged urban communities generally.[62]

The syndemics approach is also consistent with the Policy, Systems, and Environmental Change (PSE) framework. The PSE framework promotes the development of a systems approach in various settings, including communities, schools, and workplaces, that involves policy and environmental changes.[63] Multisectoral partnerships are critical to a successful PSE approach and offer the potential to bring safety to a more central and prominent role in obesity interventions.

We identified several communities around the United States that are forging community-based partnerships to simultaneously address rising levels of obesity and safety-related concerns. Communities are piecing together grant funding to develop innovative programming and large collaborative partnerships that help build neighborhoods' capacity to address these overlapping public health issues. There are formal partnerships such as the Convergence Partnership, which is committed to a place-based approach to support initiatives with the express goal of making sure communities have fresh, local, healthy food and safe places to play and exercise.[64] The Convergence Partnership promotes and supports the coordination and connections among government officials, funders, advocates, and practitioners across multiple fields and sectors.

Another example is the Northeast Neighborhoods Health Action Network in Denver, the local coalition behind LiveWell Northeast Denver, which is a collaborative effort of nonprofits, businesses, government agencies, schools, and individual residents working toward high-impact, sustainable health outcomes in Northeast Denver.[65] Their mission includes a focus on increasing public safety, and as a result, they have developed a unique partnership with the Denver Safe City Office's Gang Reduction Initiative of Denver. Collaborative partners gather regularly to discuss and develop targeted and measurable strategies that overlap efforts to reduce violence with obesity prevention strategies. Another example of partnerships that broadly address various community health problems is Transform Baltimore, a comprehensive rewriting of the city's zoning code.[66] This effort entailed significant collaboration across multiple groups and sectors, including public health officials, city planners, community leaders, researchers and academics, local business representatives, and various advocacy groups. This collaborative effort sought to develop a new master plan and zoning code that would provide opportunities for economic development, mitigate crime and violence, and improve walkability, pedestrian safety, and access to healthy food.[66,67]

These successful partnerships and collaborative efforts point to the importance of comprehensive and multisectoral interventions for reducing obesity, improving public safety, and promoting healthy neighborhoods. With future attention to systematically chronicling the development and implementation of these multifaceted strategies, coupled with rigorous process and outcome evaluations, we stand to address the current gaps in the knowledge needed for sustained and widespread adoption of innovative and comprehensive interventions.

Conclusions

The need for new knowledge regarding the connection between public safety and obesity is all too evident. Efforts to improve public safety have great potential to address several public health problems concurrently, such as injury, physical activity, and obesity. Over time, public health practitioners and researchers have begun to examine interventions in the built environment to improve traffic safety, increase physical activity levels, and reduce the risk of injury and obesity. Public health practitioners interested in improving safe access to physical activity and nutrition should become familiar with the criminal justice system and the evidence-based practices of public safety that will permit them to advocate for effective injury prevention methods and interventions to improve community safety.

There is a need not just for improved practice in this area but also for better research that explores both objective and subjective measures of public safety and the various pathways between safety, perceptions, and health behaviors and outcomes. Nationwide, studies are being conducted on ways to reduce community-level violence; obesity prevention researchers should utilize these natural experiments to examine the impact on physical activity and weight outcomes. The connections between safety, physical activity, and obesity are apparent, but other potential connections also warrant further attention. Specifically, future studies should explore how physiological stress responses resulting from unsafe environments may relate to obesity. The potential links between safety issues, the food environment, dietary intake, and obesity also should be explored.

The literature provides growing support for better integration of strategies to modify built and social environments so as to improve public safety, increase physical activity, and reduce the burden of obesity. Intersectoral collaborations to create safer neighborhoods may not only affect obesity risk for African Americans and other racial/ethnic subpopulations, such as Hispanics, at high risk of obesity; they may also promote livable and healthy communities that support improvements in population health for all.

Acknowledgment

This work was supported in part by grant no. 5R49CE001507 from the Centers for Disease Control and Prevention to the Johns Hopkins Center for Injury Research and Policy. The views expressed in this chapter are those of the authors and do not necessarily represent the position of the Centers for Disease Control and Prevention.

References

1. Gordon-Larsen P, Nelson MC, Page P, et al. Inequality in the built environment underlies key health disparities in physical activity and obesity. Pediatrics. 2006 Feb;117(2):417–24.

2. Powell LM, Slater S, Chaloupka FJ, et al. Availability of physical activity–related facilities and neighborhood demographic and socioeconomic characteristics: a national study. Am J Public Health. 2006 Sep;96(9):1676–80. Epub 2006 Jul 27.

3. Ross CE, Mirowsky J. Neighborhood disadvantage, disorder, and health. J Health Soc Behav. 2001 Sep;42(3):258–76.

4. Rossen LM, Pollack KM. Making the connection between zoning and health disparities. Environ Justice. 2012 Jun;5(3):119–27.

5. Slater SJ, Ewing R, Powell LM, et al. The association between community physical activity settings and youth physical activity, obesity, and body mass index. J Adolesc Health. 2012 Nov;47(5):496–503. Epub 2010 May 26.

6. Pollack KM. An injury prevention perspective on the childhood obesity epidemic. Prev Chronic Dis. 2009 Jul;6(3):A107. Epub 2009 Jun 15.

7. Cohen L, Davis R, Lee V, et al. Addressing the intersection: preventing violence and promoting healthy eating and active living. Oakland, CA: Prevention Institute, 2010. Available at: http://preventioninstitute.org/press/highlights/404-addressing-the-intersection.html.

8. Carver A, Timperio A, Crawford D. Playing it safe: the influence of neighbourhood safety on children's physical activity: a review. Health Place. 2008 Jun;14(2):217–27. Epub 2007 Jun 27.

9. Roman CG, Chalfin A. Fear of walking outdoors: a multilevel ecologic analysis of crime and disorder. Am J Prev Med. 2008 Apr;34(4):306–12.

10. Casagrande SS, Whitt-Glover MC, Lancaster KJ, et al. Built environment and health behaviors among African Americans: a systematic review. Am J Prev Med. 2009 Feb;36(2);174–81.

11. Larson NI, Story MT, Nelson MC. Neighborhood environments: disparities in access to healthy foods in the U.S. Am J Prev Med. 2009 Jan;36(1):74–81.

12. Powell LM, Wada R, Krauss RC, et al. Ethnic disparities in adolescent body mass index in the United States: the role of parental socioeconomic status and economic contextual factors. Soc Sci Med. 2012 Aug;75(3):469–76.

13. Flegal KM, Carroll MD, Kit BK, et al. Prevalence of obesity and trends in the distribution of body mass index among US adults, 1990–2010. JAMA. 2012 Feb 1;307(5):491–7.

14. Odgen CL, Carroll MD, Kit BK, et al. Prevalence of obesity and trends in the distribution of body mass index among US children and adolescents, 1990–2010. JAMA. 2012 Feb 1;307(5): 483–90.

15. Ham SA, Ainsworth BE. Disparities in data on Healthy People 2010 physical activity objectives collected by accelerometry and self-report. Am J Public Health. 2010 Apr 1;100 Suppl 1:S263–8.

16. Centers for Disease Control and Prevention. Healthy People 2010: final review. Atlanta, GA: Centers for Disease Control and Prevention / National Center for Health Statistics, 2013 Jan 22. Available at: http://www.cdc.gov/nchs/data/hpdata2010/hp2010_final_review.pdf.

17. Crespo CJ, Smit E, Andersen RE, et al. Race/ethnicity, social class and their relation to physical inactivity during leisure time: results from the third National Health and Nutrition Examination Survey, 1988–1994. Am J Prev Med. 2000 Jan;18(1):46–53.

18. Cooley-Strickland M, Quille TJ, Griffin RS, et al. Community violence and youth: affect, behavior, substance use, and academics. Clin Child Fam Psychol Rev. 2009 Jun;12(2):127–56.

19. Kumanyika S, Whitt-Glover MC, Gary TL, et al. Expanding the obesity research paradigm to reach African American communities. Prev Chronic Dis. 2007 Oct;4(4):A112. Epub 2007 Sep 15.

20. Must A, Spadano J, Coakley EH, et al. The disease burden associated with overweight and obesity. JAMA. 1999 Oct 27;282(16):1523–9.

21. Institute of Medicine. Accelerating progress in obesity prevention: solving the weight of the nation. Washington, DC: National Academies Press, 2012.

22. Warburton DE, Nicol CW, Bredin SSD. Health benefits of physical activity: the evidence. CMAJ. 2006 Mar 14;174(6):801–9.

23. Whitt-Glover MC, Taylor WC, Floyd MF, et al. Disparities in physical activity and sedentary behaviors among US children and adolescents: prevalence, correlates, and intervention implications. J Public Health Policy. 2009;30 Suppl 1:S309–34.

24. Siddiqi Z, Tiro JA, Shuval K. Understanding impediments and enablers to physical activity among African American adults: a systematic review of qualitative studies. Health Educ Res. 2001;26(6):1010–24.

25. Loukaitou-Sideris A, Eck JE. Crime prevention and active living. Am J Health Promot. 2007 Mar–Apr;21(4 Suppl):380–9, iii.

26. Black JL, Macinko J. Neighborhoods and obesity. Nutr Rev. 2008 Jan;66(1):2–20.

27. Sallis JF, Prochaska JJ, Taylor WC. A review of correlates of physical activity of children and adolescents. Med Sci Sports Exerc. 2000 May;32(5):963–75.

28. Gómez JE, Johnson BA, Selva M, et al. Violent crime and outdoor physical activity among inner-city youth. Prev Med. 2004 Nov;39(5):876–81.

29. Molnar BE, Gortmaker SL, Bull FC, et al. Unsafe to play? Neighborhood disorder and lack of safety predict reduced physical activity among urban children and adolescents. Am J Health Promot. 2004 May–Jun;18(5):378–86.

30. Centers for Disease Control and Prevention. Barriers to children walking to or from school—United States, 2004. MMWR Morb Mortal Wkly Rep. 2005 Sep 30;54(38): 949–52.

31. Ries AV, Gittelsohn J, Voorhees CC, et al. The environment and urban adolescents' use of recreational facilities for physical activity: a qualitative study. Am J Health Promot. 2008 Sep–Oct;23(1):43–50.

32. Grow HM, Saelens BE, Kerr J, et al. Where are youth active? Roles of proximity, active transport, and built environment. Med Sci Sports Exerc. 2008 Dec;40(12):2071–9.

33. Zhu X, Lee C. Walkability and safety around elementary schools economic and ethnic disparities. Am J Prev Med. 2008 Apr;34(4):282–90.

34. Boyington JE, Carter-Edwards L, Piehl M, et al. Cultural attitudes toward weight, diet, and physical activity among overweight African American girls. Prev Chronic Dis. 2008 Apr; 5(2):A36. Epub 2008 Mar 15.

35. Ainsworth BE, Wilcox S, Thompson WW, et al. Personal, social, and physical environmental correlates of physical activity in African-American women in South Carolina. Am J Prev Med. 2003 Oct;25(3 Suppl 1):23–9.

36. Eyler AA, Baker E, Cromer L, et al. Physical activity and minority women: a qualitative study. Health Educ Behav. 1998 Oct;25(5):640–52.

37. King AC, Castro C, Wilcox S, et al. Personal and environmental factors associated with physical inactivity among different racial-ethnic groups of U.S. middle-aged and older-aged women. Health Psychol. 2000 Jul;19(4):354–64.

38. Rohm Young D, Voorhees CC. Personal, social, and environmental correlates of physical activity in urban African-American women. Am J Prev Med. 2003 Oct;25(3 Suppl 1):38–44.

39. Sanderson BK, Foushee HR, Bittner V, et al. Personal, social, and physical environmental correlates of physical activity in rural African-American women in Alabama. Am J Prev Med. 2003 Oct;25(3 Suppl 1):30–7.

40. Day K. Active living and social justice: planning for physical activity in low-income, black, and Latino communities. J Am Plann Assoc. 2006;72(1):88–99.

41. Bjorntorp P, Rosmond R. The metabolic syndrome—a neuroendocrine disorder? Br J Nutr. 2000 Mar;83 Suppl 1:S49–57.

42. Tull ES, Sheu YT, Butler C, et al. Relationships between perceived stress, coping behavior and cortisol secretion in women with high and low levels of internalized racism. J Natl Med Assoc. 2005 Feb;97(2):206–12.

43. Vicennatti V, Pasqui F, Cavazza C, et al. Stress-related development of obesity and cortisol in women. Obesity (Silver Spring). 2009 Sep;17(9):1678–83. Epub 2009 Mar 19.

44. Bose M, Olivan B, Laferrere B. Stress and obesity: the role of the hypothalamic-pituitary-adrenal axis in metabolic disease. Curr Opin Endocrinol Diabetes Obes. 2009 Oct;16(5):340–6.

45. Institute of Medicine, National Research Council. From neurons to neighborhoods: an update: workshop summary. Washington, DC: National Academies Press, 2012.

46. Björntorp P. Do stress reactions cause abdominal obesity and comorbidities? Obes Rev. 2001 May;2(2):73–86.

47. Gibson EL. The psychobiology of comfort eating: implications for neuropharmacological interventions. Behav Pharmacol. 2012 Sep;23(5–6):442–60.

48. Adam TC, Epel ES. Stress, eating and the reward system. Physiol Behav. 2007 Jul 24;91(4):449–58. Epub 2007 Apr 14.

49. Scott AJ, Wilson RF. Upstream ecological risks for overweight and obesity among African American youth in a rural town in the Deep South, 2007. Prev Chronic Dis. 2011 Jan;8(1):A17. Epub 2010 Dec 15.

50. Dulin-Keita A, Casazza K, Fernandez JR, et al. Do neighbourhoods matter? Neighbourhood disorder and long-term trends in serum cortisol levels. J Epidemiol Community Health. 2012 Jan;66(1):24–9. Epub 2010 Aug 24.

51. Wrigley N, Warm D, Margetts B. Deprivation, diet, and food-retail access: findings from the Leeds "food deserts" study. Environ Plann. 2003;35(1):151–88.

52. Gittlelsohn J, Franceshini MCT, Rasooly IR. Understanding the food environment in a low-income urban setting: implications for food store interventions. J Hunger Environ Nutr. 2008;2(2–3):33–50.

53. Bowes DR. A two-stage model of the simultaneous relationship between retail development and crime. Econ Dev Q. 2007 Feb;21(1):79–90.

54. Burns DJ, Manolis C, Keep WW. Fear of crime on shopping intentions: an examination. Int J Retail Distribution Manage. 2010;38(1):45–56.

55. Neff RA, Palmer AM, McKenzie SE, et al. Food systems and public health disparities. J Hunger Environ Nutr. 2009;4(3–4):282–314.

56. Heath GW, Brownson RC, Kruger J, et al. The effectiveness of urban design and land use and transport policies and practices to increase physical activity: a systematic review. J Phys Act Health. 2006;3 Suppl 1:S55–76.

57. McDonald NC, Brown AL, Marchetti LM, et al. U.S. school travel, 2009 an assessment of trends. Am J Prev Med. 2011 Aug;41(2):146–51.

58. Kerr J, Rosenberg D, Sallis JF, et al. Active commuting to school: associations with environment and parental concerns. Med Sci Sports Exerc. 2006 Apr;38(4):787–94.

59. Sherman LW, Farrington DP, Welsh BC, et al, eds. Evidence-based crime prevention. New York, NY: Taylor and Francis, 2002.

60. Harpham T. Urban health in developing countries: what do we know and where do we go? Health Place. 2009 Mar;15(1):107–16. Epub 2008 Mar 25.

61. Milstein B. Introduction to the syndemics prevention network. Atlanta, GA: Centers for Disease Control and Prevention, 2002. Available at: http://www.nmpreventionnetwork.org/cdcnetworkintro.pdf.

62. Diez Roux AV. Complex systems thinking and current impasses in health disparities research. Am J Public Health. 2011 Sep;101(9):1627–34. Epub 2011 Jul 21.

63. National Association of County and City Health Officials. Healthy communities, healthy behaviors: using policy, systems, and environmental change to combat chronic disease. Washington, DC: National Association of County and City Health Officials, 2011 Oct. Available at: http://www.naccho.org/topics/HPDP/mcah/loader.cfm?csModule=security/getfile&PageID=218029.

64. Convergence Partnership. Convergence Partnership website: the healthy eating active living convergence partnership. Portland, OR: Convergence Partnership, 2010. Available at: http://www.convergencepartnership.org/site/c.fhLOK6PELmF/b.3917581/k.C802/About_Us.htm.

65. LiveWell Colorado. Northeast neighborhoods health action network in Denver. Denver, CO: LiveWell Colorado, 2012. Available at: https://about.livewellcolorado.org/livewell-northeast-denver.

66. Johnson Thonrton R, Fichtenburg C, Greiner A, et al. Zoning for a healthy Baltimore: a health impact assessment of the Transform Baltimore comprehensive zoning rewrite. Baltimore, MD: Johns Hopkins University, 2010. Available at: http://www.hopkinsbayview.org/pediatrics/zoning/files/FullReportColor.pdf.

67. Ransom MM, Greiner A, Kochtitzky C, et al. Pursuing health equity: zoning codes and public health. J Law Med Ethics. 2011 Mar;39 Suppl 1:94–7.

CHAPTER 9

Military and Civilian Approaches to the U.S. Obesity Epidemic

Robert S. Levine, MD, Barbara J. Kilbourne, PhD, Courtney J. Kihlberg, MD, MSPH, Janice S. Emerson, PhD, Irwin Goldzweig, MS, Paul Juarez, PhD, and Roger Zoorob, MD, MPH

More than 50 years ago, public health scientists observed a lethal association between the U.S. environment and heart disease. They warned about poor dietary choices[1] and were also concerned about levels of physical fitness in the young. The evidence about physical conditioning[2] so shocked President Dwight D. Eisenhower that he established his own fitness council, the President's Council on Physical Fitness and Sports.[3] President Eisenhower charged the council in a way that continues to shape civilian responses to the obesity epidemic: "I believe you and I share the feeling that more and better coordinated attention should be given to this most precious asset—our youth—within the Federal government. By this I do not mean that we should have an over-riding Federal program. The fitness of our young people is essentially a home and local community problem; your deliberations also reveal a need for arousing in the American people a new awareness of the importance of physical and recreational activity."[3] [p. 41] In other words, individual households and local communities were to be inspired by federal leadership and motivated to embrace the intrinsic value of physical fitness. The chairman of the council, Fred Seaton, echoed this charge in 1958, stating that the council must remain "a stimulator, a catalyst. Neither the President nor ourselves intended that the Council develop into a centralized, bureaucratic agency, with regional, state, and local offices doling out federal funds to 'hand down' a uniform code for fitness and to prescribe to every community in the Nation what should be done to improve the state of fitness of its young people."[3] [p. 44] In 2006, council historians Julie Sturgeon and Janice Meer concluded that "for 50

Robert S. Levine, Paul Juarez, and Roger Zoorob are professors, Barbara J. Kilbourne is an associate professor, and Courtney J. Kihlberg and Irwin Goldzweig are assistant professors in the Department of Family and Community Medicine, Meharry Medical College. Janice S. Emerson is associate director of the Center for Prevention Research, Tennessee State University.

years, the Council has remained constant in adhering to President Eisenhower's original vision—to serve as a stimulator and a catalyst. By activating resources within the public, private, and nonprofit spheres of American life, the President's Council on Physical Fitness and Sports continues to confront a pressing health problem, sedentary behavior, in creative ways that allow for both bipartisanship and continuity."[3] [p. 63]

However harmonious and sustainable, civilian handling of the Eisenhower doctrine is associated with what may be one of the most serious U.S. public failures of the twentieth century. In 2000–2001, the publication of a set of maps by the U.S. Centers for Disease Control and Prevention (CDC) and the Surgeon General's warning that obesity had become a national epidemic brought obesity to the forefront of the national policy agenda.[4] As of 2009–10, however, the sum total of U.S. efforts was associated with an overall adult obesity prevalence of 36%.[5] According to a 2011 report, the prevalence of obesity grew in 16 states during 2010 and declined in none.[6]* In 2012, the CDC reported seemingly lower percentages of self-reported obesity in several states during 2011, but it cautioned that data from 2011 forward could not be compared with previous years due to changes in methodology. According to the 2012 report, no U.S. state had a prevalence of adult obesity of under 20%, while 39 states had a prevalence of 25% or more, and 12 of these states were at 30% or more.[7] As for youth fitness, less than one-third of all children aged 6–17 were recently found to engage in vigorous activity daily, even if a minimal definition was used (at least 20 minutes of physical activity that makes the child sweat and breathe hard, at least five days a week).[6] Adding possible insult to injury, the establishment of the U.S. Interstate Highway system, which President Eisenhower signed into law in 1956, has been estimated by some researchers to account for 13% of the U.S. obesity burden,[8] although others discount the association as an ecological fallacy.[9]

The U.S. military may be an important exception to these national failures. Although between 25% and 30% of potential U.S. military recruits are rejected because of obesity, less than 1% of those accepted fail to fulfill their military obligations because of obesity.[10] And in 2002, early separations for persistent failure to meet weight and body composition standards totaled just over 1,400 people, or about 0.1% of the active-duty force of 1.4 million personnel.[11] This figure may represent an underestimate, however, since some military personnel are allowed to complete current obligations if obese but are not allowed to re-enlist.[11] Furthermore, there are some who challenge overall estimates, in part by documenting discrepancies between official records of "in standard" adherence and actual body measurements.[12] One study of

---

* More recent reports suggest that the sharp rise in obesity and overweight, at least among children and young people, is leveling out or declining. As described in a CDC report in 2013, "During 2008–2011, statistically significant downward trends in obesity prevalence were observed in 18 states and the U.S. Virgin Islands. Florida, Georgia, Missouri, New Jersey, South Dakota, and the U.S. Virgin Islands had the largest absolute decreases in obesity prevalence, each with a decrease of ≥1 percentage point. Twenty states and Puerto Rico experienced no significant change, and obesity prevalence increased significantly in three states."[99] [p. 629] Also see the 2013 report by Iannotti and Wang.[100]

4,979 active-duty Air Force personnel found that 20% exceeded maximum allowable weights, costing $22.8 million per year in medical care and lost work days.[13] Nonetheless, recent overall active-duty obesity estimates range from 12% to 17%,[9] which is well below civilian levels, and estimates from 2002 included rates of obesity of 14.2% for Army men, 6.2% for Army women, 16.2% for Navy men, and 7.4% for Navy women.[11]

Given that military success in fighting obesity is real, further study of the military experience may provide some idea of the scope of activity needed to counteract the factors that promote overweight, obesity, and poor physical fitness in the present environment. In this chapter we review the historical development of the military weight management program, show how its implementation foreshadowed current civilian models, and discuss how a better understanding of the military experience might be helpful to the civilian population.

Historical Development of U.S. Military Approaches to Obesity and Fitness

Recognition of the importance of health for U.S. soldiers is as old as the nation itself. Dr. Benjamin Rush, in his position as physician general to the military hospitals of the United States, noted the following in a 1777 pamphlet: "an attention to the health of your soldiers is absolutely necessary to form a *great* military character. Had it not been for this eminent quality, Xenophon would never have led ten thousand Greeks for sixteen months through a cold and most inhospitable country; nor would Fabius have kept that army together, without it, which conquered Hannibal, and delivered Rome."[14] [pp. 14–15] The same pamphlet recommended a diet consisting chiefly of vegetables and cited Julius Caesar's exclusive reliance on wheat to feed his army during the campaign for Gaul.[14] The importance of physical fitness, in particular, was also a key factor in the rise to prominence of General Thomas ("Stonewall") Jackson. Partly because of its rigorous training programs, the Stonewall Brigade was able to march 28 miles, with each soldier carrying a 60-pound pack, across the Cacapon River and the western Shenandoah Mountains in a driving sleet, arriving ready to fight and seize a key communications center in Romney, Virginia.[15]

Such examples were more the exception than the rule, however,[16] and while military height and weight tables were first published during the Civil War,[11] organized diagnoses of healthy and unhealthy weight did not begin on a large scale until implementation of the Selective Service Act in 1917. These efforts, while at first nonspecific and largely subjective assessments of "underweight" or "overweight" by draft board examiners,[16] formed the basis for movement toward more rigorous and objective standards. Once again, progress was gradual. In the 1950s, for example, there is evidence that examining physicians were still given considerable leeway for subjective assessment.[16,17] In 1976, however, the Army Physical Fitness and Weight Control Program (AR 600-9) marked a transition to more complex, system-wide, multilevel approaches. This regulation mandated that all soldiers younger than 40 years of age be weighed and tested for physical fitness annually, with the caution that soldiers failing to comply could suffer the consequences of poor evaluation reports, barriers to re-enlistment, and even involuntary separation.[18] The regulation also marked the introduction of the body mass index (BMI) calculation—weight in kilograms divided by height in meters squared—into Army standards. Then as now, this measure is employed as a useful (though increasingly questioned) estimate of health and body fat composition.[19,20] Today, while there are differences among the Army, Navy, Marines, and Air Force, all branches of the military still maintain gender-specific standards of weight and physical fitness. There are generally two sets, one for accession of recruits into initial entry and training and another equivalent or more stringent set of standards that must be met for retention in the service.[11]

Several driving forces played a role in the progression toward more rigorous physical standards. Early influences included readiness to fight[18,21] and evidence of the long-term effects of hypertension.[22] Sarnecky's contemporary history of the U.S. Army Nurse Corps[18,21] noted that declines in morale following the Vietnam War contributed to concerns about troop readiness in the 1970s and 1980s: if soldiers were not fit to fight, readiness was unlikely at either the personal or the unit level.[18] A foundational study by Shields[22] showed an association between obesity in recruits and subsequent development of hypertension. Hypertension, a silent killer, is not something that would regularly prevent soldiers from performing well during their initial years of service, so in part, attention to this detail reflected a broader sense of responsibility for active-duty military personnel and veterans. As time went on, a continuing and growing concern developed about costs, not only for premature separation from military service, but also for medical care for obesity-related illness. The Mission Readiness document *Too Fat to Fight*,[10] endorsed by a large group of retired generals, noted the high cost of replacing recruits who failed to complete initial obligations because of obesity, as well as the high Department of Defense costs for obesity-related health care and additional costs attributable to recruitment and retention, obesity-related comorbidities, and associated absenteeism.[23] High costs related to obesity were also reported for the U.S. Air Force.[13] More recently, there has been growing pessimism within the military about civilian efforts to combat the growing obesity epidemic; the supply of physically qualified teenagers is dropping, while the demand for soldiers is not. [21,24] Finally, Littman et al.[25] have commented on the use of appearance as partial justification for military standards—its importance deriving from public perceptions of the military and a belief that a fit appearance provides an *esprit de corps*.

Implementation of the Military Model: Foreshadowing Civilian Ideas

The Army Physical Fitness and Weight Control Program (AR 600-9) of 1976 took effect about 25 years before civilian public health authorities declared a national obesity emergency[26] and more than 30 years before a 2007 civilian gathering in Washington, DC, to reach a scientific consensus on how to proceed. The focus of the 2007 meeting was an operational framework for bridging factors that influence obesity-related behaviors at macro levels (that is, policies that shape and govern the food,

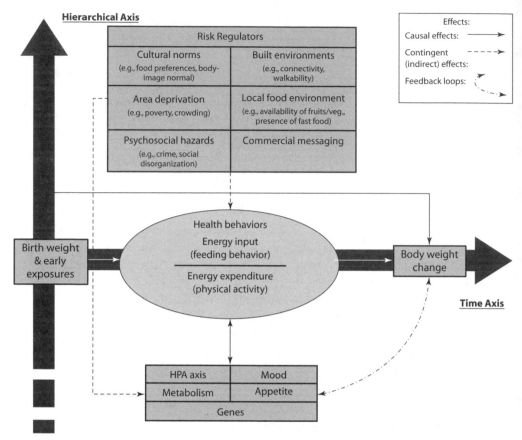

FIGURE 9.1. Hierarchical axis of biological, social, and environmental influences on obesity-related behaviors. HPA, hypothalamic-pituitary-adrenal. Source: Glass and McAtee (2006).[28] Used by permission from Elsevier.

physical, social, and economic environments) and at micro levels (factors within people or their immediate surroundings).[27] The civilian conference was supported by the National Institutes of Health (NIH: National Cancer Institute, National Institute of Diabetes and Digestive and Kidney Diseases, National Heart, Lung, and Blood Institute, Division of Nutrition Research Coordination, Office of Behavioral and Social Sciences Research, and Office of Disease Prevention), the Canadian Institutes of Health Research (Institute of Nutrition, Metabolism, and Diabetes), and the CDC.[27] A central focus of the conference was a model presented by Glass and McAtee,[28] shown in figure 9.1. The model integrates biological, social, and environmental influences on behavior. Time, on the horizontal axis, encompasses the life course; the hierarchy of systems is shown on the vertical axis.[26] A key point is that both the behaviors leading to health outcomes and the health outcomes themselves are shown to be influenced by biological, social, and environmental factors.[26]

In 2011, Barkin and Schlundt[29] presented a reformulation of the major macro- and micro-level elements of this model, identifying cascades of environmental and individual causal factors. The latter model was presented nearly 35 years after implementation of the modern military program in 1976, but as table 9.1[30–40] (based on the Barkin-Schlundt reformulation) shows, AR 600-9 fit within a systems-based multilevel envelope that foreshadowed the civilian model in all respects except food production. At no point, however, did civilian leaders seem to be aware that they were reproducing an approach that, in many respects, had already been implemented decades before.

Questions and Lessons from the Military Experience

A simple transfer of military programs to the civilian population is not feasible. In part, this is due to the closed nature of military society, its capacity for internal regulation, and its demographic characteristics. Nonetheless, several aspects of the military experience may be helpful for development of civilian responses.

Utility of Military Surveillance Data

There are major demographic and social differences between military and civilian populations. Demographically, most individuals entering the military are male (85%), and 80% of the active-duty population is between 18 and 40 years of age.[41] A greater percentage of women in the military are members of racial and ethnic minority groups; for example, 42% of Army women and 21% of Marine Corps women are Black, and 10% of Army women and 17% of Marine Corps women are Hispanic.[41] Socially, military programs begin with the requirement that the individual has reached the age of 18 years and has earned a high school degree or equivalent. Additionally, unless special waivers are granted, recruits must have no felonies or evidence of drug or alcohol abuse.[42] Despite these differences, military personnel are demographically diverse and reflect most large racial, ethnic, and socioeconomic segments of the U.S. population, except for the very poor and the very wealthy.[43,44] Overall, the proportions of Whites, American Indians/Alaska Natives, and Asian Americans/Pacific Islanders in the military are similar to those of the U.S. population as a whole, whereas the percentage of Black men is higher and the percentage of Hispanic men is lower.[41] While keeping in mind the differences, it might be helpful to make greater use of information collected during the processes of recruitment and enrollment of military populations as an indicator of civilian progress in combating the obesity epidemic.

Understanding Reasons for the Delayed Civilian Response

Further study of military responses to the problems of obesity and physical conditioning might also shed light on the profoundly slow progress of civilian programs. As mentioned above, public health scientists had identified problems related to nutrition and physical conditioning in the U.S. civilian sector by the 1950s and had brought them to the attention of government officials. By 1976, military authorities had implemented a systems-based, multilevel program to control obesity and promote physical

Table 9.1. Military analogues to civilian models for the obesity epidemic

Civilian models	Military analogues
Geophysical environment	
Interaction between people and environment	• Physical fitness regarded as a basic requirement; individuality with regard to physical fitness submerged; group cohesion stressed; superior individual performance rewarded • Capability for using environmental resources enhanced through basic recruit training • Normative experience of basic recruit training evaluated, in part, by requirements for achieving acceptable levels of competence in all basic and specialty military tasks
Built environment	• Safe indoor and outdoor physical training sites provided; library resources provided (e.g., defense digital library service makes online resources available 24 hours a day, 7 days a week)
Climate	• Undue exposure to extremes of temperature controlled by regulation
Food production	• Food programs do not generally address food production by military units
Economic environment	
Jobs	• Adherence to weight and physical fitness standards specifically linked to employment and career advancement by regulation (varies by service)
Banking/housing	• Housing or housing assistance provided
Retail	• Price advantages (commissary prices only high enough to recover item cost without factoring profit or overhead) • Food and restaurant choices left up to the individual
Political	
Public law and policy	• Uniform standards within each service branch
Media	• Internal media support regulations and policies • Commercial media maintain freedom to promote unhealthy choices
Communication systems	• Detailed procedures govern what is officially communicated and by whom it is communicated.
Community	
Local physical, social, and cultural contexts	• Interchangeability of regulations a common factor across installations
Interpersonal	
Family, friends, social networks	• Work and family benefits tied to weight and fitness
Self	
Cognitive/affective:	
1. Extrinsic (rewards and penalties)	• Extrinsic rewards and punishments clearly stated
2. Intrinsic (encouragement and barrier reduction)	• Social reinforcement in place • Medical assistance provided • Coaching available
Organ systems (medicine)	• Universal health care • Obesity testing mandated approximately every six months

Sources: U.S. Department of the Army (2012)[30]; Baseops.net (2012)[31]; Smith (2012)[32,33]; Army Basic.Org. (2012)[34]; Navy.Com. (2012)[35]; Online Computer Library Center (2008)[36]; U.S. Departments of the Army and Air Force (2003)[37]; U.S. Department of Defense (2007, 2011)[38,40]; Defense Commissary Agency (2012).[39]

conditioning. Yet, civilian public health authorities did not declare an obesity emergency for another 24–25 years,[26] and it took the NIH and the CDC another 6–7 years to reach consensus on a theoretical model,[27-29] which (at its core) duplicated what military leaders had put in place so long before. Today, the CDC notes that obesity in children was nearly three times less common in 1980 than in 2008, but not until some years after the 2007 conference did the CDC end its refusal to even use the word *obese* to describe children.[45,46] Relative to the military, both the NIH and the CDC were reactive rather than proactive in the matter of obesity, and neither the NIH nor the CDC provided acceptable protection for the civilian population. Questions remain on whether the NIH, CDC, and other government agencies have allowed similar, ongoing scenarios in relation to a wide range of specific problems (e.g., drug abuse,[47,48] breast cancer,[49] neonatal respiratory distress syndrome,[49] homicide,[50,51] and HIV disease[49,52]) as well as the health of the nation in general.[53,54] In 2006, the United States spent more per capita for health care than any other country, but it ranked 39th, 42nd, and 36th, respectively, for infant mortality, adult female mortality, and adult male mortality.[53] While civilian public health workers and health researchers can point to many twentieth-century successes,[55] the course of obesity is more consistent with the overall record. Researchers wondering, "Where is public health?" might consider (1) the accountability of military versus civilian leaders for the health of those they govern; (2) the role of civilian anti-lobbying law, which makes it a felony for public health service workers to openly challenge laws pertaining to "lawful products" unless specifically requested to do so by legislators;[49-52] (3) working relationships between public health officials and governing officials in nations with more successful health records than the that of the United States; and (4) whether such factors may have played a role in the observation that among boys and men, the United States has fallen farther behind a comparably developed nation (Australia) every year since 1974[53]—approximately the same time that the U.S. military instituted its primary obesity response.

Understanding Post-discharge Obesity among Military Personnel

While levels of obesity within the military are much lower than those found in civilian populations, there is evidence of substantial increases in obesity rates after discharge from military service,[56,57] fueled, in part, by changes in behavior on return to civilian life.[58] Behavioral Risk Factor Surveillance data adjusted for age and gender showed that obesity prevalence was similar in veterans and nonveterans, but overweight was about 3.8 percentage points more frequent in veterans.[57] Subsequent analysis of National Health and Nutrition Examination Survey data confirms comparable levels of obesity among civilians and veterans as measured by BMI, larger waist circumference among veterans than among demographically similar nonveterans, and evidence of a post–military discharge burst of weight gain.[58] However, the same study showed less excess body fat among veterans.

A recent report by Littman et al.,[25] based on the follow-up of Millennium Cohort Study participants (N = 38,686) through questionnaires administered in 2001, 2004, and 2007, provides some insight into how weight change may proceed as soldiers return to civilian life. Overall, discharge from the military was associated with a near tripling of obesity prevalence, from 12% to 31%. Weight gain seemed to be detectable three to six years prior to discharge. The authors hypothesized that this might happen once military personnel of long standing realized that further career advancement would not be tied to adherence to standards of obesity and fitness. They went on to suggest that this pattern of pre-discharge weight gain supported the hypothesis that negative consequences / extrinsic benefits were more important motivating forces than knowledge about the intrinsic values of good nutrition and physical fitness. Further support for this hypothesis came from the observation that personnel who maintained a military connection through Reserve and/or National Guard membership had a relatively lower risk of obesity. Littman et al. suggested that since Reserve and National Guard members regularly have civilian jobs and live in nonmilitary communities— except for training (one weekend per month and two weeks per year, unless actively deployed)—understanding the successful strategies employed by those who straddle the military and civilian worlds could be helpful. Analytical epidemiological studies to test these hypotheses could also be useful in formulating civilian initiatives.

Another potentially helpful area of post-discharge inquiry is the so-called *obesity paradox*. Researchers have wondered whether, in veteran populations, obesity might be protective rather than having an association with increased mortality.[59] A possible explanation was proposed in a study of 12,417 veterans by McAuley et al.: "Compared with highly fit normal-weight men, underweight men with low fitness had the highest (4.5 [3.1–6.6]) and highly fit overweight men the lowest (0.4 [0.3–0.6]) mortality risk of any subgroup. Overweight and obese men with moderate fitness had mortality rates similar to those of the highly fit normal-weight reference group."[59 [p. 115]] The authors later presented a subset analysis of 811 middle-aged men (53.3 ± 7.2 years) who had never smoked and who had no documented diabetes or cardiopulmonary disease.[60] They found no significant differences in mortality between obese and non-obese men who were physically fit and similarly observed that both obese and non-obese men who were not physically fit had approximately twice the mortality risk of a reference group. McAuley et al. concluded that cardiorespiratory fitness modified the obesity paradox, in that mortality risk was lower for both obese and non-obese men so long as they were physically fit. Useful research questions include whether a period of maintaining good physical condition and satisfactory nutritional choices in young and middle adulthood could lead to sustained behaviors and/or other health benefits that can blunt the adverse effects of later obesity and whether such observations are replicable in other groups.

Understanding What Works and What Doesn't Work in the Military Experience

Military analysts themselves have criticized the characterization of personnel by weight as one that ignores opportunities to identify and treat high-risk personnel and fails to provide a consistent or evidence-based model for early intervention and treatment of high-weight personnel.[8] Similarly, imposition of uniform regulations within the military minimizes the possibility of systematic, randomized testing of components at multiple levels of the program. The overall program may work, but it is hard to know whether any particular parts are more important than others in driving the success. It might be helpful and more feasible to investigate individual components of the military approach within civilian populations.

Military basic training (boot camp) might provide a good example for such inquiry. Social scientists recognize the importance of breaking down old behavior in order to resocialize individuals to new norms. Consistent with this view, the military employs an intense program of basic combat training. This training resocializes former civilians to military cultural norms, values, and customs.[61,62] Values alone, however, do not explain behavior. Swidler[63] argues that skills, styles, habits, and behaviors (a cultural toolbox, as it were) that are developed for survival explain more behavioral outcomes than do values or preferences. In this sense, basic combat training exchanges the cultural toolbox developed for civilian life for a new set of skills, behaviors, styles, and habits that allow for military survival. Recruits eat together, sleep together, and train together as individuals are molded into a functional unit. An individual's inability to perform by the rules affects the treatment of the entire group, resulting not only in vertical pressure but in lateral pressure (i.e., peer pressure) to perform. The training also provides graduates with a skill set that enhances self-efficacy. Unfortunately, the long-term obesity-related effects of such training, particularly in comparison with those of extrinsic benefits, are unclear. Both military and civilian efforts might benefit from a better understanding of this.

Questioning the Need for Massive Legislative Change

A vast array of legislative initiatives dealing with obesity are currently enforced or under development in the civilian world.[64] In contrast, and possibly owing to effective extrinsic motivation, millions of Americans in military service have been capable of planning and implementing successful nutrition and conditioning without such legal intrusion. This may, in part, reflect a more subtle and faithful rendering of the Eisenhower doctrine by the military. Although the doctrine's ban on central standards of physical fitness was abandoned, military leaders mostly stopped short of directly regulating what people might or might not consume. Instead, they established multilevel parameters to encourage healthy and independent individual dietary and exercise choices. Similarly, it might be helpful for civilian leaders to engage the population to identify options that could be looked upon as sufficiently beneficial extrinsic benefits for controlling obesity and promoting physical conditioning. These benefits might be scholarships or business incentives for career advancement that are tied to fitness and satisfactory nutritional choices. Companies whose profits are adversely affected by obesity might be encouraged to form alliances that support such extrinsic gains. Should these efforts be associated with consumer movement toward the purchase of healthier foods, food producers' obligations to their shareholders might mandate production changes in that industry as well. Conceptually, the efficacy of such an approach could be systematically tested along with selected legal measures. It is important that the level of evidence-based support for social and legislative experiments aimed at obesity be of comparable quality to that required for other health-related interventions. As noted above, one of the problems with understanding the military experience is that the lack of an evidence-based approach makes it difficult to know which components are driving its success—a potentially valuable lesson.

National versus Local Consensus

Military programs are characterized by national uniformity across services. Civilian programs, in accordance with the Eisenhower doctrine, rely on local consensus. This is associated with uneven civilian results. The Robert Wood Johnson Foundation, for example, recently reported that 30 states lack standards for school meals; 15 states lack nutritional standards for competitive foods (i.e., foods sold in schools outside the federal reimbursable school meals program); 29 states fail to limit access to competitive foods; 40 states and the District of Columbia lack physical activity requirements; 30 states and DC fail to record BMI or health information; 49 states and DC do not use noninvasive diabetes testing; 24 states lack a farm-to-school program; 46 states and DC lack menu-labeling laws (requiring restaurants to include calorie information on menus and menu boards and to make other written nutritional information available on request); 34 states and DC lack a complete-the-streets policy (e.g., upgrades to include safe street crossings, sidewalks, ramps, space for cyclists, and the like); and 26 states and DC lack liability laws that limit the liability of food vendors for obesity.[9] In a highly mobile society, this may be a recipe for self-defeating public confusion. In contrast, Goldzweig et al.[65] have recently described a prevention program associated with benefits to 41 million Americans that was based, in part, on application of national consensus to local context. This program may provide an example of how academic-business-community alliances can translate multilevel models to improve health.

International Experiences

In this chapter we have focused on the U.S. military, but obesity is of documented concern to military forces from countries on at least six continents, including Asia (China,[66] India,[67] Israel,[68,69] Japan,[70] Saudi Arabia,[71,72] Singapore,[73] South Korea,[74] Taiwan,[75] and Thailand[76,77]); Australia;[78] Europe (Austria,[79] Denmark,[80] Belgium,[81] Finland,[82] France,[83] Germany,[84] Great Britain,[85] Greece,[86,87] Hungary,[88] Italy,[89] Poland,[90] Portugal,[91] Spain,[92] Sweden,[93] and Switzerland[94,95]); North America (Canada[96]); and South and Central America (Brazil[97,98] and Mexico[66]). Popkin[66] suggests that in addition to threatening military security, obesity exerts a global drain on health care, workforce productivity, and economic competitiveness. Perhaps it also offers an opportunity for peaceful collaboration.

Conclusions

Military and civilian approaches to the obesity epidemic are marked by widely divergent philosophies, even taking into account the closed nature of military society. The profoundly slow and reactive course of civilian research and public health efforts is of particular concern. A better understanding of the military experience might be helpful in framing future civilian efforts, not only for obesity, but also for other health problems. At the least, military experiences show that for millions of Americans from diverse social and economic strata, obesity is not inevitable.

Acknowledgments

Funding for this work was made possible (in part) by grant no. 3P20MD000516-07S2 from the National Center on Minority Health and Health Disparities (NIH) and grant no. USDA\AFRI\NIFA 2011-68001-30113 from the U.S. Department of Agriculture. The views expressed do not necessarily reflect the official policies of the Department of Health and Human Services or the Department of Agriculture, nor does mention by trade names, commercial practices, or organizations imply endorsement by the U.S. government. Additional support for Meharry Medical College has come from the State Farm Automobile Insurance Company. Robert S. Levine is a retired member of the U.S. Army.

References

1. Keys A, Kimura N, Kusukawa A, et al. Lessons from serum cholesterol studies in Japan, Hawaii and Los Angeles. Ann Intern Med. 1958 Jan;48(1):83–94.
2. Kraus H, Hirshland RP. Muscular fitness and health. J Am Assoc Health Phys Educ Recr. 1953;24(10):17–19.
3. President's Council on Physical Fitness and Sports. The first 50 years: 1956–2006. Washington, DC: President's Council on Physical Fitness, 2006. Available at: http://www.fitness.gov/pdfs/50-year-anniversary-booklet.pdf.
4. Kersh R. The politics of obesity: a current assessment and look ahead. Milbank Q. 2009 Mar;87(1):295–316.
5. Ogden CL, Carroll MD, Kit BK, et al. Prevalence of obesity in the United States, 2009–2010. NCHS Data Brief. 2012 Jan;(82):1–8.
6. Levi J, Segal LM, St. Laurent R, et al. F as in fat: how obesity threatens America's future. Washington, DC: Trust for America's Health, 2011. Available at: http://www.healthyamericans.org/assets/files/TFAH2011FasInFat10.pdf.
7. Centers for Disease Control and Prevention. Adult obesity facts: obesity is common, serious and costly. Atlanta, GA: Centers for Disease Control and Prevention, 2012. Available at: http://www.cdc.gov/obesity/data/adult.html.
8. Zhao Z, Kaestner R. Effects of urban sprawl on obesity. J Health Econ. 2010 Dec;29(6):779–87.
9. Eid J, Overman HG, Puga D, et al. Fat city: questioning the relationship between urban sprawl and obesity. J Urban Econ. 2008 Mar;63(2):385–404.

10. Christeson W, Taggart AD, Messner-Zidell S, et al. Too fat to fight: retired military leaders want junk food out of America's schools: a report by Mission: Readiness. Washington, DC: Mission Readiness, 2010 Apr. Available at: http://cdn.missionreadiness.org/MR_Too_Fat _to_Fight-1.pdf.

11. National Research Council. Weight management: state of the science and opportunities for military programs. Washington, DC: National Academies Press, 2004.

12. Gantt CJ, Neely JA, Villafana IA, et al. Analysis of weight and associated health consequences of the active duty staff at a major Naval medical center. Mil Med. 2008 May;173(5): 434–40.

13. Robbins AS, Chao SY, Russ CR, et al. Costs of excess body weight among active duty personnel, U.S. Air Force, 1997. Mil Med. 2002 May;167(5):393–7.

14. Rush B. Directions for preserving the health of soldiers: addressed to the officers of the Army of the United States. Philadelphia, PA: Thomas Dobson, Fry and Kammerer Printers, 1808. Pp. 14–15.

15. Krause MD. History of U.S. Army soldier physical fitness: national conference on military physical fitness (Proceedings Report). Washington, DC: U.S. Department of Health and Human Services, 1990. Available at: http://www.ihpra.org/col_krause.htm.

16. Johnson NA. The history of the Army weight standards. Mil Med. 1997 Aug;162(8):564–70.

17. U.S. Department of the Army. Height and weight standards: Army regulations (40–503). Washington, DC: U.S. Department of the Army, 1956 May 9.

18. Sarnecky MT. Readiness challenges. In: Contemporary history of the U.S. Army Nurse Corps. Washington, DC: Borden Institute / Walter Reed Army Medical Center, 2010. Pp. 59–77.

19. Wildman RP, Muntner P, Reynolds K, et al. The obese without cardiometabolic risk factor clustering and the normal weight with cardiometabolic risk factor clustering: prevalence and correlates of 2 phenotypes among the US population (NHANES 1999–2004). Arch Intern Med. 2008 Aug;168(15):1617–24.

20. Stefan N, Kantartzis K, Machann J, et al. Identification and characterization of metabolically benign obesity in humans. Arch Intern Med. 2008 Aug;168(15):1609–16.

21. Sarnecky MT. Preparing for action. In: Contemporary history of the U.S. Army Nurse Corps. Washington, DC: Borden Institute / Walter Reed Army Medical Center, 2010. Available at: http://www.bordeninstitute.army.mil/other_pub/nurse/NurseCorpsch4.pdf.

22. Shields CE. Evaluation of age and weight of recruits on their blood pressure. Mil Med. 1980 May;145(5):326–8.

23. Dall TM, Zhang Y, Chen YJ, et al. Cost associated with being overweight and with obesity, high alcohol consumption, and tobacco use within the military health system's TRICARE prime-enrolled population. Am J Health Promot. 2007 Nov–Dec;22(2):120–39.

24. Thompson AJ. Physical fitness in the United States Marine Corps: history, current practices and implications for mission accomplishment and human performance. Monterrey, CA: Naval Postgraduate School, 2005. Available at: http://www.dtic.mil/cgi-bin/GetTRDoc ?AD=ADA443310.

25. Littman AJ, Jacobson IG, Boyko EJ, et al. Weight change following US military service. Int J Obes. 2012 Apr 10. doi: 10.1038/ijo.2012.46 [Epub ahead of print].

26. Kersh R. The politics of obesity: a current assessment and look ahead. Milbank Q. 2009 Mar;87(1):295–316.

27. Huang TT, Drewnosksi A, Kumanyika S, et al. A systems-oriented multilevel framework for addressing obesity in the 21st century. Prev Chronic Dis. 2009 Jul;6(3):A82.

28. Glass TA, McAtee MJ. Behavioral science at the crossroads in public health: extending horizons, envisioning the future. Soc Sci Med. 2006 Apr;62(7):1650–71.

29. Barkin S, Schlundt D. The challenge facing translation of basic science into clinical and community settings to improve health outcomes. Environ Health Perspect. 2011 Oct;119(10): A418–9.

30. U.S. Department of the Army, U.S. Army Training and Doctrine Command. Training: enlisted initial entry training policies and administration (TRADOC Regulation 350–6). Fort Monroe, VA: U.S. Department of the Army, U.S. Army Training and Doctrine Command, 2012 Jul. Available at: http://www.tradoc.army.mil/tpubs/regs/tr350-6.pdf.

31. Baseops.net. U.S. Air Force basic training. Lackland Air Force Base, TX: Baseops.net, 2012. Available at: http://www.baseops.net/basictraining/airforce_fitness.html.

32. Smith S. Navy physical readiness test (PRT) overview. Military.com, 2012. Available at: http://www.military.com/military-fitness/navy-fitness-requirements/navy-basic-training -pft.

33. Smith S. Coast Guard fitness requirements. Military.com, 2012. Available at: http://www .military.com/military-fitness/coast-guard-fitness-requirements/coast-guard-fitness.

34. Army Basic.Org. Your guide to Army basic training. Washington, DC: Army Basic.Org, 2012. Available at: http://www.armybasic.org/portal/index.php.

35. Navy.Com. Working to be healthy, fit and ready. Millington, TN: Navy.Com, 2012. Available at: http://www.navy.com/inside/fitness/physical-training.html.

36. Online Computer Library Center. The U.S. Army brings worldwide library access to soldiers on the front line. Dublin, OH: Online Computer Library Center, 2008. Available at: http:// www.oclc.org/services/brochures/212426usc_E_questionpoint_us_army.pdf.

37. U.S. Departments of the Army and Air Force. Heat stress control and heat casualty management. Washington, DC: U.S. Departments of the Army and Air Force, 2003. Available at: http://www.usariem.army.mil/pages/download/tbmed507.pdf.

38. U.S. Department of Defense. A primer on basic allowance for housing for the uniformed services. Washington, DC: U.S. Department of Defense, 2011. Available at: www.defense travel.dod.mil/Docs/perdiem/BAH-Primer.pdf.

39. Defense Commissary Agency. Prices and savings. Fort Lee, VA: Defense Commissary Agency, 2012. Available at: http://www.commissaries.com/documents/contact_deca/faqs /prices_commissary.cfm.

40. U.S. Department of Defense. Task force on the future of military health care. Washington, DC: U.S. Department of Defense, 2007. Available at: http://www.dcoe.health.mil/Content /Navigation/Documents/103-06-2-Home-Task_Force_FINAL_REPORT_122007.pdf.

41. Segal DR, Segal MW. America's military population. Washington, DC: Population Reference Bureau, 2004 Dec. Available at: http://www.prb.org/Publications/PopulationBulletins/2004 /AmericasMilitaryPopulationPDF627KB.aspx.

42. Powers R. US military enlistment standards. About.Com, 2012. Available at: http://usmilitary .about.com/od/joiningthemilitary/a/enldrugs.htm.

43. Congressional Budget Office. The all-volunteer military: issues and performance. Washington, DC: Congressional Budget Office, 2007 Jul. Available at: http://www.cbo.gov/sites/default /files/cbofiles/ftpdocs/83xx/doc8313/07-19-militaryvol.pdf.

44. Congressional Budget Office. Social representation in the U.S. military. Washington, DC: Congressional Budget Office, 1989 Oct. Available at: http://www.cbo.gov/sites/default/files /cbofiles/ftpdocs/67xx/doc6746/89-cbo-044.pdf.

45. Kuczmarski RJ, Ogden CL, Grummer-Strawn LM, et al. CDC growth charts: United States. ADV Data. 2000 Jun 8;(314):1–27.

46. Centers for Disease Control and Prevention. Overweight and obesity: basics about childhood obesity. Atlanta, GA: Centers for Disease Control and Prevention, 2012. Available at: http://www.cdc.gov/obesity/childhood/basics.html.

47. Sloboda Z, Stephens RC, Stephens PC, et al. The adolescent substance abuse prevention study: a randomized field trial of a universal substance abuse prevention program. Drug Alcohol Depend. 2009 Jun;102(1–3):1–10.

48. Kulis S, Nieri T, Yabiku S, et al. Promoting reduced and discontinued substance use among adolescent substance users: effectiveness of a universal program. Prev Sci. 2007 Mar;8(1): 35–49.

49. Levine RS, Rust GS, Pisu M, et al. Increased black-white disparities in mortality following lifesaving innovations: a possible consequence of US federal laws. Am J Public Health. 2010 Nov;100(11):2176–84.

50. Levine RS, Goldzweig I, Kilbourne B, et al. Firearms, youth violence and public health. J Health Care Poor Underserved. 2012 Feb;23(1):7–19.

51. Hennekens C, Drowos J, Levine R. Mortality from homicide among young Black men: a new American tragedy. Am J Med. 2013 Jan 16 [Epub ahead of print].

52. Levine R, Williams J, Kilbourne B, Juarez P. Tuskegee redux: evolution of legal mandates for human experimentation. J Health Care Poor Underserved. 2012 Nov;23(4 Suppl):104–25.

53. Murray CJ, Frenk J. Ranking 37th—measuring the performance of the U.S. health care system. N Engl J Med. 2010 Jan;362(2):98–9.

54. House JS, Schoeni RF, Kaplan GA, et al. The health effects of social and economic policy: the promise and challenge for research and policy. In: Shoeni RF, House JF, Kaplan GA, et al., eds. Making Americans healthier: social and economic policy as health policy. New York, NY: Russell Sage Foundation. 2008 Feb. Pp. 3–26.

55. Rust G, Satcher D, Fryer GE, et al. Triangulating on success: innovation, public health, medical care, and cause-specific US mortality rates over a half century (1950–2000). Am J Public Health. 2010 Apr;100 Suppl 1:S95–104.

56. Almond N, Kahwati L, Kinsinger L, et al. Prevalence of overweight and obesity among U.S. military veterans. Mil Med. 2008 Jun;173(6):544–9.

57. Koepsell TD, Forsberg CW, Littman AJ. Obesity, overweight, and weight control practices in U.S. veterans. Prev Med. 2009 Mar;48(3):267–71.

58. Koepsell TD, Littman AJ, Forsberg CW. Obesity, overweight, and their life course trajectories in veterans and non-veterans. Obesity (Silver Spring). 2012 Feb;20(2):434–9.

59. McAuley PA, Kokkinos PF, Oliveira RB, et al. Obesity paradox and cardiorespiratory fitness in 12,417 male veterans aged 40 to 70 years. Mayo Clin Proc. 2010 Feb;85(2):115–21.

60. McAuley PA, Smith NS, Emerson BT, Myers JN. The obesity paradox and cardiorespiratory fitness. J Obes. 2012;2012:951582. Epub 2012 Feb 20.

61. Bradley C. Veteran status and marital aggression: does military service make a difference? J Fam Violence. 2007;22:197–209.

62. Jones AD. Intimate partner violence in military couples: a review of the literature. Aggression Violent Behav. 2012 Mar–Apr;17(2):147–57.

63. Swidler A. Culture in action: symbols and strategies. Am Sociol Rev. 1986 Apr;51(2):273–86.

64. Dietz WH, Benken DE, Hunter AS. Public health law and the prevention and control of obesity. Milbank Q. 2009 Mar;87(1):215–27.

65. Goldzweig IA, Schlundt DG, Moore WE, et al. An academic, business, and community alliance to promote evidence-based public health policy: the case of primary seat belt legislation. J Health Care Poor Underserved. 2013 Aug;24(3):1364–77.

66. Popkin BM. Is the obesity epidemic a national security issue around the globe? Curr Opin Endocrinol Diabetes Obes. 2011 Oct;18(5):328–31.

67. Ray S, Kulkarni B, Sreenivas A. Prevalence of prehypertension in young military adults & its association with overweight & dyslipidaemia. Indian J Med Res. 2011 Aug;134:162–7.

68. Grotto I, Aarka S, Balicer RD, et al. Risk factors for overweight and obesity in young healthy adults during compulsory military service. Isr Med Assoc J. 2008 Aug–Sep;10(8–9):607–12.

69. Bar Dayan Y, Elishkevits K, Grotto I, et al. The prevalence of obesity and associated morbidity among 17-year-old Israeli conscripts. Public Health. 2005 May;119(5):385–9.

70. Sakuta H, Suzuki T. Physical activity and selected cardiovascular risk factors in middle-aged male personnel of self-defense forces. Ind Health. 2006 Jan;44(1):184–9.

71. Al-Qahtani DA, Imtiaz ML, Shareef MM. Obesity and cardiovascular risk factors in Saudi adult soldiers. Saudi Med J. 2005 Aug;26(8):1260–8.

72. Al-Qahtani DA, Imtiaz ML. Prevalence of metabolic syndrome in Saudi adult soldiers. Saudi Med J. 2005 Sep;26(9):1360–6.

73. Lee L, Kumar S, Leong LC. The impact of five-month basic military training on the body weight and body fat of 197 moderately to severely obese Singaporean males aged 17 to 19 years. Int J Obes Relat Metab Disord. 1994 Feb;18(2):105–9.

74. Bae KK, Kim H, Cho SI. Trends in body mass index and associations with physical activity among career soldiers in South Korea. J Prev Med Public Health. 2011 Jul;44(4):167–75.

75. Chao JK, Hwang TI, Ma MC, et al. A survey of obesity and erectile dysfunction of men conscripted into the military in Taiwan. J Sex Med. 2011 Apr;8(4):1156–63.

76. Nillakupt K, Viravathana N. A survey of metabolic syndrome and its components in Thai medical cadets. J Med Assoc Thai. 2010 Nov;93 Suppl 6:S179–85.

77. Napradit P, Pantaewan P, Nimit-arnun N, et al. Prevalence of overweight and obesity in Royal Thai Army personnel. J Med Assoc Thai. 2007 Feb;90(2):335–40.

78. McLaughlin R, Wittert G. The obesity epidemic: implications for recruitment and retention of defence force personnel. Obes Rev. 2009 Nov;10(6):693–9.

79. Wallner A, Hirz A, Schober E, et al. Evolution of cardiovascular risk factors among 18-year-old males in Austria between 1986 and 2005. Wien Klin Wochenschr. 2010 Mar;122(5–6):152–8.

80. Dahl S, Kristensen S. Health profile of Danish army personnel. Mil Med. 1997 Jun;162(6): 435–40.

81. Mullie P, Clarys P, Hulens M, et al. Distribution of cardiovascular risk factors in Belgian army men. Arch Environ Occup Health. 2010 Jul–Sep;65(3):135–9.

82. Mikkola I, Keinanen-Kiukaanniemi S, Jokelainen J, et al. Aerobic performance and body composition changes during military service. Scand J Prim Health Care. 2012 Jun;30(2): 95–100.

83. Bauduceau B, Baigts F, Bordier L, et al. Epidemiology of the metabolic syndrome in 2045 French military personnel. EPIMIL study. Diabetes Metab. 2005 Sep;31(4 Pt 1):353–9.

84. Toschke AM, Lüdde R, Eisele R, et al. The obesity epidemic in young men is not confined to low social classes—a time series of 18-year-old German men at medical examination for military service with different education attainment. Int J Obes (Lond). 2005 Jul;29(7):875–7.

85. Sundin J, Fear NT, Wessely S, et al. Obesity in the UK Armed Forces: risk factors. Mil Med. 2011 May;176(5):507–12.

86. Mazokopakis EE, Papadakis JA, Papadomanolaki MG, et al. Overweight and obesity in Greek warship personnel: prevalence and correlations. Eur J Public Health. 2004 Dec;14(4): 395–7.

87. Doupis J, Dimesthenopoulos C, Diamanti K, et al. Metabolic syndrome and Mediterranean dietary pattern in a sample of young, male, Greek navy recruits. Nutr Metab Cardiovasc Dis. 2009 Jul;19(6):e7–8.

88. Grösz A. Tóth E, Péter I. A 10-year follow-up of ischemic heart disease risk factors in military pilots. Mil Med. 2007 Feb;172(2):214–9.

89. Loviselli A, Ghiani ME, Velluzzi F, et al. Prevalence and trend of overweight and obesity among Sardinian conscripts (Italy) of 1969 and 1998. J Biosoc Sci. 2010 Mar;42(2):201–11.

90. Koziel S, Szklarska A, Bielicki T, et al. Changes in the BMI of Polish conscripts between 1965 and 2001: secular and socio-occupational variation. Int J Obes (Lond). 2006 Sep;30(9): 1382–8.

91. Padez C. Trends in overweight and obesity in Portuguese conscripts from 1986 to 2000 in relation to place of residence and educational level. Public Health. 2006 Oct;120(10): 946–52.

92. Portero MP, León M, Andrés EM, et al. Comparison of cardiovascular risk factors in young Spanish men between the 1980s and after the year 2000: data from the AGEMZA study. Rev Esp Cardiol. 2008 Dec;61(12):1260–6.

93. Neovius K, Rasmussen F, Sundström J, et al. Forecast of future premature mortality as a result of trends in obesity and smoking: nationwide cohort simulation study. Eur J Epidemiol. 2010 Oct;25(10):703–9.

94. Saely CH, Risch L, Frey F, et al. Body mass index, blood pressure, and serum cholesterol in young Swiss men: an analysis on 56784 army conscripts. Swiss Med Wkly. 2009 Sep 5;139(35–36):518–24.

95. Staub K, Rüü FJ, Woitek U, et al. BMI distribution / social stratification in Swiss conscripts from 1875 to present. Eur J Clin Nutr. 2010 Apr;64(4):335–40.

96. Jetté M, Sidney K, Lewis W. Fitness, performance and anthropometric characteristics of 19,185 Canadian Forces personnel classified according to body mass index. Mil Med. 1990 Mar;155(3):120–6.

97. Costa FF, Montenegro VB, Lopes TJ, et al. Combination of risk factors for metabolic syndrome in the military personnel of the Brazilian Navy. Arq Bras Cardiol. 2011 Dec;97(6): 485–92.

98. Neves EB. Prevalence of overweight and obesity among members of the Brazilian army: association with arterial hypertension. Cien Saude Colet. 2008 Sep–Oct;13(5):1661–8.

99. Centers for Disease Control and Prevention. Vital signs: obesity among low-income, preschool-aged children—United States, 2008–2011. MMWR Morb Mortal Wkly Rep. 2013 Aug 9;62(31):629–34.

100. Iannotti RJ, Wang J. Trends in physical activity, sedentary behavior, diet, and BMI among US adolescents, 2001–2009. Pediatrics. 2013 Oct;132(4):606–14. Epub 2013 Sep 16.

CHAPTER 10

A Healthy Weight Disparity Index and Reducing Rates of Obesity and Overweight in the United States

Wendell C. Taylor, PhD, MPH, and Leah S. Fischer, PhD

*D*isparity is defined as a marked difference or inequality between two or more population groups defined on the basis of race or ethnicity, gender, education level, or other criteria.[1] One indication of the national commitment to address disparities is found in the U.S. Department of Health and Human Services' *Healthy People* documents, which have outlined goals and objectives for health promotion and disease prevention for all people in the United States since the initiative was first launched in 2000.[2-4] In a subtle yet important way, the goal of addressing health disparities has shifted, from *reducing* disparities in *Healthy People 2000* to *eliminating* disparities in *Healthy People 2010*. For *Healthy People 2020*, the overarching goal is to achieve health equity, eliminate disparities, and improve the health of all communities.[4] Based on the goals of the *Healthy People* documents, eliminating disparities and achieving equity is central to contemporary public health. Moreover, an understanding of health disparities is essential to reducing rates of overweight and obesity among underserved populations.

In this chapter we provide a brief review of disparities related to obesity, present disparity indices, and propose the new Healthy Weight Disparities Index (HWDI). This work is relevant to much of what is clearly established in previous chapters: racial, ethnic, gender, regional, and socioeconomic disparities in obesity and overweight and their sequelae in the health of individuals, their families, and communities. To underscore the constructive intent of the work presented here—and in keeping with the orientation of this volume as a whole—we also present a new perspective to illustrate how the HWDI contributes to disparities research and can be

Wendell C. Taylor is an associate professor of health promotion and behavioral sciences at the School of Public Health, Center for Health Promotion and Prevention Research, the University of Texas Health Science Center at Houston. At the time this work was conducted, Leah S. Fischer was a postdoctoral fellow at the University of Texas Health Science Center at Houston.

instrumental in developing effective interventions to reduce obesity risk and the disparities associated with obesity.

Disparities and Obesity

We first offer a brief recap of the central facts on disparities in obesity and overweight (more thoroughly presented and discussed in chapters 1–9). The Centers for Disease Control and Prevention (CDC)[5] defines *being obese* as having a body mass index (BMI) greater than $30\,\mathrm{kg/m^2}$ and *being overweight* as having a BMI between 25 and $29.9\,\mathrm{kg/m^2}$. The prevalence of obesity and overweight has greatly increased across the United States in recent years,[6,7] which has significant implications for public health. Increasing levels of obesity lead to more chronic disease and disability, lower productivity levels, and higher costs of health care at both the local and national levels.[8] Importantly, the rising trend in obesity prevalence differs across and within racial/ ethnic groups, socioeconomic strata, gender, and educational levels and is influenced by contextual factors such as how the built environment affects opportunities for physical activity and access to healthy food.[9–15] Obesity research consistently indicates that obesity and overweight are more common among non-Hispanic Blacks, Hispanics, Native Americans, and Native Hawaiians / Pacific Islanders than among non-Hispanic Whites.[16–20] Evidence suggests that BMI and socioeconomic status tend to be inversely related among racial/ethnic minorities,[21] although other studies report a convergence in levels of obesity among those with low and high socioeconomic status.[6,7,22]

There is a growing body of research suggesting that location and place are important factors when examining associations between BMI and socioeconomic indicators such as income, education, and occupation.[23]* One study estimated models to predict BMI trajectories for Black and White women and adjusted for neighborhood disadvantage and racial composition over a period of 16 years. The models indicated that neighborhood disadvantage at baseline was associated with BMI and slightly reduced racial disparities in BMI but did not predict changes over time.[23] Another study using data from the 2003–6 National Health and Nutrition Examination Surveys investigated the relationships among household participation in the Supplemental Nutrition Assistance Program (SNAP), adiposity, and metabolic risk factors in a representative sample of low-income adults. Controlling for sociodemographic characteristics, the study found a positive association between SNAP participation and obesity (prevalence ratio = 1.58; 95% CI = 1.08 to 2.31).[24]† Overall, the literature is consistent in documenting obesity-related disparities; however, all the nuances and complexities related to obesity and disparities associated with race and ethnicity, in-

---

* See also chapters 8, 11, 12, 17, and 18 for more on the significance of place in this connection.

† See the reference list in this book's introduction (references 112–16) for some important work on the federal Supplemental Nutrition Assistance Program (SNAP, often called the Food Stamp program) and the possibilities for its role in reducing obesity and overweight in low-income populations.

come, education, and gender—and above all, the root causes of the disparities—are far from clearly understood.*

Disparity Indices
Definition of an Index

Before reviewing the disparity indices reported in the public health literature, it is important to know what an index is. The term has multiple meanings. We adhere to the New Oxford American dictionary's definition: "an *index* is a number giving the magnitude of a physical property or another measured phenomenon in terms of a standard."[25] [p. 858]

Overview of Disparity Indices

Current disparity indices are primarily measures of income inequality and include the following: the Robin Hood index, the Gini coefficient, the Relative Index of Inequality, and the Health Disparity Index. The definitions for these indices range from straightforward to complex.

The *Robin Hood index* is defined as the proportion of aggregate income that must be redistributed from households above the mean to those below the mean to achieve equality in the distribution of income.[26,27] This measure of income inequality has been associated with individual and population health, including heart disease.[26,27] The *Gini coefficient* is a measure of income inequality, both as a raw measure and one adjusted for taxes, cash transfers, and differences in household composition.[28] The Gini coefficient represents the area between the 45° line produced by equally distributed income on a graph of cumulative population income versus percentage of population and the curve on the same graph produced by unequal income distribution.[28,29] This is an example of a more complicated measure. The theoretical range of the Gini coefficient is from 0.0, representing income equality, to 1.0, representing maximum inequality. This measure of income inequality has been associated with mental health problems such as depression and alcohol dependence[28,29] and with premature cardiovascular disease (CVD) mortality.[28] The *Relative Index of Inequality* was computed by four different measures on inequality: occupation, education, net household income, and housing index.[30] This index has been studied in relation to all-cause and cause-specific mortality risk (e.g., stomach cancer, CVD, chronic obstructive pulmonary disease).[30] The *Health Disparity Index* represents the ratio of excess Black mortality to the White mortality per 100,000 individuals for a single disease process (e.g., cancer, diabetes, or infant mortality) in a specific state.[31] The comprehensive Health Disparity Index was calculated for each of seven years by using the following formula:

$$HDI_{2003} = (HDI_{cancer\ in\ 2003} + HDI_{CVD} + HDI_{diabetes} + HDI_{HIV} + HDI_{infant\ mortality}) / 5$$

---

* See chapters 1–4 and 6–8 for more discussion of these central issues.

A state HDI score of 1.00 represents racial health disparities equivalent to those existing among the entire U.S. population. An HDI score of 0.00 would represent racial health parity, and states with HDI scores of 0.01–0.99 experience less racial health disparity in mortality than is found in the U.S. population at large. States with HDI scores exceeding 1.00 exhibit more racial health disparity than U.S. averages, indicating larger differences in Black and White mortality for the selected conditions. In Webb et al.'s 2011 study,[31] Massachusetts (0.35), Oklahoma (0.35), and Washington (0.39) had the lowest HDI scores; Michigan (1.22), Wisconsin (1.32), and Illinois (1.50) had the highest HDI scores. Our *Healthy Weight Disparity Index* extends the literature on disparity indices by proposing an index to specifically assess obesity risk and disparities.

Healthy Weight Disparity Index—New and Unique

None of the indices reviewed above focused on place (geographic location), weight status (e.g., obesity), and sociodemographic characteristics related to disparity, such as income, education, gender, and racial and ethnic identity. Therefore, we propose a Healthy Weight Disparity Index that emphasizes location, obesity, and disparities related to sociodemographic factors such as income, education, gender, and racial/ethnic identity. The HWDI shines a spotlight on the greatest disparities, informs the development of interventions, and tracks progress over time. As an example of our HWDI, we developed a formula that stipulates, for each state, city, or location, a threshold that can be designated for high-, middle-, and low-income groups. The mean BMI for each income level can be identified. The CDC has identified a BMI range of $18.5–24.9 \, kg/m^2$ as a healthy standard. Based on the literature, the high-income group will most likely have the healthiest BMI[8] (therefore, we use the high-income group as the reference group).

We developed a HWDI related to income. The specific algorithm used to calculate this index is as follows:

HWDI related to income = (S BMI – High-income BMI) + (Middle-income BMI – S BMI) + (Low-income BMI – S BMI), where $S \, BMI = 25 \, kg/m^2$

Conceptually, the HWDI will reveal disparities among income levels, by location, related to weight status anchored in the designated healthy standard, $BMI < 25 \, kg/m^2$. In addition to income, we propose that the HWDI be extended to gender, education, and other sociodemographic factors between and within racial and ethnic groups.

Place is critically important to understanding obesity,[32] particularly obesity-related disparities. The behaviors most related to weight status, such as physical activity and healthy eating, are influenced by place and social context. Several authors have emphasized the neighborhood context and its influence on behaviors related to obesity.[33] A subset of place is the built environment. In fact, environmental justice principles (disproportionate impact of the environment on low-income communities and communities of color) have been applied to active living and healthy eating, with the built environment as the focal point.[14,15] Given the solid evidence for the importance of place and the built environment as it relates to obesity and concomitant behaviors, place is a central focus for the HWDI.

Application of the Healthy Weight Disparity Index: Houston, Texas
Data Source

We used data from the Health of Houston Survey 2010 (HHS 2010) to illustrate an application of the HWDI. The HHS 2010 is an address-based household survey that collects extensive information from multiple segments of the population on health status, conditions, behaviors, insurance coverage, and access to health care. The HHS 2010 sample is representative of Harris County and the City of Houston's non-institutionalized population living in households. Detailed information about the HHS 2010 methodology is given in *Health of Houston Survey, HHS 2010: Methodology Report.*[34]

Variables of Interest

We used three variables from the HHS 2010 dataset to develop a practical example of the HWDI: adult BMI, household income, and a geographic area variable. Adult BMI was calculated from height and weight variables provided by survey respondents, using the following equation: $BMI = [mass\ (lbs) \times 703] / [height\ (inches)^2]$. The categories were: $BMI < 25\,kg/m^2 = normal$; $BMI \geq 25$ but $< 30\,kg/m^2 = overweight$; and $BMI \geq 30\,kg/m^2 = obese$. The universe for this variable included all adult respondents aged 18 and older. Missing cases included children and adults who did not provide information to calculate BMI. We excluded all BMI measurements greater than $60\,kg/m^2$ (n = 16) because the highest value in BMI charts is 54.

The second HHS 2010 variable we used was household income. Interviewers asked respondents to estimate their household's combined annual income from all sources for 2009. Income sources for household income included money from such sources as jobs, Social Security, retirement income, unemployment payments, and public assistance. The income estimate also included funds from interest and dividends, net income from business, farm, or rent, and any other money income, with the exception of gifts. We classified income into the following categories (as in an earlier study)[35]: low (< $25,000 per year), middle ($25,000 to < $75,000), and high (≥ $75,000).

The variable for place was a derived aggregation from a survey question asking about the person's main residence zip code and a follow-up question to confirm Harris County as the county of residence. Based on respondents' zip codes, participating households were grouped into 28 familiar neighborhood areas, allowing researchers to draw valid conclusions about each area based on the sampled households while protecting the anonymity of individual respondents. Each of the 28 areas represents an aggregation of five or more zip codes.

Mean BMI was calculated for each of the 28 neighborhood areas. Then we ranked the neighborhoods from lowest to highest. For each neighborhood, we derived mean BMI values across the three income categories. We chose neighborhoods where the high-income group had BMI values closer to 24.9 kg/m² (the standard established by the CDC) than the middle- and low-income groups. The purpose of this illustration was to examine income disparities.

Using BMI values for each income category, we calculated the Healthy Weight Disparity Index. We used Stata 12 to perform all data analyses, with appropriate weights to take account of the HHS 2010's complex sampling design.[36]

Neighborhood Rankings by BMI, HWDI, and Concordance

Mean BMI for the 10 selected neighborhoods in Greater Houston ranged from 26.0 to 30.4 kg/m² (table 10.1). The HWDI ranged from 2.0 to 10.5, revealing disparities among income levels related to mean BMI and neighborhoods. We used a kappa statistic to assess the level of agreement between the BMI rankings and HWDI rankings. Absence of agreement would indicate that income disparities and BMI rankings present divergent perspectives on the obesity crisis and that factors related to income may be critical in understanding obesity rates in the geographic area. Agreement among the rankings would indicate that income disparity may not be the most effective target for interventions to reduce obesity risk in this geographic area. In our illustration, there was agreement between the rankings, as indicated by a significant kappa statistic [kappa (10) = 0.33; p = .0008]. This application of the HWDI focused

Table 10.1. Neighborhood rankings for mean body mass index (BMI) and Healthy Weight Disparity Index (HWDI), based on income and BMI

Houston neighborhoods	BMI, kg/m²			HWDI	HWDI rank	Mean BMI, kg/m²	BMI rank
	Low-income	Medium-income	High-income				
Medical Center–West University–Bellaire	26.41	26.22	25.61	2.02	1	26.05	1
Edgebrook–Ellington	28.02	27.67	27.20	3.50	2	27.67	2
Tomball–Cypress	27.07	29.91	27.04	4.95	3	27.99	3
Central Southwest–Fort Bend	28.34	29.47	24.69	8.11	7	28.51	4
Downtown–East End	28.67	29.84	26.60	6.91	4	28.87	5
Champions–Willowbrook	28.21	31.50	27.08	7.62	6	29.11	6
Atascosita–Lake Houston	30.90	30.35	27.96	8.29	8	29.58	7
Northline–Eastex	29.49	30.77	24.77	10.48	10	29.71	8
Near Northside–Fifth Ward	31.18	28.78	27.96	7.01	5	30.14	9
East Houston–Settegast	30.13	32.02	27.79	9.36	9	30.43	10

on income, but other sociodemographic variables can be used to assess other types of disparities.

Healthy Weight Disparity Index—Why We Need It
Broadening the Perspective of Disparities Research

Webb et al.[31] evaluated five focus areas (cancer, CVD, diabetes, HIV/AIDS, and infant mortality) of greatest racial disparities in health (i.e., disparities in Black and White mortality for the selected conditions) and compiled state health disparities index scores. Taking a similar approach, we devised the Healthy Weight Disparity Index as a measure to compare states, cities, or any designated locations on a continuum related to obesity disparities. For example, there are maps for obesity rates by state and other geographic areas. We recommend these obesity maps be accompanied by obesity disparity rate maps (HWDI scores) to more fully convey obesity trends. By viewing both maps, a more complete picture emerges. States or geographic locations with the lowest obesity rates may have the highest disparity rates. On the other hand, a state with a moderate level of obesity may have low disparity rates. The goal would be for all states to have low obesity rates and low disparity rates. The HWDI can be used to help achieve this goal by making clear comparisons.

Monitoring Progress over Time

The HWDI can be used not only for comparative purposes but to track progress over time. For example, if states or locations implement interventions, then changes in obesity and disparity rates can be assessed at short- and long-term intervals. States that are successful in reducing obesity and disparity rates can be exemplars for other locations.

Design and Development of Interventions

The HWDI can be useful in developing an intervention. To reduce disparities, an assessment of disparity rates can be implemented using the HWDI. For example, if, in a particular location, the analysis finds disparities related to income groups and no disparities for gender, education, or other sociodemographic factors, then the differences by income groups can be a focus of interventions. What are the behaviors, physical and social environments, and attitudes that differ by income groups and could be modified by interventions to reduce obesity risk? In other words, an analysis by income categories could investigate behaviors (physical activity, healthy eating, and sedentary behavior), transactions with and perceptions of the environment, social support, social cohesion, social capital, outcome expectations, self-efficacy, and barriers to healthy living. Differences by income groups in any of these domains could be targets for intervention.

With respect to designing interventions, zip codes with low rankings for BMI but medium or high rankings for HWDI could learn from zip codes with low ranks on BMI and HWDI with regard to ways of addressing the obesity epidemic. Similarly, zip codes with a low HWDI rank but a high rank for BMI might learn from zip codes ranked medium or low on BMI. Differences among the zip codes could be related to school policies on healthy eating and physical activity, characteristics of the built environment, effectiveness of advocacy organizations, infrastructures to support healthy living, vocal local champions, advertising and marketing related to lifestyles, the priorities of elected officials, and the presence or absence of community-based grassroots movements to promote healthy lifestyles. These targeted differences among zip codes could be the focus for developing interventions in designated zip codes.

Conclusions

The obesity crisis disproportionately affects low-income and racial and ethnic minority groups. To address this disparity, measures or indices are needed to assess, monitor, and track changes related to obesity risk and obesity rates. To fill a gap in the literature that indicates the clear need for an obesity disparity metric, we developed the Healthy Weight Disparity Index, and in this chapter we presented an example of how the index can be used. The HWDI can be a useful tool to assess, monitor, and track changes over time so as to promote equity and reduce disparities related to obesity risk.

The uniqueness of the HWDI derives from its focus on place and on sociodemographic factors related to weight status in order to address the obesity crisis among underserved populations in the United States. The HWDI is flexible, useful, and has multiple purposes. We hope researchers and practitioners will use this index to fully develop its potential and to explore its strengths and limitations. Our goal here was to propose a useful tool for researchers and practitioners to effectively reduce health disparities and obesity rates and improve the public health of all communities.

References

1. Pearcy JN, Keppel KG. A summary measure of health disparity. Pub Health Rep. 2002 May–Jun;117(3):273–80.
2. Centers for Disease Control and Prevention, National Center for Health Statistics. Healthy People 2000. Hyattsville, MD: Centers for Disease Control and Prevention / National Center for Health Statistics, 1990 Sep. Available at: http://www.cdc.gov/nchs/healthy_people /hp2000.htm.
3. Centers for Disease Control and Prevention, National Center for Health Statistics. Healthy People 2010. Hyattsville, MD: Centers for Disease Control and Prevention / National Center for Health Statistics, 2000 Jan. Available at: http://www.cdc.gov/nchs/healthy_people /hp2010.htm.
4. Centers for Disease Control and Prevention, National Center for Health Statistics. Healthy People 2020. Hyattsville, MD: Centers for Disease Control and Prevention / National Center for Health Statistics, 2010 Dec. Available at: http://www.cdc.gov/nchs/healthy_people /hp2020.htm.

5. Centers for Disease Control and Prevention. CDC: saving lives, protecting people. Atlanta, GA: Centers for Disease Control and Prevention, 2012. Available at: www.cdc.gov.

6. Singh GK, Siahpush M, Hiatt RA, et al. Dramatic increases in obesity and overweight prevalence and body mass index among ethnic-immigrant and social class groups in the United States, 1976–2008. J Community Health. 2011 Feb;36(1):94–110.

7. Clarke PJ, O'Malley PM, Johnston LD, et al. Differential trends in weight-related health behaviors among American young adults by gender, race/ethnicity and socioeconomic status: 1984–2006. Am J Public Health. 2009 Oct;99(10):1893–901.

8. Institute of Medicine. Accelerating progress in obesity prevention: solving the weight of the nation. Washington, DC: Institute of Medicine, 2012 May. Available at: http://www.iom .edu/~/media/Files/Report%20Files/2012/APOP/APOP_insert.pdf.

9. Floyd MF, Taylor WC, Whitt-Glover M. Measurement of park and recreation environments that support physical activity in low-income communities of color: highlights of challenges and recommendations. Am J Prev Med. 2009 Apr;36(4 Suppl):S156–60.

10. Suminski RR, Pyle S, Taylor WC. Environmental characteristics and physical activity in racial/ethnic minority and Euro-American college students. Percept Mot Skills. 2009 Apr;108(2):465–78.

11. Taylor WC, Hepworth JT, Lees E, et al. Obesity, physical activity, and the environment: is there a legal basis for environmental injustices? Environ Justice. 2008 Mar;1(1):45–8.

12. Lees E, Taylor WC, Hepworth JT, et al. Environmental changes to increase physical activity: perceptions of older urban ethnic minority women. J Aging Phys Act. 2007 Oct;15(4): 425–38.

13. Taylor WC, Sallis JF, Lees E, et al. Changing social and built environments to promote physical activity: recommendations from low income, urban women. J Phys Act Health. 2007 Jan;4(1):54–65.

14. Taylor WC, Floyd MF, Whitt-Glover MC, et al. Environmental justice: a framework for collaboration between public health and parks and recreation fields to study disparities in physical activity. J Phys Act Health. 2007;4 Suppl 1:S50–63.

15. Taylor WC, Poston WSC, Jones L, et al. Environmental justice: obesity, physical activity, and healthy eating. J Phys Act Health. 2006;3 Suppl 1:S30–54.

16. Anderson SE, Whitaker RC. Prevalence of obesity among US preschool children in different racial and ethnic groups. Arch Pediatr Adolesc Med. 2009 Apr;163(4):344–8.

17. Flegal KM, Carroll MD, Ogden CL, et al. Prevalence and trends in obesity among US adults, 1999–2008. JAMA. 2010 Jan;303(3):235–41.

18. Ogden CL, Carroll MD, Kit BK, et al. Prevalence of obesity and trends in body mass index among US children and adolescents, 1999–2010. JAMA. 2012 Feb;307(5):483–90.

19. Schoenborn CA, Adams PE. Health behaviors of adults: United States, 2005–2007. Vital Health Stat. 2010 Mar;245(10):1–132.

20. Moy KL, Sallis JF, David KJ. Health indicators of Native Hawaiian and Pacific Islanders in the United States. J Community Health. 2010 Feb;35(1):81–92.

21. Freedman DS, Centers for Disease Control and Prevention. Obesity—United States, 1988–2008. MMWR Surveill Summ. 2011 Jan;60 Suppl:73–7.

22. Chang VW, Lauderdale DS. Income disparities in body mass index and obesity in the United States, 1971–2002. Arch Intern Med. 2005 Oct;165(18):2122–8.

23. Ruel E, Reither EN, Robert SA, et al. Neighborhood effects on BMI trends: examining BMI trajectories for black and white women. Health Place. 2010 Mar;16(2):191–8.

24. Leung CW, Willett WC, Ding EL. Low-income Supplemental Nutrition Assistance Program participation is related to adiposity and metabolic risk factors. Am J Clin Nutr. 2012 Jan;95(1): 17–24.

25. McKean E, ed. Index 2005: new Oxford American dictionary. 2nd Ed. New York, NY: Oxford University Press, 2005 May.

26. Kennedy BP, Kawachi I, Prothrow-Stith D. Income distribution and mortality: cross sectional ecological study of the Robin Hood index in the United States. BMJ. 1996 Apr;312(7037): 1004–7.

27. Kawachi I, Kennedy BP. The relationship of income inequality to mortality: does the choice of indicator matter? Soc. Sci. Med. 1997 Oct;45(7):1121–7.

28. Ross CE. Neighborhood disadvantage and adult depression. J Health Soc Behav. 2000 Jun; 41(2):177–87.

29. Henderson C, Liu X, Diez Roux AV, et al. The effects of US state income inequality and alcohol policies on symptoms of depression and alcohol dependence. Soc Sci Med. 2004 Feb;58(3):565–75.

30. Naess O, Calussen B, Thelle D, et al. Four indicators of socioeconomic position: relative ranking across causes of death. Scand J Public Health. 2005;33(3):215–21.

31. Webb BC, Simpson SL, Hairston KG. From politics to parity: using a health disparities index to guide legislative efforts for health equity. Am J Public Health. 2011 Mar;101(3):554–60.

32. Drewnowski A, Rehm CD, Solet D. Disparities in obesity rates: analysis by ZIP code area. Soc Sci Med. 2007 Dec;65(12):2458–63.

33. Lovasi GS, Hutson MA, Guerra M, et al. Built environments and obesity in disadvantaged populations. Epidemiol Rev. 2009;31:7–20.

34. Dutwin D, Sherr S. Health of Houston survey, HHS 2010: methodology report. Houston, TX: Institute for Health Policy / University of Texas School of Public Health, 2011. Available at: https://sph.uth.tmc.edu/content/uploads/2011/12/Methodology-Report-HHS-092011_FINAL .pdf.

35. Taylor WC, Franzini L, Olvera N, et al. Environmental audits of friendliness toward physical activity in three income levels. J Urban Health. 2012 Feb [Epub ahead of print].

36. Stata Corp. Stata 12. College Station, TX: Stata Corp.

PART III **REPORTS FROM THE FIELD**

CHAPTER 11

Obesity Management Organized by Adolescents in Rural Appalachia

Robert A. Branch, MD, FRCP, Ann L. Chester, PhD, Sara Hanks, BS, MPH Candidate, Summer Kuhn, BS, MPH Candidate, Mary McMillion, BS, MA, Catherine Morton-McSwain, MSEd, Stephanie Paulsen, Uday Kiran Para, MS, BTech, Yvonne Cannon, RN, CCRC, and Stephen J. Groark

In this chapter we describe and confirm the feasibility of implementing a novel program, called the Community Appalachian Investigation and Research Network (CAIRN) Learning Paradigm, to address the runaway epidemic of obesity that has not been halted by other contemporary approaches in rural Appalachia, West Virginia. Rural Appalachia is recognized as a medically underserved, low-income, widely dispersed community, where health care providers and health care institutions struggle to maintain acute medical services and lack the personnel to provide adequate preventive care.[1]* It is not surprising, therefore, that this region is at the epicenter of the national epidemic of obesity and its downstream complications—including type 2 diabetes and cardiovascular disease.[2,3] The longitudinal Behavioral Risk Factor Surveillance Study (BRFSS), for example, has identified West Virginia as being at the apex of obesity prevalence over the past two decades,[3] and counties in West Virginia are among the first to report decreasing life expectancy due to complications of obesity.[4] In the experience of our program, using similar sample sizes, we found a prevalence of obesity close to 50%, compared with the BRFSS's random digit dialing sample's

Robert A. Branch is a professor of medicine at the University of Pittsburgh Medical Center. Ann L. Chester is an assistant vice president / social justice and project director; Sara Hanks, a curriculum coordinator; Summer Kuhn and Mary McMillion, community resource associates; and Catherine Morton-McSwain, an education director, all at the Health Sciences and Technology Academy, Health Sciences Center, West Virginia University. Stephanie Paulsen is a project manager; Uday Kiran Para, a software developer; Yvonne Cannon, a research coordinator; and Stephen J. Groark, a systems manager, all at the University of Pittsburgh.

* See also chapter 19, in which Raynor et al. report on Cherokee Health Systems, which developed a pediatric weight management intervention in East Tennessee, another part of rural Appalachia, and chapter 20, in which Zizzi et al. describe an innovative insurance benefit to prevent and treat obesity among public employees in West Virginia.

Table 11.1.   Pragmatic objectives of the Community Appalachian Investigation
and Research Network program in rural West Virginia

- Encourage disadvantaged and minority high school students to enroll in and graduate from college.
- Teach the science that underlies health care.
- Provide new knowledge about the relevance and implications of lifestyle choices.
- Emphasize cognitive learning as a prerequisite to changing behavior.
- Target adolescents as a vehicle for family change.
- Help the community learn new ways to care for themselves.
- Train high school students in the conduct of community-based participatory research.
- Critically evaluate whether the program is effective.

prevalence of 37%.[5,6] In the current economic climate, this situation is unlikely to change.

With this void in health care resources, the community itself has the opportunity to build on its existing strengths of strong family ties and a tradition of "looking after one's own." Unfortunately, cultural customs, built around survival in times of food shortages and famines, have led to a prioritization of poor lifestyle choices with respect to diet and exercise among local families. What has evolved is a dichotomy, where lifestyle choices are conceptually separated from the health care consequences of these choices. Furthermore, this cultural constraint has proved recalcitrant to health care providers' admonitions to eat better and exercise more.

Our strategy to meet these challenges is to direct attention to the root causes of the problem: the need for community families to learn new ways to look after themselves in the twenty-first-century environment. This requires acquisition of new knowledge about the relevance and implications of lifestyle choices, which we consider to be best provided by an educational infrastructure rather than a health care provider infrastructure. We have adopted a successful program that encourages disadvantaged and minority high school students to enroll in and graduate from college[7,8] by focusing on the teaching of science that educates students about the problem of obesity in their community. In the process, we have found that the elements of this program also encompass a broader range of objectives, such as improved obesity management, that will confer far-reaching benefits on the community (table 11.1). Furthermore, these health benefits are likely to be effective even though education is provided by the educational community, not by the health care community.

A Tiered Diffusion Model of Learning: A Prospective, Formal, Pedagogical Strategy

Our novel approach builds on an existing infrastructure of a network of 76 science clubs organized in a collaboration between communities in West Virginia and West Virginia University through the university's Health Science and Technology Academy (HSTA). These clubs have successfully created a pipeline of educational opportunity for 800 students each year, identified through a selection process prioritizing high school students who are socioeconomically disadvantaged and/or members of a racial/ethnic minority group, with the goal of encouraging participants to attend and graduate from college.[7,8] In a collaboration between HSTA and the major academic medical centers (AMCs) at the University of Pittsburgh and West Virginia University, a health care educational research focal point to the science program has been developed and implemented, collectively known as the Community Appalachian Investigation and Research Network.[3,9,10]

An underlying assumption is that knowledge is sought as a way of finding novel and productive ways of interacting with a complex world.[10] Acquiring knowledge involves a complex sequential process in which new information is built onto a conceptual baseline framework by assimilation. There is a reorganization of available information, and concept development requires the complex processes of formulation, comprehension, and meaningful understanding.[4] This consolidated base provides a springboard for abstract conceptual extrapolation and expansion to new circumstances and provides a platform for subsequent behavior. This sequential process requires each person to undergo a process of individual discovery and construction that can be sustained by motivation.

We recognize that conflict arises when new and complex lifestyle information is presented to an individual who has already established poor lifestyle behaviors. If a preconceived concept is consistent with the new information offered, then concept building is emotionally acceptable and the adoption of new behavior is relatively easy to achieve. In contrast, if the preconceived model is misconceived or incorrect, when new, correct, but more complex information is provided, the emotive response may be outright rejection or soon-forgotten learning. This conflict is fundamental to explaining the clash between science and culture as a barrier to adult learning in any situation, but it is particularly relevant when core behaviors are challenged.[5] The conflict also implies that, in general, adults are more inflexible and resistant to change than adolescents, who are still at a formative stage of development.[6] Furthermore, adolescents are at a stage when prevention of obesity rather than disease management of type 2 diabetes or cardiovascular disease has a greater chance of improving community health.[11] The rigidity in handling complexity has been suggested to be less of a problem in adolescents because the late maturation of executive areas of the brain, as proposed in the "adaptive adolescent hypothesis,"[12] confers greater intellectual flexibility in understanding and applying new information during adolescence.[13]

Unique features of the CAIRN infrastructure, added to the existing HSTA science club network, include the creation of a new community research education career—training of community research associates (CRAs)—and building of the CAIRN Communication System to support community-based participatory research (CBPR).[7–9,14,15] The CRAs in the current program are four senior science teachers, originating from and living in the community, who use their educational skills to teach the science of health care. These individuals are experienced educators but have had no training

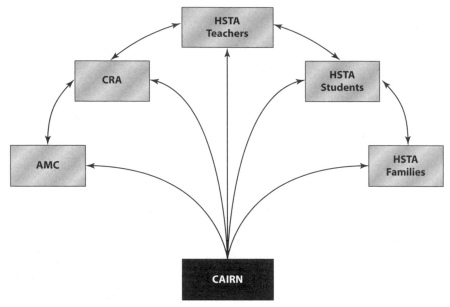

FIGURE 11.1. Schematic illustration of the Community Appalachian Investigation and Research Network (CAIRN) Tiered Diffusion Model of Learning. Each bidirectional arrow is supported by the CAIRN Communication Network. AMC, academic medical ccnter; CRA, community research associate; HSTA, Health Science and Technology Academy of West Virginia University.

in health care or community health research. With training from the University of Pittsburgh, they have responded extremely quickly and effectively in learning these skills. These are full-time, committed individuals from the community who consider family health education as their educational and career challenge. Each CRA acts as a health science educator for approximately 20 science club teachers in individual science clubs organized by HSTA. They provide the critical liaison between the families, clubs, and scientists (fig. 11.1).

A unique contribution of CAIRN is the training of HSTA club students as credentialed investigators who, with guidance, conduct credible CBPR during the annual cycle of each club, including participation in community service projects that are supported by the CAIRN Communication System to connect widely dispersed clubs.[9] Pragmatically, the opportunities revolve around the HSTA clubs' annual cycle, which in turn revolves around the high school academic year (fig. 11.2). An annual cycle of the CAIRN Learning Paradigm starts in the summer, with preparation for the major annual activity, the learning-by-doing, in each HSTA club's community project. The cycle begins with preparation of the CRAs, followed by preparation of the club teachers in intensive summer workshops. The learning-by-doing projects at each club are facilitated by the teachers. Each student is asked to use the classical sequence of the

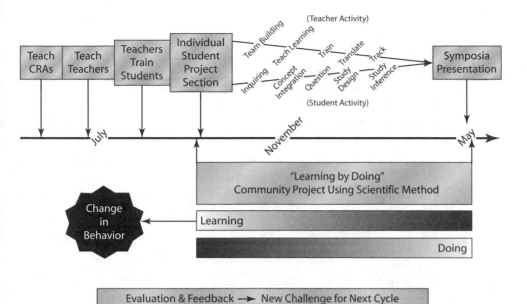

FIGURE 11.2. Annual cycle of the Health Science and Technology Academy (HSTA) clubs. CRAs, community research associates.

scientific approach to systematically address a question in prospective, small-group studies. More specifically, the tasks for each project are: build a team, learn principles of how to learn, train with the project team in the skills they need, help translate instructions and ideas into practical activities, and track the project as it is conducted to maintain timelines.

Community projects using CBPR require all involved students to be credentialed to conduct such research. Non-health-related science projects are still encouraged, as this was the initial staple of the HSTA program. Each student has to self-select his or her community project and must have between 2 and, at a maximum, 10 co-investigators (the club size limit). Each individual student is required to submit a formal project description in the form of a science question followed by a proposal of how to address that question. These submissions require approval for content and feasibility by the student's HSTA science teacher and by the regional CRA.[10,11] These projects become the hands-on focal point for learning in the community projects, extending from October to May each year, as well as providing families with the opportunity to participate actively in the learning process. Thus, in each annual cycle, the CAIRN Learning Paradigm fosters the bidirectional diffusion of concepts across the multiple tiers to ensure each teacher is also a learner (fig. 11.2):

- AMC ↔ CRA network at the University of Pittsburgh: This is supported by a series of advanced, one-day and short-course sessions designed to provide the relevant scientific concepts as well as evidence-based information on the relevant disease management, at an advanced but comprehensible level. Principles of ethics, research conduct and regulation, the scientific process, and cultural perceptions in the community are then shared.

- CRA network ↔ HSTA teachers in Teach the Teachers workshops: A biomedical summer experience—a week-long immersion training course for 18 HSTA club science teachers is followed by a practicum in which they receive practical workshop training in the program's management. In each of the following two weeks, 80 students (tenth to eleventh grade) attend a summer immersion course on CBPR and are trained by the newly trained HSTA science teachers under the oversight of the CRAs. The major objective of the course is to share principles of ethics, CBPR, and study design. In September, all 76 HSTA teachers attend a Teach the Teachers intensive weekend course to introduce the same set of common principles of the program.
- HSTA teachers ↔ HSTA students in HSTA clubs (n = 744 in 2001–12): This is conducted as a one-week summer immersion course on obesity and CBPR for students in transition between tenth and eleventh grade and the recently trained HSTA teachers. The broader information exchange is between each teacher and the club members from each grade in the weekly community project meetings (fig. 11.2).
- HSTA students ↔ HSTA families (n = 5,000+): This is encouraged by inclusion of families in community projects, by attendance at the annual symposia for HSTA clubs, and by the interest families take in their children's activities. The HSTA family members are the source for adding cultural perceptions in the community to the dialogue.

Progress Report of the CAIRN Learning Paradigm

The CAIRN's tiered diffusion learning paradigm for obesity and health and the principles of CBPR were introduced to 20 HSTA students in transition from tenth to eleventh grade and to two CRAs in the 2007–8 cycle. The 20 students represented 18 HSTA clubs. The HSTA teachers from these clubs then learned the same content material from the CRAs. That year, 180 HSTA students and 20 HSTA teachers were credentialed to conduct CBPR, and the rudiments of the CAIRN Communication Network were developed prospectively to build, collect, and organize data on obesity and diabetes prevalence. Our approach used full institutional review board (IRB)–approved written consent/assent and respected Health Insurance Portability and Accountability Act principles. This work resulted in enrollment of 976 participants from 84 families, three published, peer-reviewed manuscripts,[3,9,11] and more than 20 individual student presentations at HSTA symposia. Since then, we have added two more CRAs who live in different regions of West Virginia.

Table 11.2. Obesity-related research projects in West Virginia University's Health Science and Technology Academy (HSTA), September 2011 to May 2012

Project feature[a]	Number	% of total
Students in program	744	—
Number of projects	400	100
Obesity-related projects	224	56
Prevalence-related projects	93	23
Diet/exercise-related projects	78	20
Intervention-related projects	38	10

[a] Types of projects are not mutually exclusive.

Successful meetings have been arranged to coordinate and simplify IRB management, by involving the chairs of the respective IRBs at West Virginia University and the University of Pittsburgh. We have also refined the CAIRN Communication Network and deployed IRB-approved web-based questionnaires that use expedited consent/assent procedures and provide immediate interactive feedback to participants on estimated body mass index in the family.

In the HSTA Community Project cycle for 2011–12, activities extended, for the first time, to making the CAIRN learning program in CBPR and obesity available to all active HSTA science clubs. Thus, small-group, intensive involvement is now required. The interest in taking advantage of the CAIRN Tiered Diffusion Model of Learning has been impressive (table 11.2). The broad range of topics chosen for action in this year reflected ingenuity and entrepreneurship. The CBPR being undertaken reflects a mix of collective studies across the community, in which 224 credentialed investigators of the 400 separate projects throughout the 76 clubs chose to focus on aspects of the prevalence of obesity, type 2 diabetes, and cardiovascular disease in 224 projects (table 11.2). Of these, 42 projects address science questions related to understanding the characteristics of the prevalence of metabolic syndrome in the community, 34 relate to dietary consumption and exercise habits, and 17% are intervention studies with a pre-post design to identify potential interventions for future randomized comparative studies. This is a healthy and growing number of intervention projects that can be considered as pilot studies, seeking to learn what does and does not work in this community.

Conclusions

At the inception of the CAIRN Learning Paradigm, we knew that the HSTA program already excited adolescents' interest in science sufficiently to encourage disadvantaged and minority students to enroll and be successful in college. By providing guidance and a prerequisite infrastructure, we can now confirm adolescents' enthusiasm about the science of energy balance and weight control. We are also excited about the evidence that, with guidance, the ability of these students to conduct CBPR means that they can rigorously and critically evaluate the health care implications of their activities in their own communities.

The novelty of this approach is that it is built through education within the community, not by traditional local health care providers. It targets adolescents as the vehicle for family change and includes all families in the community, not only families with obese members, and most fundamentally, it targets cognitive understanding as a prerequisite to changing behavior. Ongoing studies are in progress to appraise whether or not this strategy is achieving its desired outcomes in changing knowledge base, behavior, and, most importantly, community health.

This program is a work in progress, and it remains to be proven that the health of the adolescents, their families, and their community is improved to a relevant and sustained extent. Thus, our report here is only descriptive; we look forward to the opportunity to evaluate the outcomes formally.

LESSONS LEARNED

Science club members in rural Appalachia can contribute and benefit in the following ways:

- Foster community trust
- Implement the Tiered Diffusion Model of Learning paradigm
- Act as community research associates (to guide the science teachers)
- Develop two-way communication
- Conduct community-based participatory research on obesity
- Launch community interventions
- Enroll in and succeed in college

Acknowledgments

The authors thank the enthusiastic Health Science and Technology Academy students and their families, without whom none of this would have been possible, and the HSTA teachers, for their dedication and the long hours they have volunteered to enhance the lives of the children they influence. They also wish to thank the National Center for Research Resources (NCRR) of the National Institutes of Health (NIH) for its support through a Science Education and Partnership Award (SEPA) to HSTA, 99001382-005; two supplemental grants to the SEPA award, one to build the Web Portal 3 R25 RR023274-04SI and the other for the Web-based SEPA-DOC questionnaire 3 R25 RR023274-05SI; and an RC4, Community-Based Participatory Research Infra-structure grant to CAIRN 1RC4RR031433-01. The content of this chapter is solely the responsibility of the authors and does not necessarily represent the official views of the NCRR or the NIH. Additional support for the program has been received from the Howard Hughes Foundation and the Claude Worthington Benedum Foundations. The authors also acknowledge the encouragement and guidance offered by the HSTA Joint Governing Board.

References

1. Adams P, Gravely M, Doria J. West Virginia diabetes strategic plan 2002–2007. Charleston, WV: West Virginia Department of Health and Human Resources, 2007. Pp. 1–37. Available at: http://www.wvdiabetes.org/Portals/12/Diabetes%20Plan.pdf.
2. Ezzati M, Friedman AB, Kulkarni SC, et al. The reversal of fortunes: trends in county mortality and cross-county mortality disparities in the United States. PLoS Med. 2008 Apr 22;5(4):e66.
3. Centers for Disease Control and Prevention. Behavioral Risk Factor Surveillance System (BRFSS) annual survey data 2001–2011. Atlanta, GA: Centers for Disease Control and Prevention, 2011. Available at: http://www.cdc.gov/brfss/technical_infodata/surveydata.htm.
4. West Virginians for Affordable Health Care. Early deaths: West Virginians have some of the shortest life expectancies in the United States. Charleston, WV: West Virginians for Affordable Health Care, 2008. Available at: http://appvoices.org/images/uploads/2011/07/WV-early -deaths-_2008.pdf.
5. Bardwell G, Morton C, Chester A, et al. Feasibility of adolescents to conduct community based participatory research on obesity and diabetes in rural Appalachia. Clin Transl Sci. 2009 Oct;2(5):340–9.
6. Pancoska P, Buch S, Cecchetti A, et al. Family networks of obesity and type 2 diabetes in rural Appalachia. Clin Transl Sci. 2009 Dec;2(6):413–21.
7. Chester A, Bowers M, Bushy A, et al. A national agenda for rural minority healthy series: recruitment and training of health professionals. Kansas City, MO: National Rural Health Associations, 2001.
8. Branch RA, Chester A. Undergraduate pipeline and community-based participatory research. Presented at: National Advisory Research Resources Council, Bethesda, MD, May 2008.
9. Branch RA, Chester A, Morton-McSwain C, et al. A novel approach to adolescent obesity in rural Appalachia of West Virginia: educating adolescents as family health coaches and research investigators. In: Zimering MB, ed. Topics in the prevention, treatment and complications of type 2 diabetes. Rijeka, Croatia: InTech, 2011. Available at: http://www.intecho pen.com/books/topics-in-the-prevention-treatment-and-complications-of-type-2-diabetes /a-novel-approach-to-adolescent-obesity-in-rural-appalachia-of-west-virginia-educating -adolescents-as.
10. Ausubel DP. A subsumption theory of meaningful verbal learning and retention. J Gen Psychol. 1962 Apr;66:213–24.
11. Patton MQ. Qualitative evaluation and research methods. 2nd ed. Thousand Oaks, CA: Sage Publications, 1990.
12. Dobbs D. Beautiful brains. Tampa, FL: National Geographic, 2011 Oct. Available at: http:// ngm.nationalgeographic.com/print/2011/10/teenage-brains/dobbs-text.
13. Fields RD. Myelination: an overlooked mechanism of synaptic plasticity? Neuroscientist. 2005 Dec;11(6):528–31.
14. Israel BA, Parker EA, Rowe Z, et al. Community-based participatory research: lessons learned from the Centers for Children's Environmental Health and Disease Prevention Research. Environ Health Perspect. 2005 Oct;113(10):1463–71.
15. Nikolajski C. Youth and community based participatory research: suggestions for future directions. Pittsburgh, PA: University of Pittsburgh, 2007. Available at: http://d-scholarship .pitt.edu/8793/1/Nikolajski_Cara_Thesis_2007.pdf.

CHAPTER 12

Winning Over Weight Wellness

A Culturally Relevant, Interactive Health Program
for Underserved Faith-Based Groups

Fern Webb, PhD, Michelle Doldren, EdD, MPH,
and Shirley Blanchard, PhD, ABDA, OTR/L, FAOTA

The Winning Over Weight Wellness (W.O.W. Wellness) program targeted Black women and their families living in Duval County (Jacksonville), Florida. The goals of W.O.W. Wellness were (1) to provide a holistic health program for Black women, (2) to improve eating practices, (3) to increase physical activity, and (4) to reduce BMI. The program was developed using themes and strategies extrapolated from an extensive review of the literature and information gleaned from numerous discussions with key collaborators and community partners. This project demonstrates innovation in design, participant recruitment, implementation, and sustainability.

Community-Based Participatory Research

A diverse team of health intervention experts and church leaders was assembled. Churches were selected primarily based on their membership being predominantly Black and on their location (i.e., Westside, Northside, and Southside of Jacksonville). A slide show presentation developed by the principal investigator explained the purposes of the project: (1) to ensure the appropriateness of W.O.W. Wellness; (2) to promote W.O.W. Wellness awareness throughout the immediate and surrounding communities; and (3) to recruit eligible Black women. An advisory council, consisting of church leaders or designees, was created for program oversight.

Fern Webb is an assistant professor in the Department of Community Health and Family Medicine, University of Florida, Jacksonville. Michelle Doldren is a research scientist at Nova Southeastern University's Institute for Child Health Policy and an adjunct assistant professor in the university's Master of Public Health Program, in Fort Lauderdale. Shirley Blanchard is an associate professor of occupational therapy in the School of Pharmacy and Health Professions and the Department of Medicine at Creighton University, in Omaha.

How Was W.O.W. Wellness Implemented?

W.O.W. Wellness was implemented at two churches and one primary care center, with significant collaboration with faith-based leaders. In addition to recruiting women from throughout the community, the churches and the primary care site made their facilities available to conduct the W.O.W. Wellness program. Each site selected at least three women who could be participants—provided they completed and submitted interest forms—to serve on the advisory council.

To be eligible to participate, a woman must (1) consider herself to be Black or African American and (2) have a desire to become healthier or lose weight. Women completed an interest form by a specified deadline, and as selected by the first 15 interest forms (stratified by site) randomly pulled from a hat, women were contacted and invited to participate. Random selection proceeded until each site had 15 women.

A train-the-trainer program was incorporated into W.O.W. Wellness to increase its likelihood of sustainability beyond the demonstration period. For the duration of each cohort, women interested in completing this program were encouraged to attend all sessions.

W.O.W. Wellness also provided childcare services and evening meals to participants, to eliminate barriers known to significantly decrease participation in lifestyle intervention programs.[1-3] As part of Kids' Play Club, participants' children increased their physical activity while mom focused on her own health. The Unwind & Dine component offered a nutritious meal that reduced competition for time and thus the likelihood that participants would arrive late, leave early, or fail to attend due to meal constraints. The scheduled meal also role-modeled the importance of eating a nutritious meal together as a family.

How Is W.O.W. Wellness Designed?

Grounded in behavioral choice[4] and social cognitive theories,[5] as well as in empirical health intervention studies implemented by Kumanyika and colleagues,[6-9] W.O.W. Wellness was developed with the premise that Black women's weight and health status are directly influenced by their eating and physical activity practices. Conducted from January through December 2010, the program consisted of 20 two-hour sessions, conducted in 10-week cohorts. Every W.O.W. Wellness session included spirituality/empowerment, nutrition, physical activity, social support, and self-accountability components.

The *spirituality* component was crafted by the ministers and addressed how to overcome barriers and readiness for change. Each session started with prayer by the ministers and encouraging words from the first ladies of each of the participating churches.

A nutritionist and/or layperson from each site facilitated the 45-minute *nutrition education* activities. Nutrition sessions focused on a variety of topics, including but not limited to using online resources, eating a variety of vegetables and fruits, eating lean protein and grains, and the importance of eating breakfast. Healthy cooking was demonstrated using sample menus and recipes, along with reading food labels and learning how to determine portion sizes. Participants visited local famers' markets and took part in at least two cooking demonstrations.

Participants engaged in at least two hours of *physical activity* each week. A certified aerobics instructor led exercises to contemporary or hip-hop gospel music and Zumba for at least one class. The other class was group-directed: the women shared their favorite exercise videos, or all chose to walk outdoors. Participants also learned FITT principles, where *F* represents frequency; *I*, intensity; one *T*, time spent exercising; and the other *T*, type of activity. Other class topics included Anywhere/Anytime Exercises, Physical Activity Action Plans, Recognizing and Avoiding Overexertion, and Relaxation Techniques.

The *social support* activities examined the positive and negative effects of having a social support network within and outside sessions. Participants selected at least one buddy by the end of week 2; the women in each subgroup were encouraged to contact each other by phone or email at least once a week and to exercise together outside class time.

Participants worked in groups to create an individual plan of action to increase *self-accountability*. During the second session, they were asked to set individual weight goals not to exceed a weight loss of more than two pounds per week. The women were encouraged to set goals for healthier eating, exercising more, and increasing self-efficacy. Program participants were required to record all foods consumed each day and to record their exercise activities in the W.O.W. weekly tracker. The type, amount of time, and intensity of each physical activity were also logged in the tracker.

What Were the Health Outcomes?

Weight was measured at the start of the program, then changes were assessed weekly and at the end of the program. Anthropometrics (height, weight, and arm, bust, waist, hip, and thigh circumferences), health behaviors (nutrition, physical activity), health behavior knowledge and attitudes, mental health (anxiety, hopelessness, depression), physiological health (general health, diabetes, hypertension, cholesterol level, cardiovascular fitness), life satisfaction and support, nutrition and physical activity self-efficacies,[10] and stages of change—all were measured at program start and end. Questions from the Centers for Disease Control and Prevention's (CDC) 2009 Behavioral Risk Factor Surveillance System survey were used.[11] Demographic characteristics (age, ethnicity, race, marital status, household children, education, working status, income) were recorded only at program start.

What Were the Results?

The first goal of W.O.W. Wellness, to provide a holistic health program for Black women in Duval County, was met. Ninety-one Black women enrolled in the program throughout its offering at two community-based and one clinical site over three cohort periods. The 91 women participated in 128 holistic health sessions, representing 1,279 health education and physical activity contacts. Sixty-four women (70%), aged 22–72 (average age of 44), completed the program.

Eating Practices

Goal 2 focused on participants' eating practices, the goal being that the proportion of participants consuming at least two daily servings of fruit would increase by 50% and the proportion consuming at least two daily servings of vegetables—at least one-third green or orange vegetables—would increase by 75%. By program end, there was little change in fruit consumption: 13% reported consuming at least two daily servings of fruit, compared with 12% at program start. The proportion of participants consuming fruit at least once a day (19% at program start; 30% at program end) or up to four times a day (0% at program start; 5% at program end) increased more substantially.

The proportion of participants consuming vegetables increased only slightly. For example, at program start, 27% reported consuming at least two servings of vegetables daily, while by program end, 32% reported consuming at least two servings daily.

Physical Activity

The physical activity (goal 3) outcomes were that the proportion of participants engaging in no leisure-time physical activity decreased, while the proportion engaging in moderate to vigorous activity consistently increased. The proportion engaging in no leisure-time physical activity decreased by 60% rather than by the projected goal of 90%; moderate activity increased by 30% rather than the projected 75%; and vigorous activity increased by 75%, more than the projected 50%. The average number of days per week that participants engaged in moderate exercise significantly increased, from 2.62 at program start to 3.68 at program end.

A large increase was observed in vigorous activities: 39% of participants reported engaging in vigorous activities at least once a week at program start, compared with 68% at program end. Participants, on average, also engaged in vigorous exercise on more days each week by program end: an average of 1.39 days at program start, but 2.58 days at program end.

Primary Outcome: Body Mass Index

Goal 4 was to reduce body mass index (BMI). Healthy weight, as defined by the CDC, is having a BMI between 18.5 and 24.9 kg/m^2.[12] The average BMI at program start was 34.87 kg/m^2, with 21% of the women being morbidly obese (BMI > 39.9 kg/m^2); 23%, significantly obese (BMI = 34.9–39.9 kg/m^2); 26%, obese (BMI = 29.9–34.9 kg/m^2); 26%, overweight (BMI = 24.9–29.9 kg/m^2); and 4% of normal weight. The average BMI at program end was slightly lower than at the start: 33.36 kg/m^2. However, the proportions of women who were morbidly obese (11%), obese (23%), and of normal weight (11%) had changed noticeably by program end. (The average BMI fails to show this apparent effect because, while the majority of individuals lost weight, seven

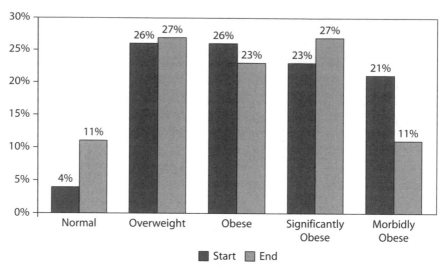

FIGURE 12.1. Distribution (percent) of participants' body mass index at the start and end of the W.O.W. Wellness program.

women had gained weight by program end.) Figure 12.1 shows the changes in BMI for participants by the end of the program.

At program start, 41% of the participants reported having high cholesterol, 17% had diabetes, and 44% had hypertension. By program end, 50% reported improvements in their cholesterol; 53%, improvements in diabetes; and 66%, improvements in hypertension. All anthropometric measurements decreased by program end: arm circumference average reduced from 13.1 to 12.8 inches; bust average, from 44.0 to 43.2 inches; hip average, from 47.1 to 46.6 inches; thigh average, from 23.8 to 23.6 inches; and waist average, from 41.6 to 40.4 inches. While decreases in anthropometric measurements were sometimes slight (except for waist circumference), all measurements were decreasing by program end.

What Worked and What Could Be Improved?

Positive change in weight and wellness requires effort, dedication, and time. The findings from the W.O.W. Wellness program emphasize the importance of remaining positive when pursuing weight loss, maintaining constant communication with community-based partners, and having an onsite team for program coordination so as to respect the faith-based organizations' time and resources. The program team checked in weekly with staff at each site; very occasionally, program sessions had to be rescheduled to another day/time or location.

On completion of the program, participants pointed out (1) the need for ongoing access to health or exercise programs; (2) their desire for continuing communication with fellow participants after the holistic health program ended; and (3) the importance of teaching other Black women how to become healthier. While the first cohort suggested that shortening the program from 12 weeks to 10 weeks would prove useful, by program end, 100% of participants wanted the program to be longer or wanted a plan for more sustainability beyond the intervention period.

Another finding was that participants preferred a simple nutritional focus on increasing the number of fruits and vegetables eaten daily or reducing portion sizes, rather than learning how to read labels, count calories, or master the various types of carbohydrates. Also, participants were more motivated when exercising in groups than when exercising outside class.

Another important sign of the program's success was the participation rate: 70% of the women who started the program finished it, which provides additional evidence that culturally relevant health education and intervention results in increased participation for this population. Having the Kids' Play Club and providing nutritious meals contributed to the high participation rate. Another asset was having church liaisons, which was essential to maintaining organizational structure and program logistics. For example, liaisons (1) informed everyone about changes in church or holistic health program schedules, (2) shared any participant or program difficulties, (3) completed and submitted weekly session evaluation forms, (4) contacted participants absent from class, and (5) collected participant tracking logs for monitoring accountability. Lastly, at least 12 women completed the train-the-trainer program to promote sustainability of W.O.W. Wellness in their respective churches.

Conclusions

All outcomes of the W.O.W. Wellness program were positive and were progressing toward the projected goals. Average BMI and anthropometric measurements, as well as self-reports about chronic health conditions, improved for the Black women participating in this holistic health program. The overall feedback from participants was that they enjoyed being a part of the program and only wished that the program provided an opportunity to continue learning about healthier eating and exercising within the group settings.

LESSONS LEARNED

On program design:
- Recognize that attaining a positive change in health status requires effort, dedication, and time.
- Remain positive when tackling weight.
- Keep nutrition and physical activity education materials simple.
- Learn what motivates the majority of participants, and implement those techniques early.

On program implementation:
- Maintain constant communication with community-based partners.
- Have liaisons for program coordination, to respect faith-based organizations' time and resources.

- Check weekly with each partnering site, given the many conferences and activities taking place.
- Provide resources (e.g., childcare and evening meals) to foster participation.

On participants' continued success and program sustainability:
- Identify low-cost or free health or exercise programs for ongoing, continued access.
- Create mechanisms for participants to communicate after the program is complete.
- Share strategies on how participants can teach other Black women how to become healthier.

References

1. Henderson KA, Ainsworth BE. A synthesis of perceptions about physical activity among older black and American Indian women. Am J Public Health. 2003 Feb;93(2):313–7.
2. Bopp M, Lattimore D, Wilcox S, et al. Understanding physical activity participation in members of an African American church: a qualitative study. Health Educ Res. 2007 Dec; 22(6):815–26.
3. Young DR, He X, Harris J, et al. Environmental, policy, and cultural factors related to physical activity in well-educated urban African American women. Women Health. 2002;36(2): 29–41.
4. Prochaska JO, DiClemente CC. Stages and processes of self-change of smoking: toward an integrative model of change. J Consult Clin Psychol. 1983 Jun;51(3):390–5.
5. Bandura A. Health promotion by social cognitive means. Health Educ Behav. 2004 Apr; 31(2):143–64.
6. Kumanyika SK, Shults J, Fassbender J, et al. Outpatient weight management in African Americans: the Healthy Eating and Lifestyle Program (HELP) study. Prev Med. 2005 Aug; 41(2):488–502.
7. Kumanyika SK, Espeland MA, Bahnson JL, et al. Ethnic comparison of weight loss in the Trial of Nonpharmacologic Interventions in the Elderly. Obes Res. 2002 Feb;10(2):96–106.
8. Kumanyika SK, Wadden TA, Shults J, et al. Trial of family and friend support for weight loss in African American adults. Arch Intern Med. 2009 Oct;169(19):1795–804.
9. Kumanyika SK, Obarzanek E, Stettler N, et al. Population-based prevention of obesity: the need for comprehensive promotion of healthful eating, physical activity, and energy balance: a scientific statement from American Heart Association Council on Epidemiology and Prevention, Interdisciplinary Committee for Prevention (formerly the Expert Panel on Population and Prevention Science). Circulation. 2008 Jul 22;118(4):428–64.
10. Sallis JF, Pinski RB, Grossman RM, et al. The development of self-efficacy scales for health-related diet and exercise behaviors. Health Educ Res. 1988;3(3):283–92.
11. Centers for Disease Control and Prevention. Behavioral Risk Factor Surveillance System survey questionnaires, 2009 survey questions. Atlanta, GA: U.S. Department of Health and Human Services, 2011. Available at: http://www.cdc.gov/brfss/questionnaires/english.htm.
12. Centers for Disease Control and Prevention. Defining overweight and obesity. Atlanta, GA: U.S. Department of Health and Human Services, Centers for Disease Control and Prevention, 2012. http://www.cdc.gov/obesity/adult/defining.html.

CHAPTER 13

Latino Migrant Middle School Students as Videographers
Learning about Healthy Choices

Jill F. Kilanowski, PhD, APN, CPNP, FAAN

The most rapidly growing ethnic minority in the United States is the Latino population; 28 million American residents are of Mexican birth or have parents of Mexican birth.[1,2] There are approximately 3–5 million migrant farmworkers in the United States; 90% are of Latino ethnicity, with the majority originating in Mexico.[3–5] As a group, migrant farmworkers have worse health status than the majority population.[6,7] In chapter 2 of this volume, Ramirez and coauthors review literature on Latino childhood obesity generally, with a focus on interventions. The intervention described here specifically targets the children of Mexican migrant farmworkers.

The Migrant Middle School Media Nutrition Project
Many migrant farmworkers have children; estimates indicate that there are at least 2 million migrant children in the United States.[8] While the majority of these children are U.S. citizens, they represent a marginalized and vulnerable group that suffers disproportionately poor health. Rates of unhealthy weight in Latino youths are higher than in the majority population, but the rate for the subpopulation of Latino migrant farmworker children is even higher.[8] There is an insufficiency of interventions that have been specially designed for vulnerable populations and tested in children from ethnic and racial minority groups. There is a gap in the literature about the effectiveness of existing migrant student programs for conducting health promotion interventions for this vulnerable and marginalized population.

The purpose of the Migrant Middle School Media Nutrition Project, a community-based pilot intervention, was to test the effectiveness of a middle school multimedia module curriculum intervention for healthy eating and physical activity. This research endeavor was an academic and community collaboration and was approved by the

Jill F. Kilanowski is a nurse scientist and assistant professor at Cincinnati Children's Hospital Medical Center.

university institutional review board through expedited review. The study's health curriculum intervention was embedded in a seven-week summer Migrant Education Program. The Migrant Education Program is funded through formula grants from the Education of Migratory Children, Title I, Part C, and supports education programs for migrant farmworker children to ensure that these children are provided with appropriate educational services.[9] In this summer school, children receive remedial instruction supported by the original No Child Left Behind legislation.[10] The goal of the Migrant Education Program is to promote students' success and meet the unique needs of migrant children. This federal program is offered free of charge to qualifying families and is accompanied daily by two meals and a snack, provided under the U.S. Department of Agriculture Summer Food Service Program.[11] There is no standardized Migrant Education Program curriculum. Local domains and classroom teachers control the curriculum content with reference to state educational grade-level standards.

No single, dominant theory for nutrition education has been developed, and Achterberg and Miller[12] concluded that no one theory can serve all people under all conditions. They suggested that a poly-theoretical model might be the best model to embrace. The theories of three disciplines contributed to the research model: transcultural nursing,[13] child development,[14-16] and education. Education theory contributed *student integrated understanding* to the methodology used for this pilot intervention. Integrated learning occurs when the learner builds connections between ideas and blends personal experiences with formal knowledge.[17,18] The intervention content of the pilot study combined hands-on learning exercises with structured lesson plans to yield a transformational approach. This dynamic approach to teaching and learning helped students make sense of the materials presented, rather than simply memorize facts about nutrition and physical activity.

The study was conducted in the largest summer Migrant Education Program in a Midwest state. The program operated for eight hours a day, five days a week, for seven weeks. Teachers and aides in the Migrant Education Program are often of Latino ethnicity and frequently return to the programs year after year. The university-based nurse researcher developed a collaborative relationship with the migrant summer school. Previous studies had pilot-tested the feasibility of introducing a nutrition and physical activity curriculum into the Migrant Education Program for grades 1–8. Organizations such as the American Academy of Pediatrics[19] and the National Association of Pediatric Nurse Practitioners[20] have established clinical practice guidelines in the identification, prevention, and treatment of childhood overweight, and these were used to guide the development of objectives and content that were ethnically tailored, suitable to the migrant lifestyle, and developmentally appropriate. The classroom objectives addressed nine tenets: (1) understand the food pyramid and My Plate,[21] (2) eat more fruits and vegetables, (3) eat a healthy breakfast, (4) eat more family meals, (5) decrease television and electronic game time to two hours per day, (6) be physically active every day for at least one hour, (7) limit sugar-sweetened drinks, (8) consider food serving portion sizes, and (9) read food labels.

In daily block periods of 45 minutes, students learned about the science of healthy eating, following a pilot-tested curriculum guide developed by the researcher. A state-certified science teacher delivered the healthy eating, nutrition, and physical activity content. Similar 45-minute block periods of physical activity were part of the students' day. In addition, two media specialists led a daily 45- to 60-minute block period on photography and videography skills. This study was conducted in English in the middle school classrooms, and students were challenged to become engaged in videography to produce infomercials on healthy eating and exercise, as reinforcement of the classroom science content. Two chapters of *Media-Smart Youth* from the We Can! study[22] (supported by the National Institute of Child Health and Human Development and the National Heart, Lung and Blood Institute) provided the background curriculum content to educate students on media awareness and the power of media in public consumption and media production. The program goals of the *Media-Smart Youth* curriculum are (1) to help middle school students become aware of and think critically about how media can affect their nutrition and physical activity choices; (2) to help young people build the skills to make good decisions about being physically active and eating nutritiously in daily life; and (3) to encourage young people to establish healthy habits that will last into adulthood.[22] The media teachers instructed the students in photographic techniques and the proper use and care of the digital and video cameras.

The middle school students were responsible for the creation of health infomercials, from storyboard to video editing. All digital and video cameras, camera accessories, supplies, and funds for props were supplied by the study, as were classroom nutrition and physical activity equipment. The salary of the media specialist was part of the grant funding support, and the Migrant Education Program provided the science teacher, physical activity teacher, and classroom space. Anthropometric measures, muscle strength and flexibility, and knowledge and attitudes were assessed at the beginning of the Migrant Education Program (baseline pre-intervention) and at its conclusion (exit post-intervention). Outcome variables were body mass index (BMI), BMI percentile, categories of BMI percentiles, muscle strength, muscle flexibility, nutrition and physical activity knowledge, and behaviors and attitudes toward healthy choices. Student pre- and post-intervention assessments used evaluation materials from We Can! that have established reliability. Muscle strength was measured by the number of "student push-ups that are a barometer of fitness and muscle strength and test the whole body by engaging muscle groups in the arms, chest, abdomen, hips and legs."[23] Muscle flexibility was assessed by the sit-and-reach test, the most widely used research measure of flexibility and a primary component of most physical fitness tests.[23]

Outcomes

In the summer of 2011, 64 middle school students in grades 6–8 were enrolled in the program (girls, n = 31; boys, n = 33; J. F. Kilanowski, unpublished data). All

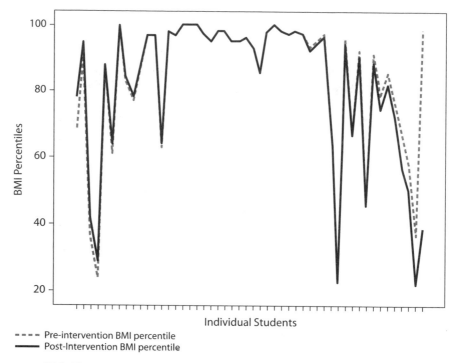

FIGURE 13.1. Changes in students' body mass index (BMI) percentiles from pre- to post-intervention in the Migrant Middle School Media Nutrition Project.

students were children of qualifying migrant workers. Migrant workers are commonly defined as persons who travel at least 75 miles during a 12-month period to obtain a farm job.[24] The majority of families identified their permanent residence as in Florida or Texas. Ninety-six percent of the students self-reported Hispanic/Latino ethnicity, 3% other, and 1% White. Students were enrolled in the 34-day program for an average of 28.32 days (SD = 6.801; range = 14–34 days) and attended classes for an average of 24.35 days (SD = 8.921; range = 5–34 days). For the 64 students enrolled in the Migrant Education Program, the average attendance, and therefore the attendance at the intervention, was 86%. Forty-one percent of the students attended 30 days or more. Eight students attended only 10 or fewer classes, and this was most likely due to age-eligible students working in the fields to harvest blueberries.

Categories of participants' BMI percentiles (underweight, normal weight, overweight, or obese) at baseline showed that 20% were overweight and 45% were obese. No child was underweight. A comparison of the students' first and second BMI percentile categories shows a positive change toward a healthy weight category. Students also showed a healthy trend toward decreasing their BMI percentiles (fig. 13.1).

Table 13.1. Positive student outcomes post-intervention in the Migrant Middle School
Media Nutrition Project

Student assessment	Outcomes
Anthropometric measurements	Changes in body mass index percentile categories toward a healthier category
We Can! CATCH Kids Club	Healthy behaviors to reduce fat in diet
	Healthy behaviors to eat more fruits and vegetables
	Healthy behaviors to read food labels
	Increased sense of self-efficacy regarding diet
	Increased food attitudes to reduce fat in diet
	Attitude to increase physical activity
	Decreased student television watching—weekday
We Can! Media-Smart Youth	Increased knowledge in physical activity needs
	Increased nutrition knowledge
	Intent to eat fewer sugar snacks
	Attitude to increase physical activity to at least one hour next month
Physical activity	Increase in push-ups
Classroom teachers' assessment	Increase in nutrition knowledge

Source: Information on We Can! CATCH Kids Club and Media-Smart Youth from National Heart Lung
and Blood Institute (2012).[22]

Students who changed their behaviors and included more fiber in their diets and
students who learned more about nutrition demonstrated greater healthy changes in
BMI percentiles. Students who had a higher BMI appeared to be more receptive to
the lessons learned in the intervention. At the close of the Migrant Education Program and completion of the video projects, improvements were seen in outcomes for
15 student assessments (table 13.1). Girls and boys showed improvement in different
assessments at post-intervention.

At the conclusion of the seven weeks, five student infomercials were completed;
one was in Spanish. The themes of the infomercials were: "Diabetes and Diabetes
Prevention"; "The New My Plate"; "El Plato de Buen Comer (Spanish video with students discussing MiPiramede [My Pyramid] and the new Plato de Buen Comer [My
Plate]); "Exercise for 60 Minutes Every Day"; and "Smart Consumers" (a video centered on healthy eating, discussing antioxidants and other nutrition concepts). Students were actively engaged in the activity of health promotion videography, and
students, faculty, and staff enjoyed the showcase of the videos. Post-intervention,
the Migrant Education Program distributed more than 100 copies of the digital
video discs to involved students and teachers and to local, regional, and national
Latino leaders in education, legislation, and health. Although causation cannot be
attributed for the improvements in students' knowledge and their positive changes
toward healthy attitudes and behaviors, the use of a multimedia project to create an

Table 13.2. Challenges and lessons learned from conduct of the pilot study

Component	Challenge	Lesson learned
Personnel	When students were actively engaged in the uploading and editing of videos, they needed direction by the media teacher.	Engage an additional classroom teacher or aide to assist in classroom dynamics and the needs of students.
Constraints of budget	One student digital camera was dropped, and a second was lost on a field trip.	Consider purchase of equipment protection plans and incorporate the cost into future budgets.
Equipment	Battery life was not sufficient for use of cameras.	Purchase additional batteries.
	Voice dialogues in some videos were difficult to hear.	Incorporate lapel microphones in the next budget.
Communication	Distance of researcher's location to study site	Along with a minimum of weekly telephone and email exchanges, three 3-day site visits were made during the 7 weeks for assessing intervention fidelity. This facilitated communication with the team and encouraged the maintenance of team dialogues.
Participants	Varied attendance of some migrant students due to the ability to pick crops and earn money	Support all students in the program and incorporate those with varied attendance into tasks that make them feel part of the team but will not affect timely completion of the video projects.

integrated learning experience demonstrated the active learning of nutrition and physical activity classroom objectives.

Conclusions

The summer school environment was effective for the delivery of health promotion lessons to a vulnerable student population, despite the program's short duration. Challenges and lessons learned, as shown in table 13.2, will provide direction for improvements in the conduct of the next study incorporating videography. Future research is planned to evaluate the modality of this health promotion delivery in a larger sample size and with a diverse ethnic and racial population of students. In addition, the research design of future projects needs to include an assessment of whether the knowledge and healthy attitudes and behaviors acquired are maintained over time. This project will serve as a prototype for middle school health interventions and can provide guidance for health promotion interventions for Latino and other immigrant student populations.

LESSONS LEARNED
See table 13.2.

Acknowledgments

The Sigma Theta Tau International, the Honor Society of Nursing Small Grants, provided funding support for this research project. The principal investigator acknowledges Maureen Anway and Crystal Elissetche (intervention teachers) and the administration, staff, students, and families of the study's summer Migrant Education Program.

References

1. U.S. Census Bureau. Table 7.2. Nativity by sex and Hispanic origin, type. Washington, DC: U.S. Census Bureau, Ethnicity and Ancestry Statistics Branch, Population Division, 2009. Available at: http://www.census.gov/population/socdemo/hispanic/cps2006/2006_tab7.2.xls.
2. U.S. Department of State's Bureau of International Information Programs. U.S. minorities will be the majority by 2042, Census Bureau says. Washington, DC: U.S. Department of State's Bureau of International Information Programs, 2008. Available at: http://www.america.gov/st/diversityenglish/2008/August/20080815140005xlrennef0.1078106.html?CP.rss=true.
3. Migrant Health Promotion. Farmworkers in the United States. Ypsilanti, MI: Migrant Health Promotion, 2012. Available at: http://www.migranthealth.org/index.php?option=com_content&view=article&id=38&Itemid=30.
4. National Center for Farmworker Health. Demographics. Buda, TX: National Center for Farmworker Health, 2002. Available at: http://www.ncfh.org/?pid=79.
5. U.S. Department of Labor, Employment and Training Administration. National Agricultural Workers Survey executive summary. Washington, DC: U.S. Department of Labor, Employment and Training Administration, 2010. Available at: http://www.doleta.gov/agworker/report9/summary.cfm.
6. Kandula NR, Kersey M, Lurie N. Assuring the health of immigrants: what the leading health indicators tell us. Annu Rev Public Health. 2004;25:357–76.
7. Rubalcave LN, Teruel GM, Thomas D, et al. The healthy migrant effect: new findings from the Mexican Family Life Survey. Am J Public Health. 2008 Jan;98(1):78–84.
8. National Center for Farmworker Health. Maternal and child health sheet. Buda, TX: National Center for Farmworker Health, 2009. Available at: http://www.ncfh.org/docs/fs-MATERNAL%20FACT%20SHEET.pdf.
9. U.S. Department of Education. Migrant education—basic state formula grants. Washington, DC: U.S. Department of Education, 2009. Available at: http://www2.ed.gov/programs/mep/index.html.
10. U.S. Department of Education. Building on results: a blueprint for strengthening the No Child Left Behind Act. Washington, DC: U.S. Department of Education, 2007. Available at: http://www2.ed.gov/policy/elsec/leg/nclb/buildingonresults.pdf.
11. U.S. Department of Agriculture. Schools / child nutrition USDA food programs. Washington, DC: U.S. Department of Agriculture, Food and Nutrition Service, 2012. Available at: http://www.fns.usda.gov/fdd/programs/schcnp.
12. Achterberg C, Miller C. Is one theory better than another in nutrition education? A viewpoint: more is better. J Nutr Educ Behav. 2004 Jan–Feb;36(1):40–2.

13. Leininger M, McFarland M. Transcultural nursing: concepts, theories, and practices. New York, NY: McGraw-Hill Professional, 2002.

14. Piaget J. The origins of intelligence in children. New York, NY: W.W. Norton & Company, 1963.

15. Erikson EH. Childhood and society. New York, NY: W.W. Norton & Company, 1963.

16. Sullivan HS. The interpersonal theory of psychiatry. New York, NY: W.W. Norton & Company, 1953.

17. Bransford J, Brown A, Cocking R, eds. How people learn: brain, mind, experience, and school. Washington, DC: National Academy Press, 1999.

18. Krajcik JS, Czernaik CM, Berger C. Teaching children science: a project-based approach. New York, NY: McGraw-Hill College, 1998.

19. Council on Sports Medicine and Fitness, Council on School Health. Active healthy living: prevention of childhood obesity through increased physical activity. Pediatrics. 2006 May;117(5):1834–42.

20. National Association of Pediatric Nurse Practitioners (NAPNAP). Healthy Eating and Activity Together (HEAT): identifying and preventing overweight in childhood clinical practice guideline. Cherry Hill, NJ: NAPNAP, 2010.

21. U.S. Department of Agriculture. ChooseMyPlate.gov. Washington, DC: U.S. Department of Agriculture, 2012. Available at:www.choosemyplate.gov.

22. National Heart Lung and Blood Institute. We Can! background. Bethesda, MD: National Heart Lung and Blood Institute, National Institute of Diabetes and Digestive and Kidney Diseases, the Eunice Kennedy Shriver National Institute of Child Health and Human Development, and the National Cancer Institute, 2012. Available at: http://www.nhlbi.nih.gov /health/public/heart/obesity/wecan/about-wecan/background.htm.

23. YMCA of the USA. YMCA fitness assessment. In: YMCA fitness testing & assessment manual. Champaign, IL: Human Kinetics, 2000. Available at: http://www.exrx.net/Testing /YMCATesting.html.

24. Employment and Training Administration. The National Agricultural Workers Survey. Washington, DC: U.S. Department of Labor, 2010. Available at: http://www.doleta.gov /agworker/report9/chapter1.cfm.

CHAPTER 14

Creating Healthy Environments in Los Angeles through Joint Use of School Facilities

Martha V. Cortes, MA

The built environment—including the availability and accessibility of parks, retailers of healthy food, and adequate transportation systems—can directly affect well-being.[1] In Los Angeles, certain communities are disproportionately affected by poor community design that does not support healthy and active lifestyles. Research has found that areas with high poverty rates have less access to and availability of recreational facilities than more affluent areas, directly affecting the levels of physical activity among members of these communities.[1-3] A study conducted by the Los Angeles County Department of Public Health found a strong correlation between race, economic hardship, and higher rates of childhood and adult obesity.[4] Given the environmental realities of low-income communities of color, urging residents to make lifestyle changes without simultaneously removing larger systemic barriers to health may result in unsuccessful interventions. To improve the effectiveness of health promotion and disease prevention among high-need populations, it is critical to develop and implement policies and programs that address underlying environmental factors, are culturally relevant, and include a broad base of stakeholders.* In Los Angeles, the Alliance for a Better Community (ABC), a policy advocacy organization, promotes joint use as a strategy to address pressing health concerns in low-income communities, providing residents with the tools they need to advocate for improved opportunities to live healthier, more active lives.†

Martha V. Cortes is affiliated with the Alliance for a Better Community, in Los Angeles.

* Several other chapters also work with the observation that inequities in the built environment—including inequities in neighborhood safety—have a strong bearing on the distribution of obesity and overweight. See, for example, chapters 2, 6–8, 10, 12, 13, 18, 22, 29, and 31 (especially chapter 8).

† The Alliance for a Better Community is a policy and advocacy organization dedicated to promoting equity for Latinos in Los Angeles in health, education, economic development, and civic engagement. The Los Angeles Unified School District defines joint use as a legally binding agreement entered by and between the district and a third party for the utilization of school facilities. In this chapter, *joint use* refers to the more commonly used definition that describes the use of school facilities by the community outside school hours.

Joint Use of School Facilities as a Healthy Solution

Los Angeles has devoted limited city land to parks and open spaces (approximately 10%), with distribution favoring certain areas within the city.[5] Although the standard provision in Los Angeles is four total acres of neighborhood and community parkland per 1,000 residents,[6] inner-city state assembly districts, predominantly comprising Latino communities, have less than one acre of parkland per 1,000 residents.[7] Research and practice recognize joint use of public facilities—specifically, school sites—as a viable and effective strategy for high-density urban communities that are working to prevent chronic diseases resulting from inactivity.[8] Particularly where parkland is expensive and time for park development is long, increasing access to safe, open spaces through joint-use partnerships can increase participation in physical activity and help rectify inequities.

Schools as Health Hubs

Due to insufficient park space in Los Angeles, public spaces such as schools become a viable alternative for recreation and access points for health resources and programs. As one of the largest landowners in the city of Los Angeles, the Los Angeles Unified School District (LAUSD) operates more than 700 schools and serves more than 660,000 students.[9] Because many of these schools are neighborhood-based, they have the potential to serve as centers for communities. While some communities are able to leverage these public resources, there are many school facilities that remain closed to residents after school hours, on weekends, and during the summer months. In 2010, ABC designed the J.U.G.A.R. (Joint Use Generating Activity and Recreation) initiative (*jugar* is the Spanish word for "to play") in response to a community health assessment conducted in Boyle Heights and East Los Angeles to identify critical health needs and solutions. Through community input, it had become evident that both of these communities lacked adequate safe and accessible spaces for residents to engage in physical activity. To address this issue, J.U.G.A.R. sought to streamline LAUSD's joint-use policies and procedures to enhance community partnerships for increased opportunities for physical activity at school sites, while simultaneously developing pilot projects to inform model practices for district-wide replication.

Policy and Systems Change

Existing state and local joint-use policies in California guide districts on the proper protocol for accessing school facilities by third parties such as government agencies, service providers, and community members. These procedures, developed to facilitate partnerships for shared access to school properties, have a level of complexity that has often impeded the establishment of joint-use agreements. To implement a district-wide systems change in LAUSD, ABC convened a broad-based coalition of district officials, county agencies, state and local organizations, service providers, and residents to assess the district's existing joint-use policies and procedures to develop recommendations for improving access to school facilities. Some of the recommendations identified by the coalition included providing guidance to school-site leadership on proper third-party access protocol; developing a centralized source that all potential partners and school-site administration could access for more information on joint use; and issuing updated information district-wide, effectively and efficiently. These recommendations led to the following district-wide tools:

1. 2011 *Principal's Handbook: A Guide for Principals to Successfully Operate a School*, a tool used by principals to guide school-site decisions, updated to include information for principals on how to establish joint-use partnerships.
2. *Healthy Spaces, Healthy People*, a webpage housed within the Facilities Division of LAUSD, created to provide the public with examples of model joint-use partnerships and practices and centralized information on establishing a joint-use agreement.
3. *Creating Healthy and Safe Environments through Shared Use*, a one-page bilingual (Spanish and English) document stating the importance of access to safe, open spaces for improving health through physical activity. The document also includes model advocacy practices.
4. *Procedures for Use of School Facilities*, an administrative policy tool outlining state and local joint-use policies and procedures to be routed by the central office to all district administrators potentially in the upcoming year.

These multiple tools were created to ensure that all stakeholders—from community members to principals to service providers—are provided with clear information on the roles and responsibilities of all individuals in the development of joint-use partnerships.

J.U.G.A.R. Pilot Project: Mendez Learning Center in Boyle Heights

An important component of the J.U.G.A.R. initiative was using these tools at the school-site level. ABC developed school-based pilot projects to ensure that the policy recommendations described above would address the opportunities and challenges faced during implementation by school personnel and service providers. J.U.G.A.R. targets schools in two high-need Latino communities in central Los Angeles; one of those is Boyle Heights.*

Boyle Heights is a high-density area east of downtown Los Angeles in which 62% of households are low-income.[10] Like many low-income communities of color, Boyle Heights suffers from high rates of obesity and overweight (35% and 36%, respectively).[10] Boyle Heights has about 1.46 acres of open space available per 1,000 residents, much less than the standard provision of 4 acres.[11] Though lacking access to

---

* Though the J.U.G.A.R. initiative is being piloted in four schools in two communities (Pico Union and Boyle Heights), this chapter focuses on the Mendez Learning Center to provide a deeper analysis of the project.

park spaces, Boyle Heights is home to 18 LAUSD schools that can serve as access points for health services and resources for the community.

A rigorous assessment of existing school-based partnerships, available facilities, school capacity, and community need was conducted in Boyle Heights to identify which schools would be the best fit for a pilot project. Felicitas and Gonzalo Mendez Learning Center (Mendez) was chosen for its unique role within the community. Mendez is a high school located in Pueblo del Sol, a redevelopment of the Aliso Village Housing Project, which was once the second largest low-income housing project in Southern California. Mendez opened its doors in 2009 as the first new high school to be built in Boyle Heights in more than 80 years.

In the preliminary analysis of existing joint-use partnerships within LAUSD, ABC found that partnerships that originate at the district level, without community input, often do not address the needs and interests of the community. For the J.U.G.A.R. initiative, a different approach is used. To develop the appropriate joint-use partnership, ABC has worked closely with school leadership, community service providers, and residents to direct the types of programs to be implemented on the Mendez school campus.

Through these efforts, ABC is partnering with Urban Strategies, a national nonprofit organization overseeing the Pueblo del Sol Community Service Center (the Center), which is located next door to Mendez. Together, the two organizations assessed the school's capacity to maximize resources to best serve the community. As a new school, Mendez seeks to enhance its efforts to engage parents and the community to create a more inclusive culture for its students and families. The school's goal to serve families better is aligned with Urban Strategies' need to provide them with programs and services. Urban Strategies previously offered women in the community Zumba classes at the Center in the afternoon, to provide them with time and space to take care of themselves.* Classes were held in the Center's carpeted multipurpose room, where chairs and tables had to be rearranged before and after every class. Due to its popularity the class was almost always at capacity, with 30 participants; a proper workout room was needed. Through the J.U.G.A.R. initiative, ABC and Urban Strategies worked with Mendez leadership to move the classes from the Center's cramped multipurpose room to the school's spacious dance room, which had been underutilized after school. Now located in the dance room, the classes' capacity has doubled. Since the move, more than 150 participants have attended the pilot Zumba class at Mendez.

In conversations with the convened coalition, many agreed that maintenance and operations were the two main challenges faced at the site. Site administrators reported that with the increase in users, schools required additional cleaning and upkeep. To provide oversight for the pilot, ABC implemented a committee comprising Urban Strategies and Mendez staff and leadership that meets quarterly to discuss the successes and challenges of the program. During the pilot phase, ABC has convened

---

* Zumba is a high-intensity aerobic activity inspired by Latin dance. Classes at Mendez are held during after-school hours, led by a certified instructor, and provide 60 minutes of exercise.

and facilitated these meetings. In between quarterly meetings, ABC encourages leadership to communicate frequently to address problems as they arise.

By engaging a broad base of community stakeholders and decision makers to select the types of joint-use partnerships to be implemented in their local school, J.U.G.A.R. has increased the types of relevant activities offered to families at Mendez. A preliminary evaluation of the impact of J.U.G.A.R. on physical activity has been conducted at Mendez, and continued evaluation will address the long-term impact of J.U.G.A.R. on community health.

Sustainability and Scalability

Development of a successful joint-use partnership requires collaboration among stakeholders. Through the pilot projects, ABC has identified the critical role each stakeholder plays in the execution of the program at the school site. Model practices have been developed for all stages of the partnership—development, implementation, and sustainability—to provide guidance to stakeholders for replication district-wide. (The model practices are listed under "Lessons Learned," below.) These model practices were published both in print and online and were disseminated widely across various networks. Community presentations were also held. Further analysis must be conducted to identify the impact of these tools on joint-use partnerships. Nonetheless, tools such as the *Healthy Spaces, Healthy People* webpage currently provide unprecedented streamlined access to information.

In developing these model practices and efforts at the school-site level, it was critical to simultaneously develop a community engagement strategy to ensure sustainability of the joint-use partnerships. ABC employed a community health training strategy to provide residents with the skills to transform the places in which they live. To introduce the J.U.G.A.R. initiative, ABC engaged more than 80 residents throughout the course of a year and invited them to participate in a health taskforce. This taskforce addresses the pressing health concerns identified by the community health assessment and develops solutions through school-based partnerships. Of these residents, a core group of 10–15 community members are participating in ongoing health trainings at Mendez to build awareness, increase capacity, and develop leadership to improve health outcomes in their home and community.

It is through the leadership of the community that an initiative such as J.U.G.A.R. can be successful. Nonetheless, there are specific challenges to this strategy. One of them is difficulty in recruiting and retaining community members for long-term engagement strategies such as trainings. In the communities that ABC serves, many of the residents have tremendous responsibilities, resulting in limited time to participate in additional activities. To overcome this particular challenge, ABC has met regularly with residents to build relationships and to align the trainings to their interests and needs. ABC is committed to evaluating this initiative in the next couple of years to assess its impact on leadership development. In the upcoming year, ABC will continue to support the work by expanding the school-based pilots and health trainings in Boyle Heights.

Although the J.U.G.A.R. initiative has identified the critical need for policies and programs to address the underlying environmental inequity—lack of access to safe places to be physically active—the engagement of the people most affected is vital to sustaining these changes. Community residents have proven resilient when faced with staggering public health concerns and remain the key to creating healthy communities. The J.U.G.A.R. initiative utilizes joint use as a strategic grassroots strategy for increasing activity opportunities in a city grappling with rising health concerns and issues of equity and access. Collaboration among residents and stakeholders in this initiative has resulted in policies and programs that have benefited all parties involved. School districts will always be vital partners in the development of active environments. It is critical that stakeholders come together to address common concerns and develop strategies such as these to create healthy communities.

LESSONS LEARNED

Model practices for school staff include:

- Collaborate with students, parents, and community organizations to identify their needs and interests.
- Engage potential program operators to identify opportunities for joint-use collaboration.
- Develop a strategic plan for the school that outlines the roles and responsibilities of school staff, partners, and the community.
- Convene school staff, program operators, and participating community members quarterly to discuss successes and challenges, and provide updates on how best to continue the partnership.

Model practices for program operators include:

- Engage the school principal, parents, and students to assess community needs and interests.
- Develop a strategy for successful development, implementation, and sustainability of the program.
- Reach out to the community to garner support for new partnerships and to promote activities.
- Communicate often across stakeholder groups to ensure a successful partnership.

Model practices for community residents include:

- Partner with other community members, parents, and students to identify the activities that are wanted on campus.
- Engage with the principal, after-school providers, and parents' center to identify organizations willing to provide after-school activities in partnership with the school.
- Support the identified community partner organization through the development process.

- Advocate for changes in the community to help improve the availability and accessibility of recreation space.

Acknowledgments

This work was made possible by funding from the United States Department of Health and Human Services through the Los Angeles County Department of Public Health.

References

1. Kerr J. Designing for active living among adults. San Diego, CA: San Diego State University, Active Living Research, 2008. Available at: https://folio.iupui.edu/bitstream/handle/10244 /621/Active_Adults.pdf.
2. Gordon-Larsen P, Nelson MC, Page P, et al. Inequality in the built environment underlies key health disparities in physical activity and obesity. Pediatrics. 2006 Feb 1;117(2):417–24.
3. Farley TA, Meriwether RA, Baker ET, et al. Safe places to promote physical activity in inner-city children: results from a pilot study of an environmental intervention. Am J Public Health. 2007 Sep;97(9):1625–31.
4. County of Los Angeles, Department of Health Services Public Health. LA health: obesity on the rise. Los Angeles, CA: Department of Health Services, 2003. Available at: lapublichealth .org/ha/reports/habriefs/lahealth073003_obes.pdf.
5. Harnik, P. Inside city parks. Washington, DC: Urban Land Institute, 2000.
6. City of Los Angeles, Department of City Planning. Mangrove estates site mixed use development environmental impact report. Los Angeles, CA: City of Los Angeles, Department of City Planning, 2010. Available at: http://cityplanning.lacity.org/EIR/MangroveEstates/FEIR /FEIR%20TOC.htm.
7. Garcia R, Strongin SH, Brakke A. Healthy parks, schools and communities: green access and equity for Los Angeles county 2011. Los Angeles, CA: City Project, 2011. Available at: http://www.mapsportal.org/thecityproject/socalmap/images/LosAngelesENGLISH.pdf.
8. Cooper T, Vincent JM. Joint use school partnerships in California: strategies to enhance schools and communities. Berkeley, CA: Centers for Cities and Schools and Public Health Law and Policy, 2008. Available at: http://citiesandschools.berkeley.edu/reports/CC&S_PHLP _2008_joint_use_with_appendices.pdf.
9. Los Angeles Unified School District. Fingertip facts 2011–2012. Los Angeles, CA: Los Angeles Unified School District, 2011. Available at: http://notebook.lausd.net/portal/page?_ pageid=33,48254&_dad=ptl&_schema=ptl_ep.
10. UCLA Center for Health Policy Research and the California Endowment. Building healthy communities: Boyle Heights health profile. Los Angeles, CA: UCLA Center for Health Policy Research and the California Endowment, 2011. Available at: mycalconnect.org/boyleheights /download.aspx?id=23680.
11. UCLA Center for Health Policy Research, CDC REACH CORE. Turning data into action: focused health profile of Boyle Heights, CA. Los Angeles, CA: UCLA Center for Health Policy Research / CDC REACH CORE, 2012. Available at: www.healthpolicy.ucla.edu/uploads /CDC_REACH_CORE_Boyle_Heights_Profile_2011.07.17.pdf.

CHAPTER 15

The Idaho Partnership for Hispanic Health

Enabling Healthy Eating and Active Living in Rural Idaho

Rachel Schwartz, MSW, MPH, and Linda Powell, MS, CPT

Hispanics are the fastest growing ethnic group in Idaho, and health disparities between Hispanics and non-Hispanics are prevalent.[1,2] The Idaho Partnership for Hispanic Health (IPHH) (www.idphh.org) is a community-based participatory research (CBPR) project formed in 2005 to address these disparities. The mission of IPHH is to identify the health issues of greatest concern to Idaho's Hispanic population and implement study interventions to improve individual and community health. The CBPR approach involves the local Hispanic community in planning and conducting the project.

Through funding from the National Institute on Minority Health and Health Disparities (grant no. R24MD001711), IPHH developed a *promotor/promotora*-led community health intervention called Compañeros en Salud. *Promotores/promotoras* are health outreach workers from the target intervention group who are trained to provide education and enhance health care access within their community.[3,4]* This intervention, with the aim of reducing the risks for metabolic syndrome and associated triggers (e.g., obesity and diabetes) by improving nutrition and physical activity, engages volunteer community participants and provides educational workshops, home visits, and activities in nutrition and physical activity.

Weiser and Mountain Home, two rural communities in southwest Idaho, participate in the program. Although Census data state that 26% of Weiser residents are Hispanic, local key informants indicate the number is considerably higher. This is based on first-hand discussions with Weiser Memorial Hospital personnel, the *promo-*

Rachel Schwartz is the Breastfeeding Promotion Program manager at WithinReach and an independent public health evaluation consultant in Seattle. Linda Powell is the principal investigator of Compañeros en Salud and is employed at Mountain States Group, a nonprofit health organization, in Boise, Idaho.

* Chapters 2, 6, 16, and 17 also stress the importance of using *promotores/promotoras* for interventions in Hispanic communities. See chapters 11, 19, 20, and 27 for more on interventions in rural areas.

tores, and other community representatives who have time and again stated the Hispanic population in Weiser is much larger than census estimates.[5] Both towns are resource-limited and home to a Critical Access Hospital. These communities are economically depressed and have a dearth of infrastructure to support healthy living (key informant interviews, IPHH Compañeros en Salud, 2006).

As of spring 2012, more than 350 individuals from 148 families have participated in Compañeros. The majority of participants are Mexican immigrants or first-generation citizens. Most of the men work in the agriculture or service industries, and many of the women are stay-at-home mothers. Ninety-one percent of adult participants have a high school degree or less education, 34% less than sixth grade. At pre-intervention, 89% of participants were at risk for, or already had, metabolic syndrome, which includes a group of risk factors that increase a person's risk for heart disease and other obesity-related sequelae such as diabetes and stroke.[6] A diagnosis of metabolic syndrome is reached when a person presents with three or more of the following elevated metabolic risk factors: waist circumference, triglycerides, HDL cholesterol, blood pressure, and fasting glucose. The entire cohort had an average body mass index (BMI) of 32 kg/m^2, which is obese by national standards. Many of the youths were overweight.

The Compañeros en Salud Program
Oversight

Active, continuous involvement by the Community Advisory Board (CAB) has made this intervention effort successful. The CAB provides guidance to IPHH to ensure the program's work is culturally relevant and is carried out in partnership with the southern Idaho Hispanic community. The CAB reviews materials and votes on changes to the intervention model. Members of the CAB also serve as IPHH advocates at the local and regional level. The core team of the IPHH strategically sought membership on the CAB from diverse sectors. The board primarily includes Hispanic individuals representing eight counties. Some are long-time residents and others migrated more recently. Occupational sectors represented include health care, agriculture, social work, labor, the unemployed, the YMCA, and the media, among others. People also participate in their roles as parents, senior citizens, educators, and public health nurses, among others.

The IPHH's core team provides oversight and project management and helps facilitate the CAB's work through leadership, data analysis, and evaluation. The team consists of the four *promotores* and representatives from Mountain States Group, a nonprofit public health organization, from the Idaho Commission for Hispanic Affairs, and from the Marshfield Clinic Research Foundation.

History
Prior to implementation of the program, IPHH conducted an intensive community needs assessment, including 519 individual interviews, 2 focus groups, and 40 key

informant interviews with southwest Idaho Hispanic residents. Respondents identified several barriers to accessing health care services and adopting healthy lifestyle changes, including poverty, language limitations, racism, legal status, and divergence between indigenous and biomedical belief systems (unpublished IPHH report on Hispanic Health Disparities in SW Idaho).[7]

These community-identified barriers informed the CAB's decision-making process. The CAB was charged with identifying a single health condition, as required by the National Institutes of Health proposal. However, the data highlighted numerous health concerns for the Hispanic community, including obesity, access to care, diabetes, heart disease, and lack of physical activity. The CAB struggled to select one health condition, especially as several of these concerns were closely interrelated. The core team proposed *metabolic syndrome* as a viable choice.[8] Reducing the risks for metabolic syndrome would also reduce the risk of diabetes and heart disease, and metabolic syndrome encompasses obesity and physical activity issues.

Addressing a community-identified need helped bring credibility to IPHH and the work of the *promotores*. There is a long history in public health research of researchers entering communities to gather information and not returning to make that work of benefit to the participants, or even sharing data outcomes. IPHH has been very careful to be accountable to the communities involved and works to bring past participants together even years after the original intervention.

To settle on a model to reduce metabolic syndrome, the core team gathered information on a variety of interventions and developed a proposal for the CAB's consideration. The proposal was based on a successful *promotora* project along the Arizona-Mexico border to reduce diabetes. Given the success of the *promotora* model in addressing diverse issues in many Hispanic communities,[8,9] this model was the clear choice.

Thirty-five interviews were conducted in the first year of the intervention to gather information about participants' explanatory models around disease. These interviews incorporated questions about families' shared belief systems and traditional, culturally bound Mesoamerican health syndromes, such as *susto, mal de ojo,* and *coraje*,[9] to learn whether and how participants viewed the interaction of these conditions with allopathic conditions such as diabetes and stress. The main themes that emerged were incorporated into the *promotora* curriculum as an effort to blend this information with the biomedical model. Evaluating the usefulness and acceptability of the process of family belief mapping[9] and the blending of the explanatory and biomedical models of disease prevention education[9] was a research aim.

Structure

The CAB was adamant that IPHH efforts be family-centered, and the core team believes this approach was central to the successful outcomes. With a family-centered focus, *promotores/promotoras* dually focus on youth obesity prevention and adult obesity reduction. Compañeros en Salud has a participant age range of 12–84 years. IPHH partnered with 4H organizations to craft activities related to nutrition and

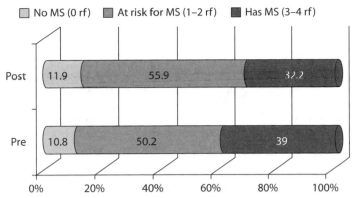

Post	11.9	55.9	32.2
Pre	10.8	50.2	39

0%   20%   40%   60%   80%   100%

FIGURE 15.1. Incidence of metabolic syndrome (MS), by number of risk factors (rf), pre- and post-intervention, in the Idaho Partnership for Hispanic Health's Compañeros en Salud program.

physical activity for children ages 6–11. Childcare is provided for children under 6 to facilitate parents' full participation.

The intervention consists of an eight-week series of group classes taught by extensively trained *promotores* at IPHH program offices. Three cohorts, each with 10 families, attended the series each year in each town. Weekly sessions included a combination of lecture presentations and conversation on healthy living and disease prevention topics. Group physical activity was also coordinated.

A substantial evaluation of the intervention was conducted. Pre- and post-intervention and annual follow-up data were gathered to assess change over time for several physiological indicators, including BMI, blood pressure, and cholesterol, glucose, and HbA1C levels, and for nutritional and physical activity behaviors. Strong partnerships with the local hospitals made this testing possible. Qualitative behavior surveys were also conducted, and structural change and social impact were assessed. In addition to significant physiological and behavioral outcomes such as reduction in the incidence of metabolic syndrome (see fig. 15.1), this program has demonstrated a long-term impact on social capital and cohesion. On average, about 65% of participants return for annual follow-up testing.

Program Outcomes and Evolution
At the time of writing, Compañeros is in its fifth and final intervention year. Throughout its lifespan, many lessons have been learned (see "Lessons Learned," below), and with an eye toward continual improvement, periodic modifications have been made.

Analysis of the results from the first two years shows a clear trend. Generally, participants had excellent outcomes from pre- to post-intervention, but they struggled to sustain those outcomes one and two years later. To improve long-term outcomes, the CAB voted to hire a fitness *promotor/promotora* to work with past participants to establish personal fitness and nutrition goals and to organize community activities.

While this position lasted just a year, its impact remains. Walking groups and Zumba classes are very popular. These gatherings are free for former participants and are coordinated by IPHH.

Early in the project, IPHH staff also took over the management of a local program that provides vouchers to low-income residents to facilitate access to health care. The Washington-Adams County Health Action Team program provides $25–$50 vouchers to low-income uninsured residents so they can access community clinicians and basic lab services. This program does not require applicants to show social security numbers or residence documentation; thus, it has been able to increase health care access and utilization for undocumented community members and has helped build credibility between the community and program staff.

Community Change and Dynamics

It was clear from the start that Weiser's social dynamics and local politics were going to be a challenge for making effective changes at the community level. The project had to confront long-standing issues in Weiser concerning immigration. The core team and CAB decided to form an integrated local council to provide an avenue for non-Hispanic White and Hispanic communities to interact. Over time, the Hispanic council members became discouraged, as it became apparent that their needs were not being considered. There is significant mistrust between the two cultures in this small town. As noted previously, local key informants consistently assert that the Hispanic population in Weiser exceeds the 26% of the total as reported in U.S. Census data. Undocumented individuals live in fear of deportation and avoid interaction with the mainstream, non-Hispanic White population, which can be discriminatory. Despite these challenges, IPHH has maintained a positive relationship with the city and local businesses by actively participating in the chamber of commerce and in meetings with the mayor.

The most important part of a successful *promotor/promotora* intervention is, indeed, the *promotores* themselves. Without the dedicated *promotores*, Compañeros en Salud's work and the long-term relationships sustained in Weiser and Mountain Home would not be possible. To facilitate staff retention and appreciation, *promotores* have been provided with opportunities for continuing education and professional development, such as English as a Second Language classes, computer software training (Excel in particular), and nutrition and medical interpretation training. Staff appreciation is accomplished through formal recognition at CAB and annual end-of-year staff meetings. Most staff have been retained over the long term.

We wanted our staff to feel invested in this program as well as empathetic toward participants. To that end, staff have tracked their own personal outcomes and accomplishments related to nutrition, physical activity, and physiological markers. By doing so, staff could serve as better role models for the changes they promote with community members. This also builds accountability within the group and facilitates compassion and respect.

In addition to teaching classes, *promotores* make weekly home visits to follow up on the lessons learned in class. Originally, the core team did not advocate for making home visits. The CAB, however, insisted that these home visits were important. While this added component is costly, it has proved to be very important to this intervention, as noted in *promotores'* journals and home visit evaluations. In the first year of the program, the *promotores* also took participants on group outings to grocery stores to discuss marketing gimmicks like shelf placement and labeling. After receiving feedback from participants that this activity created anxiety because grocery store employees seemed suspicious of a group of Hispanics wandering around, this component was eliminated.

Compañeros en Salud has effected change not only for individuals but also for the larger community. Seen through the lens of the Social Ecological Model,[10] Compañeros has made an impact at the individual, family, community, organizational, and societal levels. In towns that are not well suited to accommodate non-English-speakers, simply providing reliable materials, information, and companionship in Spanish has also been very important to participants. These tangible and intangible benefits have kept people returning, session after session.

Replication and Resource Sharing

The CAB wanted IPHH materials made available to other communities that are confronting similar challenges. Therefore, the Compañeros en Salud *promotor/promotora* curriculum and several training modules are available for download, free of charge, in English and Spanish. (This information and evaluation outcomes are available on the IPHH website, www.idphh.org.) The IPHH has highlighted both the benefits and the constraints of this community-based participatory research intervention. While the challenges to successful CBPR are numerous, this project demonstrates that the short- and long-term individual and community benefits are plentiful as well.

LESSONS LEARNED
- Researcher–*promotor/promotora* accountability to community members strongly affects trust and participants' commitment.
- Program staff must listen to participants' feedback and be willing to modify methods and approach.
- Strong group morale and cohesiveness (social capital) improve participants' health outcomes.

References

1. State of Idaho. Idaho at a glance: Hispanics: an overview. Boise, ID: Idaho Commission on Hispanic Affairs, 2010.
2. State of Idaho. Snapshot of Idaho's Latino community. Boise, ID. Idaho Commission on Hispanic Affairs, 2010.

3. New Mexico Department of Health. Border health. Santa Fe, NM: New Mexico Department of Health, 2010.

4. Migrant Health Promotion. Who are promotores(as)? Ypsilanti, MI: Migrant Health Promotion, 2010.

5. U.S. Census Bureau. 2010 Census data. Washington, DC: U.S. Census Bureau, 2011.

6. National Heart, Lung, and Blood Institute. What is metabolic syndrome? Washington, DC: National Heart, Lung, and Blood Institute, National Institutes of Health, 2012. Available at: http://www.nhlbi.nih.gov/health/health-topics/topics/ms/#.

7. Cristancho S, Garces DM, Peters KE, et al. Listening to rural Hispanic immigrants in the Midwest: a community-based participatory assessment of major barriers to health care access and use. Qual Health Res. 2008 May;18(5):633–46.

8. Cruz ML, Weigensberg MJ, Huang TTK, et al. Metabolic syndrome in overweight Hispanic youth and the role of insulin sensitivity. J Clin Endocrinol Metab. 2004 Jan 1;89(1):108–13.

9. U.S. Department of Health and Human Services. Definition of promotores de salud. Washington, DC: U.S. Department of Health and Human Services, 2010.

10. Kazak AE. Families of chronically ill children: a systems and social-ecological model of adaptation and challenge. J Consult Clin Psychol. 1989 Feb;57(1):25–30.

CHAPTER 16

Alliance for a Healthy Border
Obesity Prevention in Underserved U.S.-Mexico Border Communities

Suad Ghaddar, PhD, Cynthia J. Brown, PhD, and José A. Pagán, PhD

As is stressed throughout this volume, obesity is a major public health problem, imposing substantial costs on individuals, society, and the health care system.[1-6] Among U.S. adults, 68% are either overweight or obese.[7] Individuals who are obese are at a higher risk for developing chronic health conditions and endure cumulative disadvantage in terms of future health.[8,9] Addressing obesity among racial/ethnic minorities is most urgent, especially among Hispanics, who have a 21% greater prevalence of obesity than non-Hispanic Whites.[10] Hispanics are also more likely to suffer from higher rates of obesity-related complications.[11]*

The obesity epidemic is fueled by poor nutritional habits and sedentary lifestyles.[12] Racial/ethnic minority groups and socioeconomically disadvantaged populations are more susceptible to these influences, in part because of environments with poor access to healthy foods and physical activity venues.[13-15] Despite evidence that lifestyle interventions have the potential to promote weight loss,[16,17] few interventions have focused exclusively on low-income Hispanics[18] or integrated the resources of private and public entities. Alliance for a Healthy Border (AHB) is a public-private partnership that aimed to address obesity and its related complications among the largely Hispanic population of the U.S.-Mexico border.

In this chapter we provide an overview of the AHB initiative and its outcomes and identify some lessons learned that will be useful for others in the development of obesity prevention programs serving minority communities.

Suad Ghaddar is interim director of the South Texas Border Health Disparities Center at the University of Texas–Pan American. Cynthia J. Brown is vice provost for graduate studies at the University of Texas–Pan American. José A. Pagán is director of the Center for Health Innovation at the New York Academy of Medicine and an adjunct senior fellow at Leonard Davis Institute of Health Economics at the University of Pennsylvania.

* For reviews of the literature on Hispanic U.S. populations and obesity, see chapters 2, 4, and 6.

Location and Context

The U.S.-Mexico border is home to over seven million people who are predominantly of Hispanic descent. The region is characterized by high poverty rates and low levels of educational attainment.[19] Obesity, diabetes, and heart disease are major health challenges.[20] A 2006 report pointed out that if the 24 border counties were considered a fifty-first state, that state would rank 51st in primary health care professionals per capita, 50th in health care coverage, and 5th in diabetes-related deaths.[21]

For decades, community health centers (CHCs) have provided continuity of care to racial/ethnic minorities, low-income patients, and people without health insurance coverage.[22,23] Over the years, they have been successful at reducing racial/ethnic disparities in health status,[24] perinatal care,[25] and access to health care.[26-28] They provide an ideal platform for community-based programs targeting the adoption of healthier lifestyles to address obesity and its health risks.

Development and Implementation of the Initiative

Alliance for a Healthy Border was a three-year initiative (2006–8) funded by Pfizer Inc. and part of the company's U.S. Philanthropy Programs that aimed to reduce health disparities and expand access to health care for underserved populations. The increased interest in the U.S.-Mexico border region in the past two decades underscores the area's glaring health disparities, which were a driving force for the initiative. The alliance created partnerships between Pfizer and 12 federally qualified CHCs in the four border states of Texas, New Mexico, Arizona, and California. It also included an independent academic research team contracted by Pfizer to guide the development of the initiative and to carry out the evaluation of CHC programs.[29]

The goals of the $4.5 million initiative that funded nutritional and physical activity education programs were (1) to reduce obesity and other modifiable risk factors associated with diabetes and cardiovascular disease, (2) to establish and/or expand existing obesity and chronic disease prevention programs targeting the Hispanic population, and (3) to identify and promote best practices in the prevention of these diseases.

Two principles guided the development and implementation of AHB. First, the initiative was based on the premise that health behaviors can be influenced by culturally sensitive educational programs, which in turn can lead to improved health outcomes (fig. 16.1). Second, the initiative aimed to build on the knowledge and experience of local organizations.

A request for proposals (RFP) was issued to federally qualified CHCs located in U.S.-Mexico border communities. The RFP provided an overview of the program, its goals, and the evaluation component. It also provided information on sample programs that had already been implemented and tested in the border region, such as Su Corazón, Su Vida; Pasos Adelante; and Salud para Su Corazón (see table 16.3, below, for more information on these programs). All 12 centers that submitted a proposal

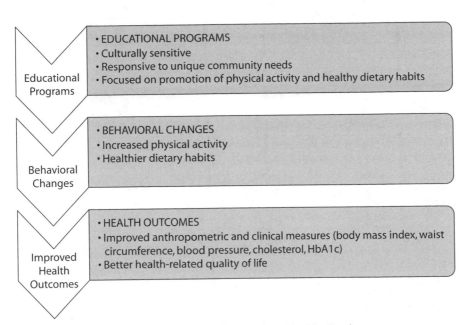

FIGURE 16.1. Conceptual framework for Alliance for a Healthy Border.

Table 16.1. Community health centers participating in Alliance for a Healthy Border

Community health center	County	State
Nuestra Clínica del Valle	Hidalgo	Texas
Gateway Community Health Center	Webb	Texas
United Medical Centers	Maverick	Texas
Centro de Salud Familiar La Fe	El Paso	Texas
La Clínica de Familia	Doña Ana	New Mexico
Ben Archer Health Center	Luna	New Mexico
Mariposa Community Health Center	Santa Cruz	Arizona
El Rio Community Health Center	Pima	Arizona
Clínicas de Salud del Pueblo	Imperial	California
Family Health Centers of San Diego	San Diego	California
La Maestra Community Health Center	San Diego	California
San Ysidro Health Center	San Diego	California

were accepted: four from Texas, two from New Mexico, two from Arizona, and four from California (table 16.1). The centers served communities of primarily Hispanic origin with high rates of poverty, uninsurance, and foreign-born residents (table 16.2) and were located in federally designated Medically Underserved Areas and/or Health Professional Shortage Areas. The centers provided a wide range of primary health care services at reduced fees based on the Federal Poverty Income level guidelines.[29]

Alliance programs were in progress from early 2006 to December 2008. Each program had its own curriculum, duration, and delivery method (table 16.3). In general,

Table 16.2. Selected characteristics of the border counties in the AHB initiative

County/sample	Percent of population				
	Hispanic	Families below poverty level	Uninsured	Foreign-born	Speak language other than English
Hidalgo, TX	89	33	31	29	83
Webb, TX	95	27	40	29	93
Maverick, TX	95	30	31	34	95
El Paso, TX	81	25	33	27	76
Doña Ana, NM	65	21	32	19	54
Luna, NM	60	29	32	19	50
Santa Cruz, AZ	81	18	24	32	81
Pima, AZ	32	10	21	13	28
Imperial, CA	76	19	20	32	69
San Diego, CA	30	8	23	23	35
U.S.	15	10	18	13	20
AHB sample	95	45	59	80	92

Sources: U.S. Census Bureau, Census 2000; 2005–7 American Community Survey; 2006 Small Area Health Insurance Estimates; and Alliance for a Healthy Border (AHB) dataset. Data sources correspond to the time period over which AHB was implemented.

programs either replicated or modified well-established, culturally appropriate programs or were developed entirely in-house. Criteria for participation in the programs varied; some centers focused on existing patients, while others recruited new people through flyers and word of mouth. Program durations ranged from five weeks to six months. The educational setting included group or individual sessions held at the CHC, in participants' homes, or in other community locations. The majority of the programs shared one key characteristic: the use of *promotores de salud* (community health workers), whose responsibilities ranged from recruiting participants to administering surveys and facilitating classes.

Alliance for a Healthy Border also featured an independent evaluation component designed (1) to assess the effectiveness of different programs in changing behaviors and improving health measures, (2) to evaluate the processes employed to deliver the educational interventions, and (3) to identify best practices. The evaluation was carried out by a research team at the University of Texas–Pan American and involved both quantitative and qualitative elements. These included (1) site visits; (2) a pre-post-post study design, involving surveys and clinical and anthropometric measures collected at the beginning and end of each program and at the six-month follow-up; and (3) focus groups of program participants.

The alliance integrated opportunities for networking and capacity building through events hosted by the AHB initiative. These included an initial grantee conference, where details of the evaluation process were provided and inputs, processes, and

Table 16.3. AHB program characteristics by community health center

Community health center and location (municipality, state)	Target population	Recruitment/promotion	Curriculum[a]	Duration	Delivery method
Nuestra Clínica del Valle, Pharr, TX	Diagnosed with diabetes	Existing clinic patients	Medir para Vivir	16 weeks	8 biweekly individual sessions
Gateway CHC, Laredo, TX	Diagnosed with diabetes and CVD; prediabetic; obese	Provider referrals (majority); flyers	Amigos en Salud	12 weeks + 12-week support	Classes + 12-week support (exercise + goal setting + support)
United Medical Centers, Eagle Pass, TX	At risk for diabetes, hypertension, and CVD; obese	Health fairs; flyers; provider referrals; word of mouth	Pasos Adelante	10 weeks	Weekly 2-hour classes
Centro de Salud Familiar La Fe, El Paso, TX	Diagnosed with diabetes	Diabetes collaborative	Salud para su Corazón + pharmacist curriculum	6 months	One-on-one vs. group (patient's choice)
La Clínica de Familia, Las Cruces, NM	Diagnosed with diabetes	Provider referrals (majority); outreach efforts	Su Corazón, Su Vida	2 months	Biweekly home visits
Ben Archer Health Center, Columbus, NM	Diagnosed with or at risk for diabetes; obese	Provider referrals (primary); health fairs / personal contacts (secondary)	Chronic Care Model: "Living with a chronic condition"	3 months	1 group session + phone contact every 2 weeks + periodic cooking class
Mariposa CHC, Nogales, AZ	At risk for diabetes, hypertension, and CVD; obese	Provider referrals (majority); clinic printouts of persons with 3 qualifying criteria	Salud para su Corazón	10 weeks	Classes
El Rio CHC, Tucson, AZ	At risk for diabetes and CVD; obese	Health fairs; flyers to existing patients	Sembrando Nuestro Futuro	5 weeks	Weekly classes
Clínicas de Salud del Pueblo, Calexico, CA	At risk for diabetes and CVD; obese	Health fairs; flyers; word of mouth	Pasos Adelante	9 weeks	Weekly 2-hour classes

(continued)

Table 16.3. (continued)

Community health center and location (municipality, state)	Target population	Recruitment/promotion	Curriculum[a]	Duration	Delivery method
Family Health Centers, San Diego, CA	At risk for diabetes; obese	Health fairs	Curriculum based on participant suggestions	8 weeks	Weekly classes
La Maestra CHC, San Diego, CA	At risk for diabetes, hypertension, and CVD; obese	Health fairs; school visits	Salud para su Corazón	8 weeks	Weekly 2-hour classes
San Ysidro Health Center, San Ysidro, CA	Children (5–12) at risk for diabetes/obese + their parents	Provider referrals	Project Salsita	6 months	Individual interaction: initial discussion then follow-up phone calls

[a] Medir para Vivir, "Measuring to Live," is a center-developed curriculum focused on developing healthy eating habits with the goal of lowering total body weight and glucose levels. The program provided participants with starter kits that facilitated measurements of food portions.

Amigos en Salud, "Friends in Health," is a comprehensive health education program designed to reach out to Hispanics with diabetes and other chronic diseases such as CVD. The program is developed by Pfizer Health Solutions. The curriculum focuses on Hispanic cultural perceptions central to successful diabetes management and uses educational materials at the appropriate literacy level.

Pasos Adelante, "Steps Forward," is a curriculum aimed at preventing diabetes, CVD, and other chronic diseases in Hispanic populations. The curriculum, based on the NHLBI's Su Corazón, Su Vida, consists of a 12-week program, facilitated by community health workers, and includes sessions on diabetes and community advocacy and incorporates walking clubs. (For more details on the program and curriculum, see http://www.borderhealthsi.org/curricula/steps/default_eng.htm.)

Salud Para Su Corazón, "Health for Your Heart," is a CVD prevention program facilitated by community health workers. The program adapted the NHLBI's Su Corazón, Su Vida to include optional diabetes health education and prevention sessions. Community health workers refer participants to health care providers for screening (blood pressure, cholesterol, blood glucose, weight, and waist circumference). The program is delivered in seven two-hour sessions over two to three months. (For details, see http://www.nhlbi.nih.gov/health/prof /heart/latino/salud.htm.)

Su Corazón, Su Vida, "Your Heart, Your Life," is a CVD prevention program developed for Latinos by the NHLBI and sponsored by the Office of Research on Minority Health at the National Institutes of Health. It is a user-friendly program that provides a manual for educators on how to lead group sessions on making simple, practical, and lasting changes to fight heart disease. The program consists of nine sessions ranging from "What You Need to Know about High Blood Pressure" to "Make Heart-Healthy Eating a Family Affair." (The manual is available in English and Spanish at http://www.nhlbi.nih.gov/health/prof/heart/latino/lat_mnl.htm.)

The Chronic Care Model is a conceptual framework incorporating multiple elements (health system, community resources, self-management support, clinical information, etc.) that need to be coordinated to care for individuals with multiple chronic conditions. (See Wagner E. Chronic disease management: what will it take to improve care for chronic illness? Eff Clin Pract. 1998 Aug–Sep;1:2–4.)

Sembrando Nuestro Futuro, "Planting Our Future," is a health education program developed for El Rio CHC by a researcher at Arizona State University. The curriculum also incorporated material from the lifestyle component of the Diabetes Prevention Program (www.bsc.gwu.edu/dpp).

Project Salsita is a prevention program that screens and educates San Ysidro Health Center Pediatric patients between the ages of 5 and 12 years old for obesity, eating and activity behaviors, family history, and lipid and glucose factors. The alliance program added information sessions for parents of youths at risk for obesity.

Abbreviations: CHC, community health center; CVD, cardiovascular disease; NHLBI, National Heart, Lung, and Blood Institute.

outcomes of the programs planned at each center were captured. Two additional AHB conferences, midway through the initiative and at its end, allowed participating CHCs to share challenges faced and lessons learned and to receive evaluation updates. Community health centers were also encouraged to participate in national conferences such as the 2007 U.S.-Mexico Border Health Association Annual Meeting and the 2007 National Promotora Conference.

Discussion
Main Outcomes

More than 4,000 individuals enrolled in the AHB programs. Of these, 2,596 (64%) and 2,134 (53%) were reached for program-end and six-month follow-up data collection, respectively. Participants were primarily Hispanic (95%), uninsured (59%), and foreign-born (80%). Almost half (45%) reported household incomes below the poverty level. Quantitative analyses of dietary and exercise habits, anthropometric measures, and clinical outcomes revealed that lifestyle interventions are effective; AHB programs positively influenced behaviors, which led to improved health outcomes and better health-related quality of life.[29] Most importantly, more than three-quarters of the participants were able to decrease their body mass index and sustain that reduction for six months following program's end (fig. 16.2). Qualitative analysis (focus groups of 226 participants) helped identify successful program components as well as challenges to adopting healthier lifestyles. The analysis revealed that curricula delivered in group settings allowed strong peer support. Strong promotora-participant relationships were also important for motivation and retention.[30]

Strengths, Challenges, and Possibilities for Replication
Alliance for a Healthy Border had several elements that were key to its success. Primarily, the initiative capitalized on existing resources in the border area, using CHCs with track records in serving the health care needs of their communities and with the capability to reach low-income, minority populations. Each center was then given the choice to develop its own educational program, promoting a sense of ownership, personnel commitment, and loyalty. This approach also allowed the programs to reflect community norms and expectations, resulting in curricula and delivery modes that were closely tailored to the culture of their own communities.

On the other hand, the setting of the initiative presented some challenges. These challenges centered around the CHCs' understanding and acceptance of the evaluation process and their limited personnel resources. The initial reaction to the evaluation process was cautious; among those CHCs that were new to evaluation (9 of the 12 centers), there were concerns about their perceived ability to be fully involved in the process. These concerns were alleviated by frequent meetings with the evaluation team, where the objectives and procedures of the evaluation were fully discussed and result updates were shared. Over time, CHC personnel came to value how incorporating evaluation can add credibility to and enhance the sustainability

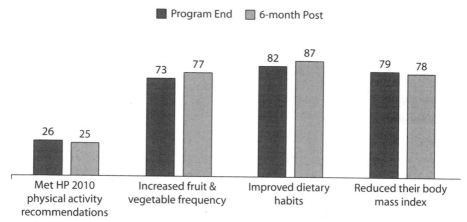

Percent of Participants Who ...

■ Program End   ▉ 6-month Post

Met HP 2010 physical activity recommendations	Increased fruit & vegetable frequency	Improved dietary habits	Reduced their body mass index
26 25	73 77	82 87	79 78

FIGURE 16.2. Main outcomes of the Alliance for a Healthy Border initiative. The Healthy People (HP) 2010 physical activity recommendations call for being moderately active for at least 30 minutes, 5–7 days a week, or vigorously active for at least 20 minutes, 3–7 days a week. Percentages indicate those who met the recommendations after not meeting them at baseline. "Dietary habits" were measured by a 12-item scale that includes statements reflecting the level of engagement in healthy dietary habits related to fat/cholesterol intake and salt/sodium intake and other general habits such as the use of nutrition labels and smaller food portions.

of their programs. Another challenge stemmed from the limited personnel and infrastructure resources that the centers could dedicate to the initiative; the externally funded project added a layer of responsibilities that stretched the workload of center personnel.

Alliance for a Healthy Border provided opportunities for CHCs to work together and share ideas in an underserved region characterized by health disparities and limited resources. Lessons were learned across different levels (summarized under "Lessons Learned," below). At the program level, there were four main commonalities among the programs of the CHCs that were more successful at consistently improving the health behaviors and outcomes of the targeted populations: (1) a clearly defined, structured curriculum; (2) a 9- to 12-week duration; (3) group sessions that enhanced peer support; and (4) active participation of *promotores*.[31] Among the less successful programs, the most common features were staff turnover and the absence of a physical activity component.

At the center level, the organizational context within which border CHCs operate brought attention to the financial pressures facing them. Border CHCs often lack adequate management and staff levels to implement new preventive health programs. Data collection efforts were particularly difficult in CHCs overwhelmed by other, competing needs. Particular attention should thus be focused on providing specific funding in this area, and this is undoubtedly necessary to guarantee program success.

Comparable to the lessons learned from similar public-private partnerships,[32,33] the AHB implementation process highlighted the importance of a clear understanding of the goals of the partnership among the different stakeholders, of constantly aligning these goals with those of individual partners, of maintaining open communication channels, and of recognizing the different organizational cultures within which each partner operates. Careful planning, starting with the assessment of community needs, then integrating an evaluation process, and continuing with constant communication and consultation with all partners, brought attention to and helped address these issues. Regular meetings and site visits clarified expectations, revealed concerns, and provided feedback on the strengths and challenges of program implementation. Collecting data on processes and outcomes at periodic intervals was also important for continuous quality improvement, program evaluation, and accountability.

While the heterogeneity of the educational programs at the various CHCs may represent a challenge to the replication of the AHB initiative, several elements that were key to its success can easily be replicated. First, AHB provided valuable networking opportunities through regular meetings and conferences. In today's more technologically advanced environment, a best-practices dialogue can easily be started among CHCs. For example, an *ask your peer* listserv can provide a forum where participants share experiences on program implementation and challenges. Second, AHB provided the opportunity to learn and to build capacity; exposure to and participation in the evaluation process furthered the understanding of a different part of program implementation and of the importance of evaluation to enhancing program credibility and sustainability. Academic institutions in border communities can serve an important role in this regard by expanding their outreach activities to promote community-based participatory research,[34] in which CHCs can be active partners in all research phases (design, implementation, evaluation, dissemination), thus promoting co-learning and capacity building.

Conclusions

Through the provision of affordable, high-quality health care to underserved minority populations, CHCs have accumulated knowledge and expertise in the unique cultural, socioeconomic, and environmental health care challenges facing these populations. Private-public partnerships can build on the outreach and experience of these centers in local communities while providing financial resources and capacity-building opportunities. Alliance for a Healthy Border is an example of a successful partnership that can serve as a model to be promoted and incorporated into public health programs, as well as into the future vision of an equitable and affordable health care system.

At the program level—researchers, in evaluating all 12 participating CHC programs, saw the importance of:

- A clearly defined, structured curriculum
- A 9- to 12-week duration
- Group sessions promoting peer support
- Active participation of *promotores*
- Inclusion of a physical activity component

At the center level—community health centers saw the need for:

- Allocation of specific funding for personnel to support initiative activities (e.g., for administrative activities and data collection)

At the partnership level—AHB partners saw the importance of:

- A clear understanding of partnership goals and alignment of these goals with those of individual partners
- Open communication channels
- Recognition of the different organizational cultures of each partner
- Frequent data collection and communication of results

Acknowledgments

The evaluation of Alliance for a Healthy Border was funded by Pfizer Inc. The authors thank Ms. Donna Jackson for her coordination efforts with program directors at the 12 community health centers and Dr. Violeta Díaz for her help with the focus groups.

References

1. Finkelstein EA, Trogdon JG, Cohen JW, et al. Annual medical spending attributable to obesity: payer- and service-specific estimates. Health Aff (Millwood). 2009 Sep–Oct;28(5):w822–31.
2. Finkelstein EA, DiBonaventura M, Burgess SM, et al. The costs of obesity in the workplace. J Occup Environ Med. 2010 Oct;52(10):971–6.
3. Gates DM, Succop P, Brehm BJ, et al. Obesity and presenteeism: the impact of body mass index on workplace productivity. J Occup Environ Med. 2008 Jan;50(1):39–45.
4. Ostbye T, Dement JM, Krause KM. Obesity and workers' compensation: results from the Duke Health and Safety Surveillance System. Arch Intern Med. 2007 Apr 23;167(8):766–73.
5. Schmier JK, Jones ML, Halpern MT. Cost of obesity in the workplace. Scand J Work Environ Health. 2006 Feb;32(1):5–11.
6. Finkelstein E, Fiebelkorn C, Wang G. The costs of obesity among full-time employees. Am J Health Promot. 2005 Sep–Oct;20(1):45–51.
7. Flegal KM, Carroll MD, Ogden CL, et al. Prevalence and trends in obesity among US adults, 1999–2008. JAMA. 2010 Jan 20;303(3):235–41.
8. Mokdad AH, Ford ES, Bowman BA, et al. Prevalence of obesity, diabetes, and obesity-related health risk factors, 2001. JAMA. 2003 Jan 1;289(1):76–9.

9. Zajacova A, Burgard SA. Body weight and health from early to mid-adulthood: a longitudinal analysis. J Health Soc Behav. 2010 Mar;51(1):92–107.

10. Centers for Disease Control and Prevention. Differences in prevalence of obesity among black, white, and Hispanic adults—United States, 2006–2008. MMWR Morb Mortal Wkly Rep. 2009 Jul 17;58(27):740–4.

11. Centers for Disease Control and Prevention. National diabetes fact sheet: national estimates and general information on diabetes and prediabetes in the United States, 2011. Atlanta, GA: U.S. Department of Health and Human Services, Centers for Disease Control and Prevention, 2011. Available at: http://www.cdc.gov/diabetes/pubs/pdf/ndfs_2011.pdf.

12. French SA, Story M, Jeffery RW. Environmental influences on eating and physical activity. Annu Rev Public Health. 2001;22:309–35.

13. Beaulac J, Kristjansson E, Cummins S. A systematic review of food deserts, 1966–2007. Prev Chronic Dis. 2009 Jul;6(3):A105.

14. Larson NI, Story MT, Nelson MC. Neighborhood environments: disparities in access to healthy foods in the U.S. Am J Prev Med. 2009 Jan;36(1):74–81.

15. Popkin BM, Duffey K, Gordon-Larsen P. Environmental influences on food choice, physical activity and energy balance. Physiol Behav. 2005 Dec 15;86(5):603–13.

16. Wing RR, Hamman RF, Bray GA, et al. Achieving weight and activity goals among diabetes prevention program lifestyle participants. Obes Res. 2004 Sep;12(9):1426–34.

17. Wadden TA, Neiberg RH, Wing RR, et al. Four-year weight losses in the Look AHEAD study: factors associated with long-term success. Obesity (Silver Spring). 2011 Oct;19(10):1987–98.

18. Drieling RL, Ma J, Stafford RS. Evaluating clinic and community-based lifestyle interventions for obesity reduction in a low-income Latino neighborhood: Vivamos Activos Fair Oaks Program. BMC Public Health. 2011 Feb 14;11:98.

19. U.S. Census Bureau. United States Census 2010: state and county quick facts. Washington, DC: U.S. Census Bureau, 2010. Available at: http://quickfacts.census.gov/qfd/index.html.

20. Fisher-Hoch SP, Rentfro AR, Salinas JJ, et al. Socioeconomic status and prevalence of obesity and diabetes in a Mexican American community, Cameron County, Texas, 2004–2007. Prev Chronic Dis. 2010 May;7(3):A53.

21. Soden DL. At the cross roads: US/Mexico border counties in transition. El Paso, TX: Institute for Policy and Economic Development, University of Texas at El Paso, 2006.

22. Forrest CB, Whelan EM. Primary care safety-net delivery sites in the United States: a comparison of community health centers, hospital outpatient departments, and physicians' offices. JAMA. 2000 Oct 25;284(16):2077–83.

23. Shi L, Lebrun LA, Tsai J, et al. Characteristics of ambulatory care patients and services: a comparison of community health centers and physicians' offices. J Health Care Poor Underserved. 2010 Nov;21(4):1169–83.

24. Shi L, Regan J, Politzer RM, et al. Community health centers and racial/ethnic disparities in healthy life. Int J Health Serv. 2001;31(3):567–82.

25. Shi L, Stevens GD, Wulu JT Jr, et al. America's health centers: reducing racial and ethnic disparities in perinatal care and birth outcomes. Health Serv Res. 2004 Dec;39(6 Pt 1):1881–901.

26. Politzer RM, Yoon J, Shi L, et al. Inequality in America: the contribution of health centers in reducing and eliminating disparities in access to care. Med Care Res Rev. 2001 Jun;58(2):234–48.

27. Regan J, Schempf AH, Yoon J, et al. The role of federally funded health centers in serving the rural population. J Rural Health. 2003 Spring;19(2):117–24; discussion 115–6.

28. Shi L, Tsai J, Higgins PC, et al. Racial/ethnic and socioeconomic disparities in access to care and quality of care for US health center patients compared with non–health center patients. J Ambul Care Manag. 2009 Oct–Dec;32(4):342–50.

29. Brown CJ, Pagán JA, Ghaddar S, Diaz V. Evaluation of Pfizer's Alliance for a Healthy Border. Presented at: 66th Annual Meeting of the United States–Mexico Border Health Association, Hermosillo, Mexico, May 2008.

30. Brown CJ, Pagán JA, Ghaddar S, Diaz V. Qualitative Evaluation of Pfizer's Alliance for a Healthy Border: a focus group study. Presented at: 67th Annual Meeting of the United States–Mexico Border Health Association, El Paso, TX, Jun 2009.

31. Wang X, Ghaddar S, Brown CJ, et al. Alliance for a Healthy Border: factors related to weight reduction and glycemic success. Popul Health Manag. 2012 Apr;15(2):90–100.

32. Buse K, Harmer AM. Seven habits of highly effective global public-private health partnerships: practice and potential. Soc Sci Med. 2007 Jan;64(2):259–71.

33. Buse K, Tanaka S. Global public-private health partnerships: lessons learned from ten years of experience and evaluation. Int Dent J. 2011 Aug;61 Suppl 2:2–10.

34. Israel BA, Schulz AJ, Parker EA, et al. Community-based participatory research: policy recommendations for promoting a partnership approach in health research. Educ Health (Abingdon). 2001;14(2):182–97.

CHAPTER 17

Comienzo Sano: Familia Saludable
Addressing Latino Childhood Obesity through a
Community-Based Participatory Research and
Bilingual Family-Focused Curriculum

Britt Rios-Ellis, PhD, Melawhy Garcia-Vega, MPH,
Gail Frank, DrPH, RD, CHES, Natalia Gatdula, MPH,
and Gino Galvez, PhD

Obesity is a major public health concern in the United States, and its prevalence has more than tripled for children and adolescents during the past three decades.[1-6] Research has shown that dietary behaviors and overweight begin tracking in early childhood, leading to chronic disease and degenerative conditions later in life.[7] Among Latino children, boys and girls have a 45.4% and 52.5% lifetime risk of developing diabetes, respectively, compared with 26.7% and 31.2% among their White male and female counterparts.[8] In addition, when compared with their African American, White, Asian / Pacific Islander, and American Indian / Alaska Native peers, Latino infants (under 12 months of age) have the highest overweight and obesity rates; these disparities continue through their school-age years into adolescence.[9] Chapter 2 of this volume reviews these and other facts.

We learned in chapter 1 that preschool is an important time for interventions designed to prevent obesity in childhood and later life. The period even before preschool is also very important in this regard. Research has shown that nutrition in early life, initiation of breastfeeding, and delayed introduction of foods are associated with reduced risk of obesity and overweight in later life.[10,11] Breastfeeding has been shown to be a sufficient source of nutrients for infant development and should be the only source of food for the first six months of life.[12] Although immigrant Latinas initiate breastfeeding more often and breastfeed for longer than more acculturated Latinas, the rate of breastfeeding among Latinas remains low.[13,14] Some cultural and family

All of the authors are affiliated with the National Council of La Raza / California State University, Long Beach (CSULB); Britt Rios-Ellis, Melawhy Garcia-Vega, Natalia Gatdula, and Gino Galvez, with the Center for Community Latino Health, Evaluation and Leadership Training; Rios-Ellis, with the Department of Health Science, CSULB; and Gail Frank, with the Department of Family and Consumer Sciences, CSULB.

beliefs and attitudes can serve as barriers to breastfeeding, such as the belief that a mother's negative feelings can turn breast milk sour or feeling embarrassed about breastfeeding in public. These beliefs and attitudes create barriers to breastfeeding that may inhibit initiation and duration and may not allow optimal health bene-fits.[15-17] Programs that promote breastfeeding have proved cost-effective and are associated with lower rates of adverse outcomes, such as childhood obesity.[15,17]

Children rely on overtaxed parents and public school systems for healthy foods but suffer from poor eating patterns, often not meeting the minimum nutrient and food group recommendations. These children experience poor physical health due to economic hardship,[18] lack of safe green spaces for exercise and recreation, and residence in food deserts.[19] Low- and middle-income parents must manage modest household budgets that may not consistently allow for essential resources, let alone seemingly expendable items like fruits and vegetables.[20] With the escalating cost of food, it is harder for parents to afford nutrient-rich fresh foods.[20-22]

Interventions using *promotores de salud* (community health workers) as a tool to encourage and empower at-risk people, in a culturally relevant manner, to participate in healthy behaviors to prevent adverse health outcomes have been well established in the literature.[23-26] *Promotores* can support culturally specific, health-reinforcing beliefs and behaviors and promote and increase knowledge in their respective communities.[27,28]* Despite the growing population of Latino students in higher education,[29] little has been done to recognize and incorporate student cultural assets in community-based participatory research (CBPR) strategies, participant recruitment, and adherence to and evaluation of interventions. Furthermore, student cultural capital[30] within a higher education community health framework is rarely acknowledged as a promising strategy for incorporation into community health program development, despite its obvious potential.

In response to this critical public health deficit and the need for culturally competent health educators, an internship was developed for Latino bilingual/bicultural nutrition and health science students at California State University, Long Beach (CSULB), to work with their communities in obesity prevention and healthy infant feeding and care.

Development of the Project

The National Council of La Raza (NCLR)/CSULB Center for Latino Community Health, Evaluation and Leadership Training received funding from the U.S. Department of Agriculture to implement the Comienzo Sano: Familia Saludable project. The project aimed to improve Latino nutrition and health by institutionalizing an educational experience. Student community health educators were recruited through in-class presentations and flyers. Students were eligible if they met the following cri-

---

* For more on the importance of *promotoras/promotores* in effective interventions in Hispanic communities, see chapters 2, 6, 15, and 16.

teria: (1) first-generation educated; (2) bilingual (Spanish-English) and bicultural; (3) in their junior year; (4) qualified for upper division directed studies or internship courses; and (5) having Latino-focused community service experience. Fourteen Latina students were interviewed and selected. They were trained in various facets of CBPR, curriculum development, and motivational interviewing (i.e., a counseling style for eliciting behavioral change by exploring and resolving ambivalence).[31] The training provided skills promoting their ability to work with the project directors to develop and implement a community-based intervention with Latina recipients of Women, Infants, and Children Supplemental Food Program (WIC) benefits in the city of Long Beach.

The internship was tailored using a *promotores* approach that recognized culture and language competency as integral elements needed in health programming to better understand and address the contexts of risks and barriers unique to Latino families. Student training focused on the development of knowledge, cultural appreciation, and health education skills necessary to deliver the curriculum.

Following an initial orientation meeting, students attended eight training sessions prior to delivering health education, followed by biweekly meetings with the project coordinator, who would provide as-needed booster training (e.g., on motivational interviewing) and support (e.g., on case management) throughout the project. The extensive training introduced the following topics: sociocultural determinants of health, institutional review boards, research ethics, CBPR, formative research methods (including focus group methodology), nutrition during pregnancy and lactation, infant nutrition in the first year of life, breastfeeding, nutrition in the preschool years, physical activity during pregnancy and lactation, lifestyle changes to prevent obesity, professional development and continuing education post-baccalaureate, and public health in practice. Furthermore, by working alongside the center's academic project faculty and staff, the students became increasingly familiar with community nuances, recruitment strategies, and issues associated with language use and curriculum development.

Using a case management approach, trained students conducted recruitment and informed consent, health education sessions, three-month follow-up interviews, data collection, and data entry and management for their caseloads. Eligible participants were recruited at collaborating WIC locations and met the following criteria: (1) Spanish-speaking Latinas; (2) at least 18 years of age; and (3) at least 20 weeks pregnant. For each student, the caseload ranged from 12 to 35 participants. Participants had the choice of receiving the sessions at the WIC site or in their homes. The educational topics included prenatal care, breastfeeding, age-appropriate introduction of foods and solids, maternal and child health, techniques for maintenance of a healthy weight, and the importance of physical activity for the family (see table 17.1). Knowledge was assessed on each topic. Students presented the topics using a flip chart and engaged participants in dialogue. During the educational sessions, students employed motivational interviewing techniques to encourage the women to make behavioral changes associated with breastfeeding, age-appropriate introduction of food,

Table 17.1. Educational topics for each session taught by students in the Comienzo Sano: Familia Saludable project

Session	Session title	Topics
Session 1	Prenatal Care	• Prenatal care • Vitamins and minerals • Recommended weight gain • Maintaining a healthy weight • Gestational diabetes
Session 2	Breastfeeding	• Benefits for mother and baby • Four breastfeeding positions • Benefits of expressing and saving milk
Session 3	Proper Nutrition	• Child nutrition from birth to the first year • Breast milk • Introduction of liquids and solid foods • Introducing new foods • USDA nutritional guidelines
Session 4	Healthy Lifestyles	• Importance of exercise in the perinatal period • Well-being and losing weight • Healthy eating • Being active • Parental role modeling • Benefits of an active child • Recreational activities for families
Session 5	Appendix	• Review of key topics • Healthy weight • Being active • Body mass index • What are food allergies? • Most common food allergies

and infant feeding practices. Lastly, students completed a survey that was designed to obtain feedback and evaluate their internship experience.

A total of 191 Latina WIC recipients participated in the intervention, and 135 (70.7%) attended the five one-hour sessions, consisting of 10 classes lasting 20–30 minutes, all held in the participants' homes. Demographic information was obtained for all participants. The women had a mean age of 27.8 years; the majority were foreign-born (67%) and were married or living with a partner (72%). Less than half had at least a high school education (45%), and only 24% had permanent employment. At the start of the project, the mean length of pregnancy was 30.7 weeks. To evaluate the intervention, surveys were administered at each session and at three months following childbirth. These surveys assessed specific knowledge related to each session and were scored for correct number of responses. Broadly, the surveys assessed knowledge retention on breastfeeding practices, proper infant feeding practices, infant health measures, and maternal health screening and guidelines. Some preliminary outcomes based on the pre- and post-session data are discussed below.

Evaluation

Our evaluation found that the project was successful in providing Latina students with research training and an opportunity to learn from and provide for their communities. Specifically, 92% reported feeling that they had learned "a lot" about their community; 62% reported learning "some" about how to solve a community need; 85% reported learning "a lot" about understanding the needs of others; and all reported that they believed the project had helped their community. On a scale from 1 to 10, students reported high levels of confidence in addressing challenges in their life (mean = 8.8, SD = 0.9), in being better prepared to pursue advanced education (mean = 8.9, SD = 1.3), and in finding a job that would fit their career interests (mean = 9.0, SD = 1.1). Open-ended responses indicated positive gains in learning on multiple topics (e.g., competence in community-based research, health education delivery, breastfeeding, and data entry and management).

Preliminary results suggest that the intervention was effective for the participants. Regarding breastfeeding and the age-appropriate introduction of foods and solids, the mean pre-session score was 6.4 (SD = 1.7) and post-session score was 8.3 (SD = 1.1). On the benefits of recreational activities with the family and children's healthy eating habits, mean pre-session score was 3.4 (SD = 1.0) and post-session score was 3.7 (SD = 0.7). Participants expressed various positive points of view regarding their behavior and confidence in feeding their infants and family in healthy ways. (The results have been analyzed for statistical significance, but the analysis is outside the scope of this chapter; results are available from the authors.)

Discussion

This project has important public health implications and serves as a model to address the inequities inherent in the escalating rates of Latino childhood overweight and obesity. *Promotores*-based models also offer great promise for tailoring education to address other health issues. The internship introduced future health professionals to community-based research. It provided an opportunity for students to engage their inherent cultural and linguistic capital while providing health education to their communities. Involving students in every part of project implementation facilitates first-hand learning and the development of effective strategies in community-based interventions.

The students' commitment was evident in their recruitment and implementation efforts. The majority of students surpassed the expected work hours and caseloads in order to meet the project's goals. The learning experience opportunity motivated them to commit beyond the expected time frame, even though grant funds limited the monetary compensation. These efforts underscore the willingness and motivation of Latina students to engage in research and professional training opportunities to further their academic careers, particularly if the experience allows the incorporation of their cultural capital by creating health interventions that directly benefit their communities.

When participants were asked whether they preferred home or WIC site settings for the sessions, they overwhelmingly reported their preference for the home setting, accentuating the participants' level of comfort with the students and the intervention. The enhanced focus on cultural values such as *personalismo* (valuing interpersonal relationships), *familismo* (the importance of family), and *confianza* (mutual trust) in conjunction with obesity-related scientific knowledge allowed students to move from the originally intended setting in WIC clinics to the participants' homes. The home setting ultimately resulted in fewer distractions, greater time to address curriculum-related questions, and an opportunity to counter myths and misunderstandings that may have impeded knowledge acquisition. Participants and students reported high levels of comfort in the sessions due to their similar ethnic backgrounds and cultural values and norms. The sharing of cultural capital allowed continued contact after the intervention, resulting in students' visits to participants at hospitals after delivery and the sharing of birth and breastfeeding experiences and baby photographs, all reflecting the level of participants' comfort and trust in the students. Comienzo Sano: Familia Saludable demonstrates the potential for the integration of cultural capital in the creation of student training and involvement in obesity prevention targeting Latino communities.

LESSONS LEARNED

- *Promotores*-based models offer great promise for tailored community education.
- Internships add to students' cultural and linguistic capital.
- Research and professional training promote future academic careers for students.
- Trust between the community and students increases when cultural values are considered.
- Development of obesity prevention demands attention to at-risk Latina communities.

Acknowledgments

This report and the project described herein were supported by Agriculture and Food Research Initiative Competitive grant no. 2009-38422-19895 from the USDA National Institute of Food and Agriculture. The authors wish to acknowledge statistical support from Enrique Ortega, PhD, and facilities at the NCLR/CSULB Center for Community Latino Health, Evaluation and Leadership Training, Long Beach, California.

References

1. National Center for Health Statistics. Health, United States, 2007, with chartbook on trends in the health of Americans. Hyattsville, MD: National Center for Health Statistics, Centers for Disease Control and Prevention, 2007. Available at: http://www.cdc.gov/nchs /data/hus/hus07.pdf.

2. Koplan JP, Liverman CT, Kraak VI, eds. Preventing childhood obesity: health in the balance. Washington, DC: Institute of Medicine, National Academy Press, 2005.

3. Ogden CL, Carroll MD, Curtin LR, et al. Prevalence of overweight and obesity in the United States, 1999–2004. JAMA. 2006 Apr 5;295(13):1549–55.

4. Singh GK, Kogan MD, van Dyck PC. A multilevel analysis of state and regional disparities in childhood and adolescent obesity in the United States. J Community Health. 2008 Apr; 33(2):90–102.

5. Singh GK, Kogan MD, van Dyck PC, et al. Racial/ethnic, socioeconomic, and behavioral determinants of childhood and adolescent obesity in the United States: analyzing independent and joint associations. Ann Epidemiol. 2008 Sep;18(9):682–95.

6. Singh GK, Kogan MD, Yu SE. Disparities in obesity and overweight prevalence among U.S. immigrant children and adolescents by generational status. J Community Health. 2009 Aug;34(4):271–81.

7. Zive MM, Berry CC, Sallis JF, et al. Tracking dietary intake in white and Mexican-American children from age 4 to 12 years. J Am Diet Assoc. 2002 May;102(5):683–9.

8. Narayan KM, Boyle JP, Thompson TJ, et al. Lifetime risk for diabetes mellitus in the United States. JAMA. 2003 Oct 8;290(14):1884–90.

9. National Council of La Raza. Profiles of Latino health: a closer look at Latino child nutrition. Issue 2: Latino trends in child overweight and obesity. Washington, DC: National Council of La Raza, 2010. Available at: http://www.nclr.org/images/uploads/pages/Jan12_Profiles_Issue _2.pdf.

10. Owen CG, Martin RM, Whinchup PH, et al. Effect of infant feeding on the risk of obesity across the life course: a quantitative review of published evidence. Pediatrics. 2005 May;115(5):1367–77.

11. Seach KA, Dharmage SC, Lowe AJ, et al. Delayed introduction of solid feeding reduces child overweight and obesity at 10 years. Int J Obes (Lond). 2010 Oct;34(10):1475–9.

12. Kolobe TH. Childrearing practices and developmental expectations for Mexican-American mothers and the developmental status of their infants. Phys Ther. 2004 May;84(5): 439–53.

13. Gill SL, Reifsnider E, Lucke JF. Effects of support on the initiation and duration of breast-feeding. West J Nurs Res. 2007 Oct;29(6):708–23.

14. John AM, Martorell R. Incidence and duration of breast-feeding in Mexican-American infants, 1970–1982. Am J Clin Nutr. 1989 Oct;50(4):868–74.

15. Bunik M, Clark L, Zimmer LM, et al. Early infant feeding decisions in low-income Latinas. Breastfeed Med. 2006 Winter;1(4):225–35.

16. Rios-Ellis B, Enguidanos SM, Espinoza-Ferrel T, et al. Early infant feeding practices of Latina immigrant mothers. Presented at: The 128th Annual Meeting of the American Public Health Association, Boston, MA, Nov 2000.

17. James WP. The epidemiology of obesity: the size of the problem. J Intern Med. 2008 Apr; 263(4):336–52.

18. National Council of La Raza. Profiles of Latino health: a closer look at Latino child nutrition. Issue 3: Food spending in Latino households. Washington, DC: National Council of La Raza, 2010. Available at: http://www.nclr.org/images/uploads/pages/Jan12_Profiles_Issue _3.pdf.

19. National Council of La Raza. Profiles of Latino health: a closer look at Latino child nutrition. Issue 4: The food environment and Latinos' access of healthy foods. Washington, DC: National Council of La Raza, 2010. Available at: http://www.nclr.org/images/uploads/pages /Jan12_Profiles_Issue_4.pdf.

20. Sealy YM. Parents' food choices: obesity among minority parents and children. J Community Health Nurs. 2010 Jan;27(1):1–11.

21. Levi J, Vinter S, Richardson L, et al. F as in fat: how obesity policies are failing in America 2009. Washington, DC: Trust for America's Health, 2009. Available at: http://healthyameri cans.org/reports/obesity2009/Obesity2009Report.pdf.

22. Capehart T, Richardson J. Food price inflation: causes and impacts. Washington, DC: Congressional Research Service, Library of Congress, 2008. Available at: http://www.schoolnutri tion.org/uploadedFiles_old/ASFSA/childnutrition/govtaffairs/CRSFoodPriceInflation4-10-08 .pdf.

23. McCloskey J. Promotores as partners in a community-based diabetes intervention program targeting Hispanics. Fam Community Health. 2009 Jan–Mar;32(1):48–57.

24. Shattell MM, Smith KM, Quinlan-Colwell A, Villalba JA. Factors contributing to depression in Latinas of Mexican origin residing in the United States: implications for nurses. J Am Psychiatr Nurses Assoc. 2008 Jun;14(3):193–204.

25. Hanks CA. Community empowerment: a partnership approach to public health program implementation. Policy Polit Nurs Pract. 2006 Nov;7(4):297–306.

26. Rodriguez VM, Conway TL, Woodruff SI, et al. Pilot test of an assessment instrument for Latina community health advisors conducting an ETS intervention. J Immigr Health. 2003 Jul;5(3):129–37.

27. Unger JB, Molina GB, Baron M. Evaluation of sweet temptations, a fotonovela for diabetes education. Hisp Health Care Int. 2009;7(3):145–52.

28. Hutchins V, Walch C. Meeting minority health needs through special MCH projects. Public Health Rep. 1989 Nov–Dec;104(6):621–6.

29. Fry R. Hispanic college enrollment spikes, narrowing gaps with other groups. Washington, DC: Pew Hispanic Center, 2011. Available at: http://www.pewhispanic.org/files/2011/08 /146.pdf.

30. Yosso TJ. Whose culture has capital? A critical race theory discussion of community cultural wealth. Race Ethn Educ. 2005 Mar;8(1):69–91.

31. Rollnick S, Miller WR. What is motivational interviewing? Behav Cogn Psychother. 1995; 23:325–34.

CHAPTER 18

Fine, Fit, and Fabulous
Addressing Obesity in Underserved Communities through
a Faith-Based Nutrition and Fitness Program

Carlos Devia, MA, Charmaine Ruddock, MS, Maxine Golub, MPH,
Loyce Godfrey, BS, Jill Linnell, MPH, Linda Weiss, PhD,
Jaime Gutierrez, MPH, Rosa Rosen, JD, Joyce Davis, BA,
and Neil Calman, MD

The Institute for Family Health is a federally qualified health center network dedicated to providing primary health services to medically underserved populations. Since 1999, the institute has led the Bronx Health REACH Coalition (the Coalition), with funding provided by the Centers for Disease Control and Prevention (CDC) REACH program (Racial and Ethnic Approaches to Community Health). The Coalition includes over 70 community and faith-based organizations dedicated to eliminating health disparities in New York City.[1] In 2007, the CDC designated Bronx Health REACH a National Center of Excellence to Eliminate Disparities.

The Coalition is based in the Southwest Bronx, a low-income urban community where 95% of the residents are African American or Latino and suffer disproportionately from asthma, HIV/AIDS, cardiovascular disease, diabetes, and obesity. Twenty-seven

Carlos Devia is the project manager for research and evaluation of Bronx Health REACH/New York Center of Excellence to Eliminate Disparities (CEED) and project coordinator of the Faith-Based Outreach Initiative. Charmaine Ruddock is the director of Bronx Health REACH/CEED. Maxine Golub is the senior vice president for planning and development at the Institute for Family Health and project administrator of Bronx Health REACH/CEED. Loyce Godfrey is the director of food and nutrition services at MidBronx Senior Center and a faith-based health coordinator; she created the Fine, Fit, and Fabulous program. Jill Linnell is the grants and contracts manager at Bronx Health REACH/CEED and the Faith-Based Outreach Initiative. Linda Weiss is the director of the Center for Evaluation and Applied Research at the New York Academy of Medicine. Jaime Gutierrez is a project director at the Center for Evaluation and Applied Research, New York Academy of Medicine. Rosa Rosen was a diabetes advocate and educator and the manager of Together on Diabetes, an initiative that helps seniors in Upper Manhattan learn how to live well with diabetes. Joyce Davis is a founding member of Bronx Health REACH/CEED and is actively involved in developing and leading the Faith-Based Outreach Initiative. Neil Calman is the president and CEO of the Institute for Family Health and principal investigator of Bronx Faith-Based Initiative to Eliminate Racial Disparities in Health and of Bronx Health REACH/CEED.

percent of residents in the southwest Bronx are obese, compared with 25% of Bronx residents and 21% of New York City residents.[2,3]

Since its inception, the Coalition has worked with religious institutions to reach at-risk populations and promote behavioral change. In communities of color, faith institutions provide infrastructure and communications systems that can be leveraged to promote health,[4,5] and studies show that faith-based health interventions can result in significant improvement in diabetes management, cardiovascular health, and obesity reduction for participants.[6-9]

In 2001, the Coalition created a Faith-Based Outreach Initiative (FBOI), which has grown to include 47 churches of various Christian denominations. The congregations range in size from 25 to 2,000 and serve primarily African American, Caribbean, West African, and Latino congregants. The FBOI has two goals: (1) to use the capacity of faith institutions to change knowledge, attitudes, and behaviors about healthy eating and physical activity, diabetes management, and how to navigate the health care system; and (2) to mobilize the clergy and congregants to promote access to equitable care, healthy food, and places to exercise through public policy.*

In each church, the pastor made a commitment to share information about health disparities and health promotion from the pulpit and selected a health coordinator who would participate in monthly meetings and implement health activities. The Coalition provides churches with health materials, an annual stipend, training, and technical assistance for coordinators. FBOI activities are evaluated by the New York Academy of Medicine and guided by a Community Research Committee (CRC) made up of community leaders, pastors, physicians, and residents. The committee meets regularly with Bronx Health REACH staff and the FBOI evaluators to discuss the design and implementation of evaluation tools and research methodologies. The committee also plays a key role in interpreting and disseminating research findings on the FBOI.

One of the most successful FBOI programs is a 12-week faith-based diabetes prevention program known as Fine, Fit, and Fabulous (FFF), which offers nutrition education and fitness activities in a spiritual context using group support. The program began at one church and developed, through a participatory and iterative process, into a broad faith-based health initiative. To date, the Coalition has implemented FFF in 10 English- and 9 Spanish-speaking churches, reaching 505 individuals. Seventy percent of all participants lost weight (n = 305) during the program period, with an average loss of 4 lbs or 3% of initial body weight. In this chapter we describe the program's implementation, its impact on individual participants and participating churches, its strengths and challenges, and how lessons learned have shaped similar initiatives in other communities.

---

* See chapter 12 for a faith-based nutrition and fitness program in Florida that is focused on African American women. The theme of culturally specific interventions (such as interventions emerging from churches of populations of interest, as seen in this chapter) recurs throughout this volume.

Program Development and Implementation

> Sisters are loving God, themselves, and each other. Sisters are sharing, laughing and praying together . . . encouraging church folks to hire their own fitness instructors, planning fancy gourmet menus, going back to basics, eating more traditional diets rather than processed fast food, taking back their temple by claiming their heritage and history.
>
> —*Loyce Godfrey*

History

In 2004, a group of women guided by Loyce Godfrey, a health coordinator with a background in food and nutrition management, started the Fine, Fit, and Fabulous ministry in partnership with Bronx Health REACH at Bronx Christian Fellowship Church. The FFF ministry aimed to help congregants gain balance in their body, mind, and spiritual life, improve weight control and physical fitness, and adopt healthy eating habits. After a promising first year, Coalition leaders decided to develop the model into a program that could be offered to other FBOI churches. For a year, Bronx Health REACH nutritionists, Loyce Godfrey, and early participants worked to formalize FFF activities into a curriculum. While much of the content of the curriculum is original and written by the Coalition, some of the evidence-based nutrition information is culled from the U.S. Department of Agriculture's *Dietary Guidelines for Americans*.[10] In addition, the program is grounded in the Diabetes Prevention Program Research Group's recommendation that lifestyle interventions are more efficient and cost-effective than drug treatments.[11,12] Funding from the New York State Department of Health's Bureau of Chronic Disease provided additional funds for the Coalition to implement the new curriculum in 10 African American churches. After four years of implementing and fine-tuning the program in English, the Coalition spent a year collaborating with pastors and congregants from Spanish-speaking churches to adapt the program linguistically and culturally for Latinos. At every stage of development, the Coalition carefully retained the unique spirit of the FFF model while creating an easily replicable program.

Description

The FFF program is best defined as spiritually driven, goal-oriented, and support group–based. The program structure includes an orientation session and 11 weekly sessions. Key concepts in the sessions include dietary guidelines, the Plate Method, portion sizes, healthy cooking techniques, and spiritual lessons (table 18.1). Each session includes two parts: a one-hour nutrition discussion followed by a one-hour exercise session taught by a fitness instructor. All activities take place in the church. The program's effectiveness and replication are directly dependent on its relevance to the faith community. Thus, every session starts and ends with a prayer. In addition, all program materials include references to scriptures as a way to link

Table 18.1. Fine, Fit, and Fabulous: group discussions overview

Session	Content
Orientation	Participants are welcomed to the program, receive program materials, and complete the baseline evaluation. The orientation is also used to pair up participants into buddies and guide them through the process of developing an action plan.
Week 1. The Food, God, and Health Connection	Participants learn about chronic diseases resulting from obesity, and their responsibility to take care of their body as a temple in order to avoid diet-related diseases is emphasized.
Week 2. The Basics of Healthy Eating and Making Lifestyle Changes	Participants discuss the benefits of healthy diets and regular physical activity along with the steps necessary to succeed in making lifestyle changes.
Week 3. Making Lifestyle Changes	Participants learn steps in how to make lifestyle changes by "taking back their body's temple," through a discussion of the article "Why Is the Church So Fat?"
Week 4. Purpose-Driven Reasons for Wanting to Be Fine, Fit, and Fabulous	Participants identify purpose-driven reasons to be Fine, Fit, and Fabulous, including a discussion on unhealthy motives like vanity or achieving nonsustainable goals.
Week 5. Dietary Guidelines for Americans–Feeding God's Flock	Participants learn about healthy diets as defined by the USDA's *Dietary Guidelines for Americans*. They discuss eating from a variety of food groups, with emphasis on vegetables, whole grains, and foods low in saturated fats, trans fats, cholesterol, sodium, and added sugar.
Week 6. Self-indulgence and Gluttony Are Sins–Are You Sinning?	Participants reflect on how people who engage in self-indulgence such as gluttony are displaying sinful behavior. They are asked to think about the link between gluttony and other forms of addiction.
Week 7. Fast Food and Overeating–Forget McDonald's, Make God's Presence Your Comfort Food!	Participants learn why most fast-food items are unhealthy and how to make healthier choices–even in fast-food restaurants. The lesson also advises on managing food portions using the Plate Method and raises awareness of how portion sizes affect our perception of food, eating habits, and overall health.
Week 8. Self-discipline, Moderation, and Self-Control–Is That Your Stomach Growling or Your Soul?	Participants discuss how their faith influences their lifestyle choices around health and can help them practice self-discipline, moderation, and self-control when faced with temptations.
Week 9. 5-A-Day the Color Way!	Participants learn about the nutrients in fruits and vegetables, including vitamins, minerals, and phytochemicals found in colored plant foods. They are encouraged to choose a variety of colored fruits and vegetables daily to obtain maximum health benefits and to achieve healthy weights.
Week 10. Honor God by Taking Care of Your Temple–Is the Holy Spirit at Home in Your Body?	Participants identify two changes they want to make to live healthier lives and discuss how one of their responsibilities toward God is to take care of the body as a temple.
Week 11. Using God's Strength to Live a Healthier Life–Trading in "Fat and Happy" for "Fit and Healthy"	Participants discuss how God can help them make healthy changes in their lives and how to use God's strength to maintain these improvements. The session includes the post-program evaluation.

spiritual values to healthy behaviors, focusing on three key points: (1) purpose-driven reasons for caring for one's body; (2) adopting a healthier lifestyle, which requires discipline, moderation, and self-control, character traits emphasized throughout the scriptures; and (3) honoring God by taking care of one's body, understood as the dwelling place of the Holy Spirit. Participants in the program are asked to develop an individual action plan with both nutrition and fitness goals, which are discussed weekly with the group. Each participant is assigned a partner or buddy for ongoing support in meeting health goals and ensuring accountability. Participants track their progress through nutrition tests and by using weight, diet, and exercise logs.

Implementation

Each church that participates in the FBOI has a health coordinator responsible for starting, leading, and maintaining health programs in the church. The FFF program begins with an initial meeting between the church health coordinator, Bronx Health REACH staff, and church leaders to discuss recruitment, materials (printed curriculum guides and a scale for weigh-ins), and other logistics. This initial meeting is also an opportunity to plan the orientation session for participants, where they will receive their program materials, meet each other, and learn about the program. For FFF to be relevant and helpful to all members of the church, health coordinators are asked to involve representatives from as many of the church groups as possible in the recruitment process. Once the church decides to sponsor FFF, a space in the church is reserved for the 12 sessions, a fitness instructor is hired for the program, and flyers and announcements at weekly services are used to publicize the program. After the program has been successfully implemented weekly for 12 weeks, the final session may be used to formally acknowledge participants' completion of the program. Alternatively, some churches choose to honor participants with certificates during a church service so that the entire congregation can share in their accomplishments. A toolkit describing detailed steps on how to implement, budget, market, and evaluate the FFF program is available for download, free of charge, at www.bronxhealthreach.org.

Outcomes

In 2005, the Coalition received funds from the National Institute on Minority Health and Health Disparities to evaluate the FBOI, including the FFF program, using a community-based participatory research (CBPR) approach. The evaluation includes 19 churches (n = 9 African American, 9 Latino, and 1 West African) from various Christian denominations (n = 6 Baptist, 3 Pentecostal, 1 Mennonite, 1 Catholic, 1 Evangelical, and 7 nondenominational), averaging 400 members per church. A total of 24 FFF programs were implemented in the 19 churches. Evaluation of the FFF program received institutional review board approval from the Institute for Family Health and the New York Academy of Medicine.

Individual Impact

Fine, Fit, and Fabulous programs averaged 21 participants. Most participants were women (92%) with an average baseline body mass index (BMI) of 31 kg/m². One-third reported having diabetes; half were identified as at high risk for developing diabetes, based on the American Diabetes Association Risk Test.[13] In total, 505 individuals participated in the 24 FFF programs. Seventy percent of all participants (n = 355) had lost weight by the end of the 12 weeks, while 21% (n = 105) maintained their original weight and 9% (n = 45) gained 1–8 lbs. As shown in figure 18.1, of the 355 participants who lost weight, the majority (n = 135) lost 1%–3% of their initial body weight, and over a quarter (n = 92) lost 5%–10% of their initial body weight. All programs resulted in improved knowledge about nutrition, as demonstrated on pre- and post-program surveys. Knowledge and behavior scores related to the benefits of eating fruits and vegetables, drinking water, reading food labels, and judging food portion sizes improved significantly compared with baseline (detailed survey results to be reported).

Qualitative evaluation results also demonstrate how the program affected the health behaviors of participants. For example, one participant started the program at 321 lbs and by the conclusion was down to 270 lbs. She continued her nutrition and fitness regimen after completing FFF and lost an additional 59 lbs. As a result, her doctor suspended her hypertension medications. She is now employed teaching nutrition to parents in her community. Stories like this demonstrate how the adoption of FFF lessons can create healthy lifestyles and improve quality of life.

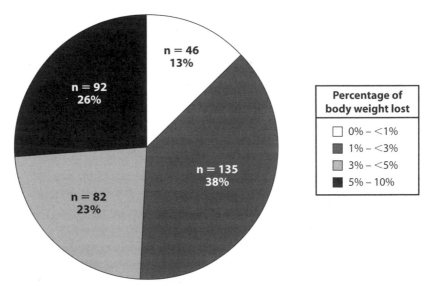

FIGURE 18.1. Distribution of the 355 participants who had lost a percentage of their initial body weight by the end of the 12 weeks of the Bronx Health REACH Coalition's Fine, Fit, and Fabulous program.

Institutional Impact

Many churches have created ways to sustain and promote FFF fitness activities by purchasing exercise machines, using fitness videos, and/or negotiating a reduced fee with a fitness instructor and dividing the cost among the group. Others have started walking clubs, weight management support groups, and a faith-based boot camp. The energy and excitement generated in FFF programs has also led to new institutional policies in churches regarding healthy eating, including serving healthy food at all church events; using the pulpit for weekly reminders about reading food labels, limiting sweetened beverages and fast food, and watching food portions; using church space for urban agriculture projects; and supporting farmers' markets, community gardens, and community-supported agriculture projects.

Discussion

The success of Fine, Fit, and Fabulous is due, in part, to the meaningful collaboration developed among Bronx Health REACH staff, faith organizations, academic partners, health care providers, community residents, and funders, all with a shared commitment to the overarching goal of eliminating disparities, not just the outcome of a single program. Along the way, the Coalition has identified several elements important to the success of a faith-based initiative focused on addressing health disparities in obesity and related comorbidities (discussed here and summarized under "Lessons Learned," below).

Church Leadership

The Coalition had previously identified the importance of pastors and church leaders in faith-based health initiatives,[14] a lesson that reemerged in FFF. Pastors' engagement is important to provide spiritual context to health initiatives, to facilitate access to communities of faith, and to support the implementation of health initiatives in church settings. In our experience, the absence of church leadership in program promotion, recruitment, and implementation signaled that FFF was not a priority and often led to logistical problems: health coordinators did not have access to the pulpit to promote the program; recruitment and attendance were lower; the scheduling of sessions was more difficult; space availability was limited; and programs were perceived as increasing utility expenses, resulting in restricted use of heat and light. Such problems were addressed at monthly FBOI meetings and follow-up meetings with pastors, but the problems highlight the importance of engaging leadership prior to program implementation.

Church Motivation

The FFF program references scriptures throughout the lessons, stressing "your body as the temple of the living God," and facilitates discussions on related spiritual and health topics. For example, participants discuss the article "Why Is the Church So

Fat?"[15] to consider how complacency toward obesity in the faith community may be related to complacency in spiritual values such as temptation, gluttony, and laziness (e.g., overeating and lack of exercise). For many years, the Coalition recognized that linking religious tenets to health messages is critical for the success of any activity in the FBOI.[16]

Program Sustainability

The Faith-Based Outreach Initiative has health coordinators responsible for implementing health programs in the churches, such as FFF. Our health coordinators are individuals committed to their church, well-regarded in the church community, and interested in the topic of health and health disparities. Bronx Health REACH Coalition staff members meet with them monthly to provide trainings to enhance their organizational, networking, and health promotion skills. However, to spark long-term and sustainable changes in churches, the health coordinators need the energy and support of a dedicated team. After hearing the feedback from our health coordinators, we have changed the FBOI goals to focus on the creation of sustainable health ministries in our churches. The health ministry is a long-term team of church members with the skills and commitment to carry on health, nutrition, and fitness activities in their church.

Using Community-Based Participatory Research to Evaluate Faith-Based Initiatives

Members of the Coalition have come to value the principles of CBPR—especially the trust built into the Coalition's research efforts, the value placed on the capacity of community members to perform research, and the commitment to capture information diligently in order to share knowledge broadly. The Coalition has built research capacity in our community by involving health coordinators and FFF facilitators in the data-collection and data-reporting process. However, we initially underestimated the difficulties of evaluation tasks. Common mistakes included distribution of the wrong surveys, missing informed consent forms, inability to match pre- and post-program data because of missing data or pages, and poor documentation of process data. The CRC suggested a training to address the administrative, data-management, and planning skills required for evaluation. Coalition staff and evaluators facilitated the training, including a presentation of preliminary FFF results. Community program facilitators were disturbed that missing or incomplete data painted an incomplete picture of the outcomes they were witnessing in participants' lifestyles and the churches' wellness practices. After the training, community members involved in FFF worked with evaluators to create a more effective data-collection process.

Investing Resources in the Community with High Returns

The Bronx Health REACH Coalition has spent six years in the planning, development, implementation, and refinement of FFF, including translating the curriculum into Spanish and disseminating the program. While this represents a substantial investment of grant funds, staff time, and community effort, the return, as they say, is priceless: a sustainable, replicable, and low-cost intervention with high success in improving participants' weight management habits. Assuming the availability of a volunteer coordinator and free space, church costs to run FFF are limited to the cost of printing curriculum guides, hiring a fitness instructor, and purchasing a scale. Based on a program with 20 individuals, this averages $60 per participant for the entire 12-week program ($5 per class). In our experience, 26% of participants (n = 92) lost 5%–10% of their initial body weight—a weight change that, depending on age, gender, and BMI, studies have associated with significant improvements in health[17] and a decrease in expected lifetime medical care costs (due to hypertension, hypercholesterolemia, type 2 diabetes, coronary heart disease, and stroke) of $2,200 to $5,300 per individual.[18] Using this cost-savings measure, we can calculate that the 92 participants who lost up to 10% of their initial body weight through FFF saved the health care system $202,400–$487,600—a substantial return on investment by any measure.

Scalability

Development of a FFF toolkit has enabled at least seven faith-based groups throughout New York, Georgia, and Virginia to successfully replicate the program, and other groups have used it for cancer patients, fitness classes at health centers, and a Gospel gym in California. Currently, the coalition is collaborating with community groups in other states to adapt the toolkit for male-only groups and non-Christian faith groups.

Conclusions

Faith-based organizations are in a unique position to address health disparities and promote wellness. The good physical health and well-being of individuals may extend far beyond medical advice, treatments, and prescriptions to include a meaningful spiritual component that the health care system is not equipped to provide. Fine, Fit, and Fabulous has successfully used faith settings to reach obese and overweight individuals of various racial and ethnic groups, leading to significant improvements in health behaviors resulting in weight loss. This evidence-based program demonstrates a culturally affirming initiative that engages churches as venues for health education and intervention and creates a low-cost, easily replicable nutrition and fitness program for high-risk communities across the country.

LESSONS LEARNED
- The role of pastors and faith-based leaders is key, in order to:
    —Provide a spiritual orientation to health information
    —Provide access to church resources
    —Promote sustainable behavioral changes in eating and fitness habits

- —Support the implementation of health programming in church settings
  - —Engage clergy from various faith denominations and racial/ethnic backgrounds to expand wellness efforts communitywide
- Providing a spiritual context to health messages contributes to the success of faith-based health initiatives because it leverages church members' beliefs and values to motivate change and adopt healthy lifestyles.
- Creating a structured health ministry with dedicated church members can amplify wellness efforts in the congregation and guarantee church commitment to funding, coordination, and sustainability of the health activities.
- Church members can gain critical evaluation skills to assess health activities, but ongoing training and technical assistance are important to ensure administrative, data-management, and planning skills required for a proper program evaluation.
- Results from these assessments can help church members continue the work (refine activities, report to their community, seek new funding).
- Community-led efforts often require long-term commitments. Development, implementation, and refinement of culturally affirming health initiatives take years but can pay off in the long run with low-cost replicable programs.
- Coalitions can help develop and sustain these efforts by integrating them into the mission of member organizations, but long-term funding is essential.
- A nutrition and fitness program that takes advantage of existing church structures can be highly cost-effective and replicable.
- A toolkit with clear steps to implement, budget, market, and evaluate the program is an effective way to disseminate these activities to faith-based communities nationally.

Acknowledgments

The authors are grateful to their funders: the Centers for Disease Control and Prevention, the New York State Department of Health's Bureau of Chronic Disease, and the National Institute on Minority Health and Health Disparities, which are committed to the overarching goal of improving the health of communities of color and reducing racial and ethnic health disparities. The authors express their appreciation to dedicated Community Research Committee members—Rev. Robert L. Foley, Sister Ellenrita Pucaro, Evalina Irish-Spencer, Toni Carter, Brenda Barretto, Sue Kaplan, Carolyn Berry, Lydia Sierra, and Kwaku Boakye—whose openness to sharing their wisdom and assistance made this project possible; previous Bronx Health REACH staff—Brooke Bennett, Bethany Gotkin, Lan Lee, and Ruchi Mathur—for their contributions in the early stages of the program; Deacon Joseph Ellis, for assisting in the implementation of the program; Suzanna Tejovic, for assisting in the cost-benefit analysis of the program; and Paula Park and Francesca Heintz, for their assistance in preparing this manuscript. The authors also thank Louise Square, New York State Department of Health, for providing technical assistance to develop and implement the program, and Rev. Dr. Suzan Johnson Cook, for supporting the pilot of the program at Bronx Christian Fellowship Church. Finally, deepest appreciation is extended to all the members of Bronx Health REACH's Faith-Based Outreach Initiative for their participation in and support of the project and their commitment to improving the health of their fellow congregants.

References

1. Calman N. Making health equality a reality: the Bronx takes action. Health Aff (Millwood). 2005 Mar–Apr;24(2):491–8.

2. New York City Department of Health and Mental Hygiene. Community health survey profiles: Take Care Highbridge and Morrisania, The Bronx. New York, NY: New York City Department of Health and Mental Hygiene, 2006. Available at: http://www.nyc.gov/html/doh/downloads/pdf/data/2006chp-106.pdf.

3. New York City Department of Health and Mental Hygiene. Community health survey profiles: Take Care Central Bronx. New York, NY: New York City Department of Health and Mental Hygiene, 2006. Available at: http://www.nyc.gov/html/doh/downloads/pdf/data/2006chp-105.pdf.

4. Sutton MY, Parks CP. HIV/AIDS prevention, faith, and spirituality among Black/African American and Latino communities in the United States: strengthening scientific faith-based efforts to shift the course of the epidemic and reduce HIV-related health disparities. J Relig Health. 2011 May 28 [Epub ahead of print].

5. Chatters LM, Levin JS, Ellison CG. Public health and health education in faith communities. Health Educ Behav. 1998 Dec;25(6):689–99.

6. Yanek LR, Becker DM, Moy TF, et al. Project joy: faith based cardiovascular health promotion for African American women. Public Health Rep. 2001;116(1 Suppl):68–81.

7. Boltri JM, Davis-Smith YM, Seale JP, et al. Diabetes prevention in a faith-based setting: results of translational research. J Public Health Manag Pract. 2008 Jan–Feb;14(1):29–32.

8. Samuel-Hodge CD, Keyserling TC, Park S, et al. A randomized trial of a church-based diabetes self-management program for African Americans with type 2 diabetes. Diabetes Educ. 2009 May–Jun;35(3):439–54.

9. Campbell MK, Demark-Wahnefried W, Symons M, et al. Fruit and vegetable consumption and prevention of cancer: the Black Churches United for Better Health Project. Am J Public Health. 1999 Sep;89(9):1390–6.

10. U.S. Department of Agriculture, U.S. Department of Health and Human Services. Dietary guidelines for Americans 2010. Washington, DC: U.S. Department of Agriculture, U.S. Department of Health and Human Services, 2010. Available at: http://health.gov/dietaryguidelines/dga2010/dietaryguidelines2010.pdf.

11. Knowler WC, Barrett-Connor E, Fowler SE, et al. Reduction in the incidence of type 2 diabetes with lifestyle intervention or metformin. N Engl J Med. 2002 Feb 7;346(6):393–403.

12. Hernan WH, Hoerger TJ, Brandle M, et al. The cost-effectiveness of lifestyle modification or metformin in preventing type 2 diabetes in adults with impaired glucose tolerance. Ann Intern Med. 2005 Mar;142(5):323–32.

13. Heikes KE, Eddy DM, Arondekar B, et al. Diabetes risk calculator: a simple tool for detecting undiagnosed diabetes and pre-diabetes. Diabetes Care. 2008 May;31(5):1040–5.

14. Kaplan SA, Calman NS, Golub M, et al. The role of faith-based institutions in addressing health disparities: a case study of an initiative in the southwest Bronx. J Health Care Poor Underserved. 2006 May;17(2 Suppl):9–19.

15. Davis K. Why is the church so fat? Charisma Magazine. 2004 Jun 30. Lake Mary, FL: Charisma Media. Available at: http://www.charismamag.com/site-archives/146-covers/cover-story/1265-why-is-the-church-so-fat.

16. Kaplan SA, Ruddock C, Golub M, et al. Stirring up the mud: using a community-based participatory approach to address health disparities through a faith-based initiative. J Health Care Poor Underserved. 2009 Nov;20(4):1111–23.

17. Wing RR, Hill JO. Successful weight loss maintenance. Annu Rev Nutr. 2001 Jul;21:323–41.

18. Oster G, Thompson D, Edelsberg J, et al. Lifetime health and economic benefits of weight loss among obese persons. Am J Public Health. 1999 Oct;89(10):1536–42.

CHAPTER 19

Changes for Life

A Primary Care–Based Multidisciplinary Program
for Obesity in Children and Families

Hollie A. Raynor, PhD, RD, Jena Saporito, PhD, and Parinda Khatri, PhD

As described repeatedly in this volume (see chapters 1–3, 13, 26, 27, and 29), the prevalence of childhood obesity has increased dramatically in the United States, and it is important to note that the most prominent increases have been seen in individuals of low socioeconomic status.[1–4] The adverse medical and psychosocial effects of pediatric obesity are well established.[5–11] To address the obesity epidemic, Healthy People 2020 has an objective to reduce the proportion of children and adolescents who are obese and has established a new developmental objective for preventing unhealthy weight gain in youths and adults.[12]

Treatment for pediatric obesity has progressed far in the past 25 years, and multicomponent, family-based behavioral interventions are now considered evidence-based treatments for obesity.[13] However, most of these types of programs are based in specialty settings serving a limited population.[13] Primary care is an ideal setting for an integrated approach to combat pediatric obesity. In the United States, children aged 2–21 years are encouraged to have well-child visits with their pediatricians annually;[14] at these visits, growth is monitored, thus allowing early identification and intervention for pediatric overweight and obesity.[15] Pediatricians report that part of their role in primary care is to address child weight status at well-child visits.[16] Finally, parents view primary care as an appropriate setting for childhood obesity treatment[17] and highly value a primary care provider's advice for health behavior management.[18–21]

Program Planning

To address the lack of pediatric obesity treatment available to families in Eastern Tennessee, Cherokee Health Systems (CHS; a federally qualified health center and

Hollie A. Raynor is an associate professor in the Department of Nutrition, University of Tennessee. Jena Saporito is a behavioral health consultant and Parinda Khatri is the director of Integrated Care, both at Cherokee Health Systems.

community health center that employs an integrated model of care in treating children and families) developed a pediatric weight management intervention to serve the needs of its families. The intervention targeted health behavior change in children and their families to improve children's weight status and reduce their risk of developing type 2 diabetes. Cherokee Health Systems has 22 clinic sites in 12 counties in Eastern Tennessee, providing care to over 57,000 patients in approximately 452,000 visits per year. Federally qualified health centers are community-based organizations that provide comprehensive primary and preventive health, dental health, and mental health / substance abuse services, regardless of a person's ability to pay.[22] The main purpose of these centers is to enhance access to comprehensive health care services in underserved urban and rural communities. The model of integrated primary care used by CHS involves embedding behavioral health providers as part of the primary care team.

To develop the program, CHS recognized the need for representation of disciplines that commonly interact in multicomponent pediatric obesity interventions. Thus, primary care providers, behavioral health consultants (independently licensed behavioral health providers, including psychologists and clinical social workers), and nurses were included in program development discussions. As CHS does not have nutrition professionals within the primary care setting, it worked with the Department of Nutrition at a local university (University of Tennessee), also involving the nutritionists in program development. This partnership led to Changes for Life, a program funded in part by the State of Tennessee, in which behaviorists and nutritionists applied evidence-based practice strategies during primary care visits. Changes for Life was implemented at CHS from 2009 to 2011.

Program Design and Implementation
Primary Care Recommendations

Evidence-based recommendations for pediatric obesity treatment in a primary care setting were established in 1997[23] and updated in 2007.[15] These recommendations encourage (1) targeting a few behaviors related to energy balance (i.e., reducing sugar-sweetened beverage consumption and screen time; increasing fruit and vegetable consumption and physical activity), using strategies to motivate families (i.e., motivational interviewing); (2) implementing behavior modification techniques (i.e., self-monitoring, goal setting, reinforcement) that assist with behavioral change, using a family-based approach; (3) establishing office systems that allow delivery of the recommendations; and (4) applying a staged approach to treatment.[15]

Program Components
Based on the recommendations for intervention in primary care, Changes for Life focused on three components: (1) eating more healthfully (i.e., reducing sugar-sweetened beverage consumption, increasing fruits and vegetables, making healthy choices at

fast-food restaurants, and making healthy food choices while shopping on a budget), (2) increasing physical activity (increasing daily activity and reducing screen time), and (3) implementing behavior modification strategies (goal setting, self-monitoring, self-management, and reinforcement) to assist with changing family eating and physical activity behaviors. Families were assessed in their readiness to change eating and activity behaviors, and motivational interviewing was used for those families with a lower readiness to change. Families established their own goals related to the eating and activity behaviors and developed their own self-management behavior modification plans to meet these goals, based on their stage of readiness to change. As Changes for Life was a multicomponent program, staff training was conducted annually so that behavioral, nutritional, and primary care team members were knowledgeable about and capable of implementing the three components of the program with families.

Implementation

At three designated CHS clinics that provide the majority of pediatric well-child visits at CHS, all children aged 2–18 years were screened at every well/sick visit for eligibility in Changes for Life. Eligibility criteria included body mass index (BMI) > 85th percentile, taking atypical antipsychotic medications, a family history of diabetes, and a family history of obesity. Height and weight were also measured at every office visit to determine the child's BMI and BMI percentile (based on the 2000 Centers for Disease Control and Prevention [CDC] BMI growth chart).[24] Primary care providers also reviewed the electronic health record (EHR) to identify whether children met any of the other three eligibility criteria for Changes for Life.

Children who were identified as eligible during office visits were immediately sent to the behavioral health consultant (usually a clinical psychologist) for a 15- to 30-minute in-person, consultation to discuss the program. During the consultation, the provider assessed the child's and parent's readiness to change and their interest in addressing the child's increased risk for developing type 2 diabetes. Families that were interested in receiving additional support were provided with education on healthy eating and/or physical activity and a readiness stage-matched behavioral intervention. Families were then offered regular follow-up appointments with the behavioral health consultant or nutritionist to provide encouragement and additional readiness stage-matched behavioral interventions. These follow-up appointments occurred as frequently as necessary (weekly if needed, with a goal to return no later than monthly); BMI was assessed at each visit.

Program Evaluation

Methods

Evaluation data included pre- and post-intervention measures. The data collected included height and weight, allowing calculation of BMI, BMI percentile, and standardized BMI (ZBMI). For children, ZBMI is calculated based on the value of the 50th BMI percentile and the standard deviation for the age- and sex-appropriate sample from the CDC growth charts.[24] ZBMI allows BMI to be compared among children of different genders and ages. Questions taken from the Youth Risk Behavior Surveillance System assessed children's fruit and vegetable intake, physical activity, and television watching.[25] Information collected was documented in the EHR. Pre-intervention measures were collected from families during their first consultation. Post-intervention measures were collected at each subsequent visit or at the end of the fiscal year in which the child had started the program for families that did not return for follow-up; thus, post-intervention data for each family were collected within one year of the first consultation. As a result, the length of time between pre- and post-intervention measures varied among families.

Outcomes

In the three CHS clinics implementing Changes for Life, according to an EHR review, there were 3,568 well-child visits, at which all children were to be screened, during the course of the program. Of the 3,568 children attending well-child visits, 1,197 were eligible for the program. Of these 1,197 children, 404 families (33.8% of families with an eligible child attending a well-child visit) completed pre-intervention measures during the initial consultation and expressed an interest in receiving additional support. The 404 participating children were aged 9.2 ± 4.3 years; 53.4% were male; 5.7% were African American and 43.0% Hispanic; and they had a BMI of $27.4 \pm 7.2 \, kg/m^2$, a ZBMI of 2.33 ± 0.58, and a BMI percentile of $96.1\% \pm 4.2\%$, indicating that the children were obese.

From these 404 families, post-intervention measures were collected on 106 children (26.2%). For these 106 children, outcomes revealed that 55.7% had a reduction in ZBMI, 57.3% increased fruit consumption, 36.9% increased vegetable consumption, 43.1% increased physical activity, and 44.5% reduced television watching on school days.

Program Modifications

Changes for Life was designed to be implemented in group sessions, in which children and their parents could attend sessions and receive education on healthy lifestyles, engage in some physical activity, and discuss the challenges and successes they were experiencing in relation to developing a healthy lifestyle. This discussion would allow families to provide support to each other. Despite scheduling the group sessions in the late afternoon and early evening on weekdays, attendance remained low. Similarly, offering incentives (e.g., a drawing for a free Wii at every group session) did not significantly affect group attendance. Thus, the delivery of Changes for Life shifted from a group format to individual family sessions. As this shift occurred, it became clear that rather than scheduling a separate appointment for families to attend, encouraging a "hand-off" (i.e., families meeting with a behavioral health provider immediately following the primary care visit) improved attendance and follow-up. This allowed families to become engaged in the program immediately after the primary care provider raised concerns about a child's risk for the development of type 2 diabetes. Similarly, attendance was improved by scheduling follow-up sessions to co-occur with other scheduled primary care appointments (e.g., for lab tests), rather than stand-alone behavioral appointments. Finally, unexpected cultural issues arose. For example, many Hispanic families reported consuming Agua Fresca (literally translated as "fresh water"), a behavior at first encouraged by providers. It was later clarified that Agua Fresca is a sugar-sweetened beverage, highlighting the need for understanding cultural differences in foods and beverages commonly consumed.

Limitations

While Changes for Life successfully improved weight status in over half of the children evaluated, as well as increasing self-reported healthy behaviors, the program had a few limitations. The first is that for the projected number of children eligible to participate in the program, the participation rate was fairly low. It is not clear whether the low rate of participation was due to lack of screening by the primary care providers, lack of interest in participating on the part of eligible families, or a combination of these two factors. Furthermore, only slightly more than a quarter of the families participating in the program completed the post-intervention evaluation. This may bias the reported outcomes due to self-selection bias, whereby families completing the evaluations may have experienced more positive outcomes. Increased documentation in the EHR regarding the screening process and the number of completed follow-up sessions by participating families would assist in understanding potential bias. Additionally, changes in consumption of sugar-sweetened beverages were not assessed in the evaluation, despite being a goal of many families.

Several factors might be important in translating this program into other primary care settings. For example, implementation of this type of program may be facilitated by EHRs (vs. paper records) for more accurate and efficient screening. Having providers who are trained in the three components of Changes for Life, particularly in behavior modification strategies, is important, and the setting at CHS afforded these opportunities.

Conclusions

A short-term, evidence-based pediatric obesity treatment program was implemented within a primary care setting and produced improvements in weight status and health behaviors in children at risk for the development of type 2 diabetes (see "Lessons Learned," below). Also noteworthy is that positive findings were evident in a traditionally underserved population—specifically, in families of lower socioeconomic status. Further work is needed to understand how participation rates for the program could be increased to better address the needs of families with children at risk for developing type 2 diabetes.

LESSONS LEARNED

- Individual family sessions that were delivered through "hand-offs" (families meeting with a behavioral health provider immediately following the primary care visit) increased participation.
- Scheduling follow-up sessions to coincide with other primary care appointments increased participation.
- Cultural issues around dietary choices can arise.
- Increased documentation in the EHR can help identify issues related to participation and follow-up.
- Provider training may be needed when providing a multicomponent program.

References

1. Hedley AA, Ogden CL, Johnson CL, et al. Prevalence of overweight and obesity among US children, adolescents, and adults, 1999–2002. JAMA. 2004 Jun 16;291(23):2847–50.
2. Ogden C, Troiano RP, Briefel RR, et al. Prevalence of overweight among preschool children in the United States, 1971 through 1994. Pediatrics. 1997 Apr;99(4):E1.
3. Ogden CL, Carroll MD, Curtin LR, et al. Prevalence of high body mass index in US children and adolescents, 2007–2008. JAMA. 2010 Jan 20;303(3):242–9.
4. Ogden CL, Carroll MD, Curtin LR, et al. Prevalence of overweight and obesity in the United States, 1999–2004. JAMA. 2006 Apr 5;295(13):1549–55.
5. Dietz WH. Health consequences of obesity in youth: childhood predictors of adult disease. Pediatrics. 1998 Mar;101(3 Pt 2):518–25.
6. Berenson GS, Srinivasan SR, Bao W, et al. Association between multiple cardiovascular risk factors and artherosclerosis in children and young adults: The Bogalusa Heart Study. N Engl J Med. 1998 Jun 4;338(23):1650–6.
7. Whitaker RC, Wright JA, Pepe MS, et al. Predicting obesity in young adulthood from childhood and parental obesity. N Engl J Med. 1997 Sep 25;337(13):869–73.
8. Guo SS, Wu W, Chumlea WC, et al. Predicting overweight and obesity in adulthood from body mass index values in childhood and adolescence. Am J Clin Nutr. 2002 Sep;76(3):653–8.
9. Sorof J, Daniels S. Obesity and hypertension in children: problem of epidemic proportions. Hypertension. 2002 Oct;40(4):441–7.
10. Freedman DS, Dietz WH, Srinivasan SR, et al. The relation of overweight to cardiovascular risk factors among children and adolescents: the Bogalusa Heart Study. Pediatrics. 1999 Jun 1;103(6 Pt 1):1175–82.
11. Latner JD, Stunkard AJ. Getting worse: the stigmatization of obese children. Obesity Res. 2003 Mar;11(3):452–6.
12. Healthy People 2020. Topics & objectives index—healthy people. Washington, DC: U.S. Department of Health and Human Services, 2012. Available at: http://www.healthypeople.gov/hp2020/Objectives/TopicAreas.aspx.
13. Epstein LH, Paluch RA, Roemmich JN, et al. Family-based obesity treatment, then and now: twenty-five years of pediatric obesity treatment. Health Psychol. 2007 Jul;26(4):381–91.
14. National Center for Biotechnology Information. Well-child visits. Bethesda, MD: A.D.A.M. Medical Encyclopedia, U.S. National Library of Medicine, 2011. Available at: http://www.ncbi.nlm.nih.gov/pubmedhealth/PMH0002655.

15. Spear BA, Barlow SE, Ervin C, et al. Recommendations for treatment of child and adolescent overweight and obesity. Pediatrics. 2007 Dec 1;120 Suppl 4:S254–88.

16. Klein JD, Sesselberg TS, Johnson MS, et al. Adoption of body mass index guidelines for screening and counseling in pediatric practice. Pediatrics. 2010 Feb;125(2):265–72.

17. Turner KM, Salisbury C, Sheild JP. Parents' views and experiences of childhood obesity management in primary care: a qualitative study. Family Prac. 2011 Aug;29(4):476–81.

18. Li V, Coates TJ, Ewart CK, et al. The effectiveness of smoking cessation advice given during routine medical care: physicians can make a difference. Am J Prev Med. 1987 Mar–Apr; 3(2):81–6.

19. Inui TS, Yourtee EL, Williamson JW. Improved outcomes in hypertension after physician tutorials: a controlled trial. Ann Intern Med. 1976 Jun;84(6):646–51.

20. Cohen M, D'Amico F, Merenstein JH. Weight reduction in obese hypertensive patients. Fam Med. 1991 Jan;23(1):25–8.

21. Sciamanna CN, Tate DF, Lang W, et al. Who reports receiving advice to lose weight? Results from a multistate survey. Arch Intern Med. 2000 Aug 14–18;160(15):2334–9.

22. Centers for Medicare and Medicaid Services. Medicare Learning Network [ICN 006397], Federally Qualified Health Center, rural health fact sheet series. Washington, DC: U.S. Department of Health and Human Services, 2011. Available at: http://www.cms.gov/Outreach -and-Education/Medicare-Learning-Network-MLN/MLNProducts/downloads/fqhcfact sheet.pdf.

23. Barlow SE, Dietz WH. Obesity evaluation and treatment: expert committee recommendations. The Maternal and Child Health Bureau, Health Resources and Services Administration, and the Department of Health and Human Services. Pediatrics. 1998 Sep;102(3):E29.

24. Kuczmarski RJ, Ogden CL, Grummer-Strawn LM, et al. CDC growth charts: United States. Adv Data. 2000;314:1–27.

25. Eaton DK, Kann L, Kinchen S, et al. Youth risk behavior surveillance—United States, 2007. MMWR Surveill Summ. 2008 Jun 6;57(4):1–131.

CHAPTER 20

The West Virginia PEIA Weight Management Program

An Innovative Approach to Obesity Prevention and Treatment in Appalachian Communities

Sam Zizzi, EdD, Christiaan Abildso, PhD, MPH, Nidia Henderson, MPA, and Kaitlyn Cobb, BS

Residents of West Virginia suffer disproportionately (higher prevalence and mortality) from many chronic illnesses, including cardiovascular diseases, diabetes, and multiple types of cancers. Not coincidentally, unhealthy behaviors (e.g., rates of smoking, not meeting recommendations for fruit and vegetable consumption and physical activity) and poor health outcomes (e.g., fair or poor self-rated health status, premature mortality) are higher than in the nation as a whole.[1] Approximately 33% of the adult population is classified as obese, for example, and nearly 12% of those over 18 are diagnosed with diabetes.*

Program Design and Implementation
History

Citing many of these poor health outcomes, the West Virginia Public Employees Insurance Agency (PEIA) began offering the Dean Ornish Program for Reversing Heart Disease as a member benefit in 2002. In July 2004, based on its experience with the Dean Ornish Program and noting a lack of offerings to meet its bariatric surgery eligibility requirement of 12 months of medically supervised weight management, PEIA developed and piloted a Weight Management Program at one approved provider.

Sam Zizzi is a professor of sport and exercise psychology at West Virginia University (WVU) and principal investigator on the contract with West Virginia PEIA. Christiaan Abildso is the program coordinator for the PEIA Weight Management Program, overseeing day-to-day operations and program evaluation. Nidia Henderson is the health promotions director at West Virginia PEIA, providing administration, oversight, and strategic management of wellness-oriented benefits. Kaitlyn Cobb coordinates all administrative functions related to the PEIA Weight Management Program, including enrollment, referrals, and all forms of participant communication.

* See chapters 11 and 19 for more work set in Appalachia.

Insurance agency administrators teamed up with Epi-Aid investigators from the Centers for Disease Control and Prevention's Division of Nutrition, Physical Activity, and Obesity to create a model of comprehensive care to provide individualized physical activity and nutrition behavioral change in community settings. The pilot was a 12-month intervention that provided access to an approved exercise facility, fitness assessments with an exercise physiologist (EP), medical nutrition therapy with a registered dietitian (RD), personal training with certified professionals (PTr), and case management with a nurse, conducted by phone.

For the pilot, insured members were eligible if their body mass index (BMI) was $\geq 30 \, \text{kg/m}^2$ or if they had a BMI between 25 and $29.9 \, \text{kg/m}^2$ and one or more concurrent chronic conditions that could be attenuated by increasing exercise and improving nutrition (i.e., heart disease, high blood pressure, cancer, diabetes, sleep apnea, metabolic syndrome). If eligible, members were required to provide informed consent, a physical activity acknowledgment, results of recent blood work, and a physician's approval to enroll. During the pilot period, enrollment was restricted to a few participants at five locations to allow a thorough evaluation of procedures and outcomes while feedback was solicited from participants, providers, and the agency. Participants consented to exercise at the designated facility at least twice a week, keep all scheduled appointments with service providers, cooperate with monthly measurement collection at the facility (height, weight, waist circumference, blood pressure, body fat percentage), maintain a food log, and submit monthly copayments to the facility. To remain in the program, participants were required to keep all appointments and to show progress in one of the outcomes measured each month by the provider. Much-needed back-end support was developed during the pilot, including a secure database that allowed providers to enter measurement data, confidentially exchange notes with other professionals, track monthly gym visits, and notify other database users about new referrals or participants' needs.

Program Growth

Following the pilot period, in which 52 people enrolled in the first four months, the program was expanded in 2005 to add seven new facilities and 356 participants, and it has steadily increased since. New program providers are solicited by a site development coordinator in conjunction with PEIA and must be approved to offer the program by PEIA. Facilities must meet strict criteria for safety (e.g., access to a defibrillator, properly maintained equipment), confidentiality (e.g., use of a private room for fitness assessments, compliance with Health Insurance Portability and Accountability Act–protected health information guidelines), and staffing (e.g., employing or contracting with a licensed/registered dietitian, employing certified fitness professionals). Providers are responsible for delivering professional services (RD, EP, PTr), documenting the services provided and the monthly measurements in the secure online database, billing PEIA for services provided, and collecting monthly member copayments. Currently approved providers include private (n = 26) and university-operated (n = 2) fitness/wellness centers, community centers (n = 8), physical therapy facilities (n = 13), a university-operated exercise physiology lab (n = 1), and hospital-affiliated wellness centers (n = 8). Further program expansion has occurred, including addition of a second year to the benefit in April 2007 and relaxation of the eligibility criteria in July 2011 to allow participation of all members with a BMI ≥ 25 kg/m² (regardless of other conditions) or a waist circumference ≥ 35 inches for women or ≥ 40 inches for men.

Service Expansion

In 2008, PEIA entered into a partnership with the College of Physical Activity and Sport Sciences at West Virginia University (WVU) to provide program evaluation and research services. This partnership has yielded numerous benefits, including a comprehensive evaluation of a single provider that provided face-to-face health behavior counseling;[2] a full evaluation of the program;[3] and a bevy of online resources, including nutrition tracking links, blog posts, and best-practice resources for both participants and providers. This partnership expanded further in July 2010 to engage WVU staff to administer the program and provide telephone-based health behavior counseling. In December 2010, an online eligibility screening and enrollment system was implemented, allowing greater efficiency in these administrative processes.

In the course of its history, the program has enrolled more than 4,000 participants who have achieved in-program weight loss of over 20 tons. As of May 21, 2012, the program included 1,063 active participants at 58 approved providers in 29 of 55 counties in West Virginia. Approximately two-thirds of participants complete at least six months in the program, and slightly less than one-half complete a year. Additionally, 47% of all participants have achieved clinically significant weight loss[2,3] (≥ 5% of body weight), and the percentage of participants meeting physical activity guidelines has doubled from pre- to post-program. Additional outcome data are available online (http://healthperformance.wordpress.com) and in our peer-reviewed articles.[4,5]

The Program Today

The current PEIA Weight Management Program benefit is a once-in-a-lifetime offering that, for a $20 monthly member copayment, provides access to the fitness facility and the following services:

1. Fitness assessments with an EP during months 1, 3, 6, and 13
2. Medical nutrition therapy with an RD during months 2, 4, 6, and 13
3. Certified PTr services for 120 minutes per month in months 1–5; 60 minutes per month in months 6–12; and 45 minutes per month in months 13–24
4. Telephone-based health behavior counseling every 45–60 days during year 1

Participants consent to comply with specific behavioral requirements or outcome goals and may be removed from the program for noncompliance. Behavioral requirements include:

1. Attending the facility at least twice per week
2. Making monthly copayments to the provider
3. Attending all meetings with professional service providers
4. Submitting food logs to the provider
5. Completing measurements monthly at the provider site

Outcome goals include (1) weight loss of 2.5% at 3 months, 5% at 6 months, 10% at 12 months and thereafter (or significant improvements in fitness or other measurements); or (2) BMI $\leq 25\,\text{kg/m}^2$ and waist circumference ≤ 35 inches (women) or ≤ 40 inches (men). WVU staff track participants' progress and assess their compliance and goal achievement each month, in conjunction with providers, to determine whether a participant should be removed from the program. Generally, participants are allowed a three-month probationary period prior to being removed if they are noncompliant or not meeting goals, but they can be removed at any time by the program administration or leave voluntarily.

Factors Promoting the Program's Success

In this section we discuss several of the replicable factors that other counties, states, or insurance agencies may want to consider in developing similar programs. In the next section we highlight the barriers encountered that continue to limit the growth of the program.

Delivering Quality Services That Promote Healthy Living after the Program

The best-practice recommendations for obesity treatment include individualized exercise and dietary modifications and behavioral counseling to support the lifestyle changes necessary to adopt and maintain these new habits.[6,7] The PEIA Weight Management Program was built on this idea—that is, to provide participants with access to trained professionals in their communities who can help teach and support participants in developing the necessary skills in fitness, nutrition, and behavioral change. Participant feedback through program evaluation surveys or during interviews or focus groups has validated the lasting impact that professionals can have on participants over the course of the program.

The Merging of the Fitness and Health Care Industries

The Weight Management Program was built upon and, subsequently, has enhanced the existing fitness and health infrastructure in West Virginia communities. This model takes an Exercise Is Medicine approach[8] that attempts to link the fitness and medical communities in the delivery of preventive services. One of the unanticipated benefits of this approach has been to identify (and in some cases to train) health professionals in underserved communities who are capable of working effectively with obese individuals with multiple comorbid health conditions. With the identification of these professionals and the facilities in which they work and, meanwhile, their association with a large insurance company, primary care physicians may be more likely to make referrals when they identify adults or children at risk for similar problems.

Finding a Cost-Effective Model for the Participant and for the Agency

Even in underserved areas, and even for participants of lower socioeconomic status, the $20 monthly price appears to be attractive to members. The shared investment of the participant (~20% of the program service cost) and the agency (~80%), along with external accountability that evaluates participants' progress, keeps participants engaged on a monthly basis and may be more effective than an access-only model, such as Silver Sneakers.[9] The Silver Sneakers program for older adults provides a basic membership in a fitness facility and access to educational resources related to healthy eating and active living. In West Virginia, there are over 60 locations to access this benefit; however, aside from occasional group exercise classes, no other professional services or external accountability are provided to help participants navigate the behavioral change process. Another factor that has been critical to the success and growth of the PEIA program is a set of administrators at the insurance agency who were willing to invest significant time, effort, and money in prevention. Given the complexity of the program and the many barriers faced, the easy road would have been to shut down the program in favor of a simpler, cheaper, watered-down approach. Their steadfast approach and the constant advocacy of the health promotions director at the agency have fueled the program's success, but with an eye toward developing a program that does not cost too much relative to participant outcomes.

Factors Limiting Program Growth or Success

The facilitative factors described above have allowed the program to have a positive impact on thousands of citizens in West Virginia. Many of those who have benefited from this program live in rural, underserved areas. However, there are many curves in the road when delivering this type of comprehensive program in the Appalachian region, and we are hopeful that future public health officials, program managers, or health insurance executives can learn from the struggles experienced in administering this program.

Limited Access to Facilities

Wide swaths of the state have no recreational or fitness facilities, and the vast majority of counties have extremely limited access (< 0.121 facilities per 1,000 residents).[10] Thus, rural residents who struggle to find proximal access to an urgent care facility, pharmacy, or hospital may also have little or no access to fitness and recreational facilities. PEIA, program development, and WVU staff constantly work to identify potential facilities and service providers in underserved areas in an effort to increase the reach of the program. Despite these efforts, many enrolled members still have to drive 30 minutes or longer to reach an approved facility to participate in this program. This driving barrier is compounded in the winter months when some participants are hesitant to drive in bad weather over mountainous terrain in some parts of the state.

Limited Access to Service Providers

The limitation in access is particularly evident in rural settings where the success of many fitness facilities hinges on one or two key health advocates in those communities. There have been several instances where small, successful sites were essentially dismantled due to the loss of one key stakeholder. There have been other examples, though, where program staff were able to intervene and provide training to support these personnel to keep a site active or to find a suitable replacement. In these underserved areas, and in similar areas all across the United States, this issue will persist. One promising trend is the growth of telehealth,[11] which may, in the near future, allow for the provision of individualized fitness and dietary services via distance technology in communities where access to trained staff is limited.

Difficulty of Standardizing Program Delivery

It is a constant struggle to provide members with a consistent benefit package across dozens of fitness facilities of different sizes that are staffed by several hundred health and fitness professionals with varying degrees of training. In many areas of this rural state, the program cannot be expected to maintain the same staffing and training standards as larger facilities in more urban areas. The coordinated care approach, facilitated by the secure web-based database, does allow all professionals to enter data and post participants' records so that all parties can share their experiences working with each participant. However, the program is not able to, nor does it aspire to, completely standardize how each RD, EP, and PTr interacts with each participant. There is no requirement for a specific type of scale for measuring body weight or a particular instrument or protocol for the measurement of body fat percentage or blood pressure. This limitation in the internal validity of the intervention is a natural consequence of adapting a complex behavior change program across multiple sites using a changing pool of health and fitness providers. These issues prevent a full understanding of the optimal dose of the intervention, for example, because we cannot compare with a control group or even make comparisons between some sites because we cannot be sure of how the program is being delivered in each case.

Fitness Facilities' Struggle in Adapting to a Professional Services Model of Payment

Health insurance companies and their associated third party providers are used to working with private entities, such as doctor's offices and urgent care clinics, that are accustomed to a pay-for-service model and have experience in navigating the insurance industry's billing process. Many of the private fitness facilities (particularly those that are not based in hospitals or housed in physical therapy clinics) have struggled to adapt to this model. These facilities make their money from monthly membership dues that are not contingent on participants' attendance. By contrast, to ensure payment for services rendered, PEIA requires facility staff to track members' visits and to submit billing receipts (in 15-minute increments) for EP, RD, and PTr services for each member for every month in the program. If a participant does not show up for a service, the facility is not paid. This model requires efficient scheduling of participants for professional services, and many providers struggle to meet the demand. Additionally, if the providers do not submit their monthly reports, they are not reimbursed for services rendered. Even when they do submit their monthly reports on time and the insurance agency reimburses them in a timely fashion (typically 30–60 days), this delay in payment is uncommon for professional services (fitness patrons are typically expected to pay immediately or even prior to receiving services). To ease the burden of this transition, PEIA provides trainings in the form of yearly meetings, web-based podcasts, and phone consultations with billing specialists.

Conclusions

We are hopeful that this report from the field inspires others to tackle the challenge of obesity prevention and treatment head on. Delivering these types of programs in underserved communities can be challenging, and many barriers will emerge. However, the potential public health impact of such an approach should not be underestimated. With vigilance and persistence, many can be served and many can reap the benefits of adopting and maintaining a healthy lifestyle.

LESSONS LEARNED
- Taking the time to identify potential locations for structured physical activity and to train motivated health professionals in rural communities appears to be a worthwhile investment of public tax dollars in the fight against obesity.
- One size does not fit all in rural communities. Given the limited access to quality facilities or trained health professionals in some communities, different strategies may be needed in each context to make the intervention most effective and sustainable.
- Most exercise facilities, with the exception of physical therapy clinics, have struggled to adapt to the fee-for-service norm in the insurance industry. Thus, though they are happy to have extra paying customers, the facility staff may require additional training to prepare for administrative requirements.

References

1. Centers for Disease Control and Prevention. Behavior risk factor surveillance system: 2009 prevalence data. Atlanta, GA: Centers for Disease Control and Prevention, 2012. Available at: http://apps.nccd.cdc.gov/brfss.

2. Wing RR, Koeske R, Epstein LH, et al. Long-term effects of modest weight loss in type II diabetic patients. Arch Intern Med. 1987 Oct;147(10):1749–53.

3. Mertens IL, Van Gaal LF. Overweight, obesity, and blood pressure: the effects of modest weight reduction. Obesity. 2000 May;8(3):270–8.

4. Abildso C, Zizzi S, Gilleland D, et al. A mixed methods evaluation of a 12-week insurance-sponsored weight management program incorporating cognitive-behavioral counseling. J Mixed Methods Res. 2010 Oct;4(4):278–94.

5. Abildso CG, Zizzi SJ, Reger-Nash B. Evaluating an insurance-sponsored weight management program with the RE-AIM model, West Virginia, 2004–2008. Prev Chronic Dis. 2010 May;7(3):A46.

6. NHLBI Obesity Education Initiative Expert Panel on the Identification, Evaluation, and Treatment of Obesity in Adults (US). Clinical guidelines on the identification, evaluation, and treatment of overweight and obesity in adults: the evidence report. Bethesda, MD: National Heart, Lung, and Blood Institute, 1998. Available at: http://www.ncbi.nlm.nih.gov/books/NBK2003.

7. Wadden TA, Stunkard AJ. Handbook of obesity treatment. New York, NY: Guilford Press, 2004.

8. American College of Sports Medicine. About Exercise Is Medicine. Indianapolis, IN: American College of Sports Medicine, 2008. Available at: http://exerciseismedicine.org/about.htm.

9. Healthways, Inc. What is the SilverSneakers fitness program? Franklin, TN: Healthways, Inc, 2012. Available at: http://www.silversneakers.com/TellMeEverything/WhatisSilverSneakers.aspx.

10. U.S. Department of Agriculture, Economic Research Service. Food environment atlas. Washington, DC: U.S. Department of Agriculture, 2012. Available at: http://maps.ers.usda.gov/FoodAtlas.

11. Maheu M, Whitten P, Allen A. E-health, telehealth, and telemedicine: a guide to start-up and success. Hoboken, NJ: John Wiley & Sons, 2001.

CHAPTER 21

SOPHE
Sustainable Solutions for Health Equity

Nicolette Warren, MS, MCHES, and Charlotte Kaboré, MS, MPH, MCHES

The Society for Public Health Education (SOPHE) is a 501(c)(3) professional organization, founded in 1950, that comprises 4,000 health education researchers and practitioners in all 50 states and in 19 chapters that cover 35 states, western Canada, and northern Mexico. SOPHE provides global leadership to the profession of health education and health promotion and eliminates health disparities through (1) advances in health education theory and research; (2) excellence in professional preparation and practice; and (3) advocacy for public policies conducive to health. SOPHE is the *only* independent professional organization devoted exclusively to health education and health promotion. Its 19 chapters provide "boots on the ground" linkages for continuing education, partnerships, networking, and advocacy at the state and local levels. Chapters are engaged in addressing health disparities through their continuing education activities, listservs, policy advocacy efforts, and collaboration with other organizations in their states or regions. Chapter outreach is complemented by SOPHE's connections to some 250 professional preparation programs in health education and public health around the country. The organization's national and chapter members are engaged in disease prevention and health promotion in both the public and private sectors. SOPHE has a rich, lengthy history of contribution to developing a research agenda for health disparities and advancing the application of evidence-based practices to improve community health. SOPHE chapters have been key partners in empowering health equity with community members to reduce diabetes and related risk factors among African American / Black (AA/B) and American Indian / Alaska Native (AI/AN) populations.

Inequalities in health status among racial and ethnic groups include the higher rates of obesity among American Indians / Alaska Natives and African Americans / Blacks than among non-Hispanic Whites. Obesity (as defined by body mass

Nicolette Warren is affiliated with the Society for Public Health Education; Charlotte Kaboré, with the Centers for Disease Control and Prevention.

index [BMI] $> 30 \, \text{kg/m}^2$) is a major factor in the high prevalence of diabetes among AA/B and AI/AN communities. Though it is not the only predictor, obesity is the best predictor of being newly diagnosed with diabetes. Age, race, and educational level are also associated with diabetes; race has an effect over and above body mass, which could be due to genetic influences or the possibility that being overweight has a more toxic effect in these groups.[1]*

According to the Office of Minority Health, AI/AN and AA/B populations are twice as likely as the non-Hispanic White adult population to have been diagnosed with diabetes by a physician.[2] The health impact of diabetes and obesity among AA/B populations in rural settings and AI/AN populations in urban settings is a major concern among public health professionals.

The Target Populations and Purposes of the Interventions
Jenkins County, Southeast Georgia

In 2006, African Americans made up 41.1% of the population of Jenkins County, located in rural southeast Georgia, compared with 29.9% in the State of Georgia.[3] Nearly 65% (64.9%) of these AA/B residents of Jenkins County were aged 20 years or older.[4] The Georgia Department of Human Resources places all of Jenkins County in the *lower middle socioeconomic status* and *lower socioeconomic status* demographic clusters.[4] In Jenkins County, African Americans aged 20 years and older accounted for 73% of all diabetes morbidity, defined as people treated for diabetes-related illness in nonfederal acute care inpatient facilities in 2006.[4]

The disproportionately high burden of diabetes morbidity in Jenkins County indicates a pressing need to address proper diabetes management as a focus for intervention(s). With diabetes morbidity in Jenkins County reaching populations 20–29 years old (the second largest age group in the county),[4] it is important that intervention activities be targeted at the greater county community to have a larger public health impact on preventing early-onset diabetes.

Northern California, San Francisco Bay Area

The San Francisco, California, Bay Area's American Indian community faces disproportionately high rates of diabetes, heart disease, obesity, and other health problems. The City of Oakland has a significantly higher rate of hospitalization for diabetes-related illness and a higher rate of diabetes-related death than the county (Alameda County).[5] Diabetes and diabetes-related illnesses are the leading causes of death for all AI/AN residents of the area.[5] Although American Indians have diabetes-related mortality rates that are three times those of all other races/ethnicities combined,[3] AI/AN populations are often not reported or recognized in Health Status Reports,

---

* See chapters 2–4, 6–8, and 10 for thorough presentations of central health disparities among subpopulations in the United States with respect to overweight and obesity. See chapter 27 for more work on obesity and overweight in American Indian children.

making it very difficult to track progress or reach community members with targeted programs.[6]

An important component of reversing the numerous challenges facing the Bay Area AI/AN community is to reconnect people to traditional, enjoyable, community-rich forms of exercise and to revitalize knowledge and interest in traditional foods, which are significantly more healthful. By creating this model at Intertribal Friendship House (IFH; a community center well versed in bridging the differences among more than 500 different tribes), IFH can weave a healthy, well-connected, and organized community that is better able to voice its needs and sustain itself.

Aims of the Interventions

The socioecological model states that the behavior of an individual is determined not only by intrapersonal characteristics such as knowledge, attitudes, beliefs, and personality traits but also by relationships with family and peers, organizational structures, social networks within the community, and public policies.[7] This model provided the framework for a collaborative partnership to encourage improved dietary habits and increased levels of physical activity among AI/AN and AA/B communities. Improved prevention, treatment, and management of diabetes and obesity will not only reduce the economic burden of diabetes but also improve health outcomes and quality of life for the AI/AN and AA/B communities. In this chapter we describe the feasibility and acceptability of SOPHE chapters' work with community-based organizations to combat diabetes and obesity among AI/AN and AA/B communities through sponsored health promotion interventions and trainings.

SOPHE Chapters and Community-Based Organizations Join Forces

This pilot project was conducted to develop a strategic, sustainable initiative to address the growing health burden of diabetes and obesity among AA/B and AI/AN communities. The goals were (1) to build SOPHE chapters' leadership and partnership capacity to facilitate community action on policy and environmental systems change; (2) to extend the lives of AI/AN populations, who suffer disproportionately from disease and disability; (3) to work with AA/B communities to develop tools, policies, and strategies to improve the social conditions that are the root cause of health inequities; and (4) to improve the lives of racial/ethnic populations that suffer disproportionately from the burden of disease and disability.

In September 2009, SOPHE's Health Equity Project was funded by the Centers for Disease Control and Prevention (CDC) to encourage SOPHE chapters to engage with Racial and Ethnic Approaches to Community Health (REACH), Centers of Excellence in the Elimination of Disparities (CEEDs), and local partners, including community-based organizations and members, to address the risk factors associated with diabetes and other chronic diseases among AA/B and AI/AN populations.

An advisory committee was established, consisting of experts in the field of minority health and working with AI/AN and AA/B populations. This committee served

Table 21.1. SOPHE Collaborative Partnerships

Georgia SOPHE	National SOPHE	Northern California SOPHE
American Cancer Society	Alliance to Reduce Disparities in Diabetes	Berkeley Farmers Market
American Heart Association	American Association for Diabetes Educators	Community members with diabetes
Bump It Up a Buck Coalition	American Diabetes Association	Community members (local businesses, grocers)
Centers for Disease Control and Prevention (CDC)	CDC Division of Diabetes Translation	Intertribal Friendship House
Community members with diabetes	Center for Managing Chronic Disease at University of Michigan	Mills College
Community members (local businesses, grocers)	Department of Health and Human Services / Office of Minority Health	Native American Health Center, Oakland
Emory University	Regional Health Equity Councils	Oakland Food Policy Council
Georgia Department of Public Health	National Association of Chronic Disease Directors	San Jose State University
Georgia Diabetes Coalition	REACH/CEED–University of Colorado in Denver	Seva Foundation
Georgia Public Health Association	SOPHE Minority Communities Advisory Committee	Slow Foods East Chapter
Georgia Rural Health Association		University of California, Berkeley
Georgia Southern University		
Georgia State University		
Georgians for a Healthy Future		
Gordon County Chamber of Commerce		
Jenkins County Diabetes Coalition		
North Georgia Health District 1–1		
North Georgia Health District 1–2		
Partner Up! for Public Health		
Policy Leadership for Active Youth		
REACH Legacy Project 2009		
State of Georgia Breast and Cervical Cancer Control Program		
Susan G. Komen, Chattanooga Affiliate		

as the oversight body for the overall project and assisted with all major project activities (e.g., request for proposals and chapter selection). Georgia and Northern California SOPHE chapters established collaborative partnerships with community leaders to assess need (table 21.1), to develop action plans, to implement culturally tailored initiatives, and to disseminate initiative efforts emphasizing the program's theory of change for addressing health disparities.[8]

Each of these chapters received $250,000 in funding for five years. SOPHE integrated shared decision-making authority among chapters and their community partners, accomplished by expecting chapters to allocate 50% of their funding to community partners. Chapter partnerships developed unique community-led strategies to address diabetes and obesity disparities in their communities. This practice supported a community-based participatory approach among SOPHE, the chapters, and their partners to prevent diabetes and reduce obesity among AI/AN and AA/B populations.[9]

Georgia SOPHE Chapter Intervention

The Georgia SOPHE project brought together chapter members at Georgia Southern University and community members to work with the rural AA/B population and the community-based Jenkins County Diabetes Coalition in Millen, Georgia, to prevent diabetes and obesity. The project focused on developing and expanding the capacity for change in Jenkins County. Georgia SOPHE and various community-based partners combined their efforts to enhance the capacity of local and regional AA/B community members who suffer disproportionately from diabetes and obesity.

The Georgia SOPHE and Jenkins County Diabetes Coalition members organized a fitness intervention during the county's largest annual community event. Approximately 150 pedometers and state fair passports (walking logs) and 100 American Diabetes Association educational brochures were distributed. The Jenkins County Diabetes Coalition employed the Coalition Effective Inventory self-assessment tool to evaluate the strengths of the coalition and its stages of development.[10] For each coalition meeting, the Coalition Meeting Checkup form was used to assess the effectiveness of the meeting.[10] The Diabetes Coalition used coalition development and evaluation tools to document effectiveness.

Pre- and post-tests were conducted on general diabetes knowledge, monitoring, medication, exercising, care for feet and eyes, blood pressure, kidney function, and better nutrition. The change in mean score for pre- and post-tests was calculated and interpreted with care due to the low sample size. With respect to the Road to Health training, pre- and post-test results for 10 of the 14 participants showed a small increase in basic diabetes knowledge. Given the small sample, statistical analysis of the difference between mean pre-test score and mean post-test score cannot be used to draw inferences. Diabetes 101 train-the-trainer sessions were conducted to increase knowledge of diabetes.

The Jenkins County Diabetes Coalition's development efforts were guided by community empowerment, Coalition Technical Assistance and Training, and capacity-building models.[10] The Coalition Development Training in Strategic Planning activities were evidence- and best practice–based to contribute to the success of the coalition activities.[10] All Coalition Development in Strategic Planning trainings were evaluated through evidence-based, best-practice tools in the form of an open-ended questionnaire. Anecdotally, the ongoing coalition facilitator noted individual changes in some of the coalition members.

Northern California SOPHE Chapter Intervention

Northern California SOPHE's goal is to build leadership and partnership capacity to implement sustainable diabetes and obesity prevention and management interventions and to monitor change among AI/AN populations in the urban Bay Area of California. The chapter (with the Seva Foundation) worked with the only community-based American Indian center in the San Francisco Bay area (Intertribal Friendship House), in Oakland. This partnership established the Health Action Collaborative team. The Seva Foundation is an international health organization working to build sustainable programs in underserved communities around the globe.

The chapter's strategy was to build organizational awareness, trust, and familiarity by attending key community events such as the Native American Health Center meeting, IFH's Harvest Auction fundraiser event and dinner, the Seva World Diabetes Day Dinner, and IFH / Seva Foundation Health Equity Kick-off Gathering meetings. This was central to the project's success and to accomplishing the community-based participatory research goals.[11]

The SOPHE chapter, Seva Foundation, and IFH coordinated a community event for partners and community residents to discuss activities/ideas for implementing the policy, systems, and environmental change approaches and tools. The Health Action Collaborative team attended biweekly meetings of the Oakland Food Policy Council and the Slow Foods East Bay Chapter to enable IFH to reduce health disparities with more environmentally based program activities. The SOPHE chapter and the Health Action Collaborative team participated in the Running Is My High event that supports Native health. This event had 586 participants. As a result, the team recruited 45 participants for the IFH community gardening program.

The chapter supported the eight-week garden-program diabetes self-management education activities, which produced substantive shifts in knowledge, skills, and abilities. In the IFH community, members expressed satisfaction about the garden and enjoyment of working in and eating the products from the garden. These activities significantly strengthened the community's advocacy to raise participants' health needs and sustain itself.

The Health Action Collaborative team used Seva's highly effective training, called Diabetes Talking Circles, at IFH. Diabetes Talking Circles helps Native people develop self-management strategies for diabetes prevention and treatment. Seva's Native American Community Health Program builds sustainable health programs focused on food justice and the prevention of diabetes. Social capital values social networks; interaction enables people to build communities, to commit themselves to each other, and to knit the social fabric. A sense of belonging and the concrete experience of social networks (and the relationships of trust and tolerance that can be involved) can bring great benefits to people.[12]

The collaborative partnerships of the Northern California SOPHE chapter in engaging urban AI/AN communities and the Georgia SOPHE chapter in engaging rural AA/B communities led to important lessons for the SOPHE Health Equity Project (see "Lessons Learned," below).

Discussion

The SOPHE project addressed the social determinants of health, using evidenced-based strategies and tools to eliminate health disparities. The project built the capacity of SOPHE chapters to effect change at the local level and to promote community empowerment through nontraditional physical activity and nutrition interventions.

The results of this pilot project show the extent to which the Georgia and Northern California SOPHE chapters helped to improve diabetes and obesity disparities in their local communities. Through this CDC cooperative agreement, SOPHE engaged Georgia and Northern California SOPHE chapters, REACH/CEEDs, national partners, community-based organizations, and community members to support a national framework to eliminate health disparities and promote health equity among AA/B and AI/AN populations, in an effort to reduce and prevent diabetes and promote health. SOPHE demonstrated the feasibility of chapters working with community-based organizations and universities to build a foundation for policy and environmental change, using nontraditional physical activity and nutrition interventions.

LESSONS LEARNED

For key project personnel, critical factors are:
- Careful selection of partners
- Management of project staff turnover
- Establishment of standard operating procedures for all chapter activities, especially policy and procedures to handle personnel compliance
- Leadership development and training of volunteers
- Staff training
- Effective communication

For collaborative partnerships, critical factors are:
- Time: community-based partnerships take at least 6–9 months to establish
- Trust and respect
- Equitable funding of partners
- Representation of community members with diabetes and other related chronic diseases in planning self-management programs
- Development of partnership agreements
- Initial needs assessments and trainings to build effective action plans
- Cultural competence

Project evaluation requires:
- Establishing clear expectations
- Technical assistance that is strategic and useful
- Developing competence-based technical assistance, requiring a team approach with experts and community involvement

- Identifying tools for reporting progress, to manage technical assistance effectively
- Managing funders' and community partners' expectations
- Evaluating dissemination efforts to assess project reach

Building and developing chapter capacity requires:

- Strong membership recruitment and retention plans
- Accountability and commitment for chapter activities (e.g., project management and implementation, evaluation, continuing education, partnerships, resource development, marketing, communication, and dissemination)
- Creating a balance between capacity building, improving individual and community health, and promoting health education
- Access to technology (e.g., website, Internet, computer, office space, electronic communication)
- A foundation to operate as an independent nonprofit organization
- Providing unique opportunities to reconnect with colleagues, thus rejuvenating commitment
- In-depth webinar content
- Sustainable funding to support capacity building, development, and project implementation

Acknowledgments

This work was supported by Cooperative Agreement Number 5U58DP002328-03 from the Centers for Disease Control and Prevention. The contents of this chapter are solely the responsibility of the authors and do not necessarily represent the official views of the Centers for Disease Control and Prevention. The authors thank the community partners and participating community members for their contributions to this project. The authors had no professional relationship with any company or manufacturer that would benefit from the results of this project.

References

1. Kuo S, Fleming BB, Gittings NS, et al. Trends in care practices and outcomes among Medicare beneficiaries with diabetes. Am J Prev Med. 2005 Dec;29(5):396–403.
2. Office of Minority Health. Diabetes data/statistics. Washington, DC: U.S. Department of Health and Human Services, 2012. Available at: http://www.minorityhealth.hhs.gov/templates/browse.aspx?lvl=3&lvlid=62.
3. U.S. Census Bureau. State and county quick facts: data derived from population estimates, American community survey, census of population and housing, state and county housing unit estimates, county business patterns, nonemployer statistics, economic census, survey of business owners, building permits, consolidated federal funds report. Suitland, MD: U.S.

Census Bureau, 2008. Available at: http://quickfacts.census.gov/qfd/states/13/13165.html and http://quickfacts.census.gov/qfd/states/13000.html.

4. Office of Health Indicators for Planning. Online Analytical Statistical Information System (OASIS). Atlanta, GA: Georgia Department of Public Health, 2012. Available at: http://oasis.state.ga.us.

5. Alameda County Public Health Department. County health status report 2006. Oakland, CA: Alameda County Public Health Department, 2006. Available at: http://www.acphd.org/media/52956/achsr2006.pdf.

6. California Diabetes Control Program. The burden of diabetes in California counties. Sacramento, CA: California Department of Health Services, 2000. Available at: http://sandiegohealth.org/disease/diabetes/stat-burdenofdiabetesca1.pdf.

7. Robinson T. Applying the socio-ecological model to improving fruit and vegetable intake among low-income African Americans. J Community Health. 2008 Dec;33(6):395–406.

8. Tucker P, Liao Y, Giles WH, et al. The REACH 2010 logic model: an illustration of expected performance. Prev Chronic Dis. 2006 Jan;3(1):A21.

9. Wallerstein NB, Duran B. Using community-based participatory research to address health disparities. Health Promot Pract. 2006 Jul;7(3):312–23.

10. Butterfoss FD. Coalitions and partnerships in community health. Hoboken, NJ: Jossey-Bass, 2007.

11. Minkler M, Wallerstein N, eds. Community-based participatory research for health: from process to outcomes. Hoboken, NJ: Jossey-Bass, 2008.

12. Smith MK. Social capital. In: The encyclopedia of informal education. London, UK: YMCA George Williams College, 2009. Available at: http://www.infed.org/biblio/social_capital.htm.

CHAPTER 22

The Prevention of Obesity in Homeless Shelter Settings

Melissa Bennett, MD, Melissa Berrios, MSW, and Karen Hudson, MSW, LSW

The Children's Hospital of Philadelphia's Homeless Health Initiative (HHI) is a multidisciplinary health outreach effort that aims to help women and children living in shelters achieve optimal health and life potential. Under the dedicated leadership of a social work program leader, medical advisor, and social work trainer, hundreds of HHI volunteers provide free, high-quality medical and dental screenings, access to health insurance, access to primary and specialty care services, and health education workshops to families living in select Philadelphia emergency housing shelters. In Philadelphia, family shelters primarily serve women and children.

Shelter staff and families enlisted HHI's expertise to assist in preventing obesity. Thanks to the three-year support of the Philadelphia Foundation, HHI developed and implemented an obesity prevention program—Operation CHOICES. This program has nutrition and physical fitness components that can be delivered separately or together and are tailored to different age groups, including adults, school-age children, and preschoolers. This chapter details the development and implementation of Operation CHOICES, specifically targeting women and children living in shelters; however, we believe that the program can be replicated in various settings.*

Obesity, Food Insecurity, and Homelessness

Nationally, obesity continues to worsen and disproportionately affects those of low socioeconomic status, including women and children experiencing homelessness. Obesity prevalence among children and adolescents has nearly tripled in the past three decades, affecting 12.5 million children.[1] One of seven low-income preschool

---

Melissa Bennett, Melissa Berrios, and Karen Hudson are affiliated with the Children's Hospital of Philadelphia Homeless Health Initiative: Operation CHOICES obesity prevention programming for families experiencing homelessness.

* See chapters 5 (on prison populations) and 9 (on members of the military) for other work on people living in controlled environments and the effect of such environments on healthy weight.

children is overweight or obese. While the national obesity epidemic receives widespread attention, little consideration is given to the impact of obesity and food insecurity on families experiencing homelessness.*

Estimates from Baltimore and New York suggest that as many as 31% of children in shelters may already qualify as overweight or obese.[2,3] Physical disorders linked to obesity include cardiovascular disease, diabetes, sleep apnea, and organ failure.[4] These comorbid disorders ultimately decrease quality of life for individuals and increase costs to society through higher utilization of medical services.[5] Furthermore, children experiencing obesity are often targets of bullying, discrimination, and poor self-esteem, exacerbating trauma experienced in shelters and compounding psychological disorders.[6] They are also more likely to become adults who struggle with obesity.[7]

Food insecurity, defined by the U.S. Department of Agriculture (USDA) as limited or uncertain access to adequate food,[8] affects an estimated 17.3 million households.[9] Two-thirds of children experiencing homelessness worry that they will not have sufficient food to eat; over one-third have been forced to skip meals; they are twice as likely as children with homes to experience hunger.[10]

In shelters, food availability becomes more certain for families, though food choices, timing of meals, and meal preparation are often not in their control. Trauma and depression, which affect many families in poverty, may also contribute to obesity. All of these factors contribute to the coexistence of food insecurity and obesity among families living in poverty, especially those experiencing homelessness.

Development and Implementation of Operation CHOICES

After learning from families and staff in shelters about the experiences of obesity and the nutrition and physical activity needs of families, HHI leadership organized a leadership team of experienced and dedicated pediatricians and social workers. The Operation CHOICES leadership team recruited and guided health care volunteers to address the nutrition and physical activity needs of families living in shelters. As a result, the Operation CHOICES team has created and implemented nutrition and physical activity curricula for families in shelters; while Operation CHOICES leadership has advocated on behalf of families at the shelter and city level.

The Shelter Environment Compounds Limitation of Choices

The Operation CHOICES team conducted interviews and focus groups with staff, women, and children (separately) to learn more about their needs. Staff and families expressed interest in nutrition education, increasing physical activity, growing fresh food, cooking classes, creating choices for families—especially children—at mealtime, and identifying community resources that would help them access fresh produce. Families described barriers to making healthy nutrition and fitness choices, includ-

---

* See chapters 1, 2, and 10, as well as other chapters in part III, on issues of childhood obesity and food insecurity.

ing limited access to the kitchen; lack of affordable fresh produce, green spaces, and transportation options; and an overabundance of fast food and corner stores that promote inexpensive, low-nutritional-value foods. All of these barriers are probably contributing to increasing rates of obesity.

Using this information, HHI health care volunteers created Operation CHOICES, a dynamic nutrition and physical fitness program, which consists of fun, hands-on nutrition and fitness education tailored to families living in shelters, as well as community advocacy. The leadership team led a multidisciplinary volunteer health care team of 15 pediatricians, nurses, dietitians, physical therapists, and social workers, all with field experience, in developing nutrition and physical activity curricula for women and children living in shelters.

Program Components

Nutrition Originally, the nutrition program consisted of a six-lesson cycle, on the same day and at the same time for six consecutive weeks, for mothers and children together. The nutrition curriculum was developed by a pediatric resident with previous experience at the USDA and a dietitian, with input and guidance from the leadership team. Based on participant feedback, the Operation CHOICES team tailored lessons for adult women, school-age children, and preschool children. The adult nutrition curriculum components include learning about basic food groups, nutrition labels, serving sizes, vitamins and minerals, eating in moderation, hypertension, and heart disease, and a field trip to a local supermarket. Similar themes are taught simultaneously to preschool and school-age groups to reinforce the lessons taught to their parents. All sessions include visual props, healthy snacks, handouts, and tip sheets. For preschoolers, lessons are made fun by reading age-appropriate books, such as *Growing Vegetable Soup*, making crafts, coloring pictures, singing songs, and helping adults make healthy snacks. Healthy snacks are offered at every interaction to expose families to tasty, healthy foods.

Physical Activity Like the nutrition program, the physical activity program occurred on the same day and at the same time for six consecutive weeks, with mothers and children together. A cardiovascular nurse developed sessions to include topics on physical activity guidelines, the importance of exercise, exercise and the heart, exercise and the lungs, the importance of hydration, and healthy eating. Based on participant feedback, the Operation CHOICES team created separate groups for women and children. The women's groups focus on health and wellness, including yoga, kickboxing, and breathing techniques. Physical therapist volunteers tailored the children's program, which is now called SPARK—Safe Physical Activity and Recreation for Kids—to provide education and safe, structured physical activities. The curriculum includes lesson plans, activities, and a how-to manual. Programming focuses on themes of flexibility, endurance, strengthening, balance, coordination, and agility. The physical activities include dancing, relay races, and exercises. All activities are based on the limited resources available to families in shelters. The leadership team believes it is important to show families how to increase their physical activity without money or resources such as fitness equipment or gym memberships.

Integration of Nutrition and Physical Activity During the second year of programming, HHI implemented families' request that the Operation CHOICES team integrate nutrition and physical activity into each session. Furthermore, the program no longer runs on six-week cycles, alternating between nutrition and fitness; rather, it runs continuously throughout the year, with weekly sessions combining nutrition and fitness lessons.

Due to the overwhelmingly positive response from families, HHI currently offers seven sessions a week at three women and children's shelters—three sessions for mothers and four sessions for children. During the past three years, over 700 mothers and children have participated in Operation CHOICES programming in the three shelters.

Volunteers

Volunteers are recruited primarily from Children's Hospital of Philadelphia and local universities and receive training from an HHI leader. In addition to learning how to teach the curriculum, volunteers are also taught to deliver programming in a trauma-informed manner. Over 100 volunteers have been trained and delivered programming during three years of Operation CHOICES.

Trauma

Trauma is an experience that produces feelings of fright, terror, or powerlessness that thwart a person's ability to cope.[11] Many of the families served by Operation CHOICES have experienced trauma.[12] HHI aims to deliver all of its programming using a trauma model of care, and volunteers, as noted above, are trained accordingly.

Challenges and Outcomes

Challenges include finding green spaces in safe, walkable proximity to the urban shelters. Communication with families about programming was initially difficult, resulting in low attendance, but once class times became routine and shelter staff and families developed positive relationships with volunteers, attendance skyrocketed from under 60 women and children to over 700 participants. Other challenges included the intensive amount of time required to recruit, train, and coordinate schedules. Initial problems related to the behavior of some children who were coping with trauma led to the formation of smaller groups based on age, which allowed volunteers to provide better supervision and support.

As Operation CHOICES is a behavioral education and prevention program for mothers and children in emergency housing, quantitative outcome measurements have been very challenging. Participants enter and exit the shelters and programs at different time points and have lives complicated by numerous confounding variables (e.g., life stressors, mental health issues, trauma, depression). Furthermore, body mass index may not change in the amount of time families are in a shelter, where they may have little control over their food and activity choices. HHI has attempted to demonstrate outcomes by increasing the numbers of participating families (increasing almost 400% over three years) and volunteers (increasing approximately 1,000% over three years). HHI is currently evaluating families' readiness to change and the impact of programming, through interviews and written surveys with mothers. This has also posed challenges, as participants often do not have protected time after programming to engage in the evaluations.

Creating Cultures That Value Healthy Choices and Fostering Community Connections

Shelter and community representatives share successful strategies regarding healthy nutrition and food choices at quarterly HHI stakeholder meetings and at special events. HHI collaborates with shelter staff, city government, and community service providers to encourage a child-friendly, culturally respectful environment that supports healthy choices. One shelter improved the dining experience for families by playing music during mealtimes. At another shelter, kitchen staff invite parents to help with food preparation and service, and families taste-test new items before they are added to the menu.

To work toward sustainability, HHI has helped its three partner shelters connect with local community agencies to offer cooking programs to families, support a garden, and offer storage space for mothers to practice shopping and preparing a healthy snack. Local universities offer volunteers and contribute the use of green field space for fitness programming. HHI encourages and supervises local schools and community groups that wish to host food drives to support a shelter's food pantry.

Conclusions

Evidence shows that behavioral and societal changes have contributed to the obesity epidemic.[13] Given the epidemic's complex roots, it is critical to address it from multiple angles and to involve stakeholders in finding solutions. Prevention through education and experiential opportunities, as offered in Children's Hospital of Philadelphia's Homeless Health Initiative's Operation CHOICES program, can assist in curbing the obesity epidemic. Experience with Operation CHOICES shows that a variety of approaches, strong leadership and relationships, and investment of time are necessary to change behavior and shift community attitudes toward healthy nutrition and fitness.

LESSONS LEARNED
- Establish dedicated program leadership to interact regularly with the city, community, program volunteers, and shelter stakeholders—both staff and families.

- Seek the WIFM (What's in It For Me) from all stakeholders, and secure their commitment to the program.
- Make obesity prevention sensitive to the context, addressing the needs of the target population and the environmental context.
- Build trusted relationships with all stakeholders; doing so requires time and consistency.
- Motivate participants through the consistency of volunteers and program delivery.
- Standardize recruitment, training, and mentoring of large groups of volunteers to deliver such consistency.
- Communicate regularly with stakeholders to inform and improve program delivery while in progress.
- Deliver messages about healthy nutrition and fitness choices frequently to reinforce healthy lifestyle lessons.
- Deliver programming using a variety of dynamic modalities and fun activities to appeal to various audiences and to encourage choices.

References

1. Ogden C, Carroll MD. Prevalence of obesity among children and adolescents: United States, trends 1963–1965 through 2007–2008. Atlanta, GA: Centers for Disease Control and Prevention, National Center for Health Statistics, 2010. Available at: http://www.cdc.gov/nchs/data/hestat/obesity_child_07_08/obesity_child_07_08.pdf.
2. Han JC, Lawlor DA, Kimm SY. Childhood obesity. Lancet. 2010 May 15;375(9727): 1737–48.
3. Finkelstein EA, Trogdon JG, Cohen JW, et al. Annual medical spending attributable to obesity: payer- and service-specific estimates. Health Aff (Millwood). 2009 Sep–Oct;28(5): w822–31.
4. Whitlock EP, Williams SB, Gold R, et al. Screening and interventions for childhood overweight: a summary of evidence for the US Preventive Services Task Force. Pediatrics. 2005 Jul;116(1):e125–44.
5. Biro FM, Wien M. Childhood obesity and adult morbidities. Am J Clin Nutr. 2010 May; 91(5):1499–505S.
6. Nord M, Andrews M, Carlson S. Household food security in the United States, 2006. Washington, DC: Economic Research Service, U.S. Department of Agriculture, 2012. Available at: www.ers.usda.gov/publications/err49.
7. Coleman-Jensen A, Nord M, Andrews M, et al. Household food security in the United States in 2010. Washington, DC: Economic Research Service, U.S. Department of Agriculture, 2011. Available at: http://www.ers.usda.gov/Publications/ERR125/err125.pdf.
8. Grant R, Shapiro A, Joseph S, et al. The health of homeless children revisited. Adv Pediatr. 2007;54:173–87.
9. Schwartz KB, Garrett B, Hampsey J, et al. High prevalence of overweight and obesity in homeless Baltimore children and their caregivers: a pilot study. MedGenMed. 2007 Mar 7;9(1):48.

10. Bassuk EL, Murphy C, Coupe NT, et al. America's youngest outcasts. Needham, MA: National Center on Family Homelessness, 2011.
11. Hopper EK, Bassuk EL, Olivet J. Shelter from the storm: trauma-informed care in homelessness services settings. Open Health Serv Policy J. 2010;3:80–100.
12. Bassuk EL, Weinreb LF, Buckner JC. The characteristics and needs of sheltered homeless and low-income housed mothers. JAMA. 1996 Aug 28;276(8):640–6.
13. Nader PR, Huang TT, Gahagan S, et al. Next steps in obesity prevention: altering early life systems to support healthy parents, infants, and toddlers. Child Obes. 2012 Jun;8(3): 195–204.

CHAPTER 23

Get FIT (Fitness Integration Training)

A Program to Reduce Obesity and Metabolic Syndrome
in People with Intellectual and Developmental Disabilities
and Their Caregivers

Laurie DiRosa, EdD, Thomas Pote, BA, Barbara Wilhite,
EdD, and Leslie Spencer, PhD

Maintaining health and wellness is important for people with disabilities and their caregivers and is neglected more frequently than average in this population. Not surprisingly, people with intellectual and developmental disabilities (IDD) tend to be more sedentary than their nondisabled counterparts. In 2009, the Centers for Disease Control and Prevention (CDC) reported that 22% of adults (aged 18 and older) with disabilities participated in no leisure-time physical activity, compared with 10% of adults without disabilities. Research also demonstrates that compared with people without a disability, people with IDD are more likely to have poor health, to be susceptible to illness, to have limited access to health care, and to be excluded from health promotion opportunities. Approximately 40% of those with disabilities rate their health as fair/poor, compared with 10% of those without disabilities.[1]

People with IDD are also at a far greater risk for health-compromising conditions secondary to their disability, such as higher rates of high cholesterol and blood pressure, along with higher rates of obesity[2–4] and metabolic syndrome.* Metabolic syndrome is a combination of risk factors for both cardiovascular disease and diabetes, which exacerbate each other. Specifically, metabolic syndrome occurs in a person who is obese, has a high fasting blood sugar (indicative of prediabetes), is hypertensive,

---

Laurie DiRosa is an adjunct professor and the nutrition and research consultant of the Get FIT program at Rowan University. Thomas Pote is founder and owner of Pulse Fitness Professionals and the fitness consultant of the Get FIT program. Barbara Wilhite has coordinated the Get FIT initiative since its inception in 2008, for all of New Jersey, through the Family Resource Network. Leslie Spencer is a professor of health and exercise science and the faculty coordinator / principal investigator of the Get FIT program.

* The facts about barriers to exercise for people with disability discussed in this chapter illustrate in a fresh way the underlying premise of much of this volume—that structural social factors must be addressed to stem the tide of overweight and obesity in underserved communities in the United States. See the introduction and chapter 7 for development of this point of view.

and shows one or more signs of atherosclerosis (high triglyceride levels, low blood HDL levels).[5]

A growing body of research also offers evidence that individuals providing care for others often neglect their own health in their devotion to caring for the family member with IDD. Caregivers describe negative physical, emotional, and functional health consequences of long-term informal caregiving. Caregivers also have higher levels of stress than non-caregivers and describe feeling frustrated, angry, drained, guilty, or helpless as a result of providing care.[6] Additionally, poor caregiver health may contribute to recurrent hospitalizations and out-of-home placements for individuals with chronic conditions and disabilities.[7]

According to the CDC's 2008 Physical Activity Guidelines for Americans and the National Center on Physical Activity and Disability, adults with disabilities need two types of physical activity each week to improve their health: aerobic and muscle-strengthening. The CDC guidelines recommend, for those that are able, 150 minutes or more of moderate physical activity per week or 75 or more minutes of vigorous physical activity per week to achieve important health benefits, as well as muscle-strengthening activities two or more days a week that work all major muscle groups. In 2006, the proportions of people with IDD who met the CDC's recommendations ranged from 17.5% to 33%.[8]

Health disparities between people with and without a disability are due, in part, to individual behaviors that contribute to secondary conditions because of inadequate knowledge about health-promoting lifestyles, cognitively inaccessible health promotion programs, and residential settings that encourage inactivity and poor nutrition.[2] While there is an emerging concept that people with disabilities can improve their health in the same manner as nondisabled people, health promotion opportunities offered in the general community often pose barriers that limit their participation, including public attitudes, uninformed and unaccommodating health providers, and inadequate health promotion programs for this population.[9-11]

In response to the urgent need for effective physical activity interventions for people with disabilities and their caregivers, the Family Resource Network developed Get FIT (Fitness, Integration, Training), in collaboration with the Department of Health and Exercise Science at Rowan University in Glassboro, New Jersey. The primary goal of Get FIT is to equip people with IDD and their caregivers with the skills, habits, and motivation to maintain regular exercise as recommended in the CDC guidelines and to implement healthy eating habits beyond the 10-week intervention. For each client with IDD, the goal is to also involve the caregiver, as he or she is very influential in the lifestyle habits of the person with the disability. Involving caregivers both improves their health and increases the program's sustainability. The program is designed to challenge the clients with IDD both physically and socially, as well as to give caregivers much needed time to focus on their own health and nutrition. To our knowledge, no other organization is providing a program similar to Get FIT in New Jersey or nearby states. A 2010 literature search on the topic of fitness and nutrition programming for people with IDD did not yield information on other, similar programs.

Program Overview

Over a 10-week period, clients in the Get FIT program attend 1.5-hour sessions, three times per week, and receive one-on-one fitness training, individual nutrition counseling, and group nutrition education in a university fitness lab. During each session, clients participate in 75 minutes of fitness training that includes three components: (1) strength training using selected equipment, (2) cardiovascular training using treadmills, elliptical trainers, and stationary bicycles, and (3) group exercise using various callisthenic types of movement. Student trainers record notes on the sessions so that the program is progressive for each client. The remainder of the session is used for nutrition education, either in a large group format or in individual counseling sessions. Group nutrition education focuses on various topics and has included discussions on portion control, reading food labels, general eating behaviors (signs of hunger, emotional eating), and modifying recipes to reduce sugar and/or fat. Individual sessions are delivered by trained student volunteers and use motivational interviewing. Motivational interviewing is a counseling technique that is individually centered to enhance intrinsic motivation to promote behavioral change, which it accomplishes by eliciting concerns about the problems and reasons for change from the individual, rather than directly confronting the client's need to change.[12,13] In these sessions, clients are encouraged to define their own goals and develop their own plan for change. They receive three individual sessions during the 10-week program.

To offer the most individualized program for each client and to keep the program cost-free, trained student staff (n = 6) and student volunteers (n = 45) serve as fitness trainers and nutrition counselors. Because the success of Get FIT is predicated on volunteers, Rowan University has built volunteering into the curriculum by awarding students contact hours (CH) for serving as a volunteer. Accumulating CH is necessary to graduate from the health promotion degree program, so we have a constant supply of volunteers every semester. We have not noted any negative effects on the participants or the volunteers by awarding CH for volunteering. In fact, because of their positive experience, many students continue to volunteer even when their CH requirement has been fulfilled

Student staff and volunteers are trained by the Get FIT professional staff on the fitness and nutrition protocols as well as on nonverbal communication and sensitivity to working with people with IDD. Most of their training on how to work with individuals with IDD occurs on the job, where they learn their own client's personal limitations and work within that framework to make adaptations. For group nutrition education, the students use visual aids and interactive discussion to encourage participation. For the counseling portion, since it is individualized, minor modifications are made by each counselor, as he or she sees fit, for the individual client. Additional training and resources are available through Rowan University's partner, the state agency Family Resource Network.

Data on clients' fitness, body composition, and nutrition components are collected at baseline and at the program's end. Fitness testing includes a VO_2 max treadmill test, a sit-to-stand test that measures lower body strength, and a plank test that measures both upper body and core strength. Data on blood lipids, glucose levels, blood pressure, and waist circumference are also collected in order to measure the effect of the program on metabolic syndrome, as defined by the American Heart Association / National Heart, Lung, and Blood Institute Scientific Statement. Weight, height, and hip circumference measures are also collected. Nutritional data collected include stage of change for eating fruits and vegetables and a general food frequency questionnaire.

Outcomes

The 2011 session that ran from October to December proved to be our largest program to date, with 45 clients participating. Most of the clients with IDD were male and ranged in age from 11 to 30. In comparison, the caregiver population was mostly female, with an average age of 52. The descriptive outcomes of the program are summarized in table 23.1. Seventy-one percent of the clients were either obese or overweight, and 33% were diagnosed with metabolic syndrome. Among those without metabolic syndrome, over 75% had either one or two risk factors for metabolic syndrome (mainly low HDL levels and elevated waist circumference).

Very few clients were in the "good to excellent" range for VO_2 max or the sit-to-stand and plank tests. The majority of clients reported being in the contemplative

Table 23.1. Results on fitness, body composition, metabolic syndrome, and nutrition for the 2011 cohort of the Get FIT program

Characteristic	Percent	
	Pre-program	Post-program
Fitness test		
VO_2 max (in range)	36	61
Sit-to-stand (good to excellent)	52	91
Plank (good to excellent)	49	71
Body composition		
Overweight/obese	71	56
Lost weight	—	38.5
Lost waist inches	—	32
Lost hip inches	—	24
Metabolic syndrome		
Diagnosed with metabolic syndrome	33	24
Intention to eat more fruits/vegetables		
Pre-contemplation/contemplation	63	47
Preparation/action/maintenance	38	53

stage of change (thinking about changing in the next six months) for increasing their intake of fruits and vegetables.

At the end of the program, we documented a 9% decrease in metabolic syndrome. At baseline, the majority of clients had low levels of HDL (high-density lipoprotein) cholesterol, a risk factor for metabolic syndrome (data not shown). High-density lipoprotein levels are typically increased by increasing physical activity. By the end of the program, almost half of the clients with low HDL increased their levels, which could be explained by the increase in VO_2 max, and 91% of clients were in the "good to excellent" range for the sit-to-stand test and 71% in the "good to excellent" range for the plank test. Additionally, of those with an elevated waist circumference, another risk for metabolic syndrome, 32% lost inches from their waistlines.

Although 38.5% of the participants lost weight, the average weight loss was only 1.0 ± 2.6 lbs over the 10 weeks. This is not a clinically significant loss (> 5% loss of body weight). However, of those with high attendance in the program, 52% lost weight, an average of 3.75 ± 15.0 lbs (data not shown). This greater weight loss indicates that adherence to the program is one of the keys to success for the client.

Program evaluations and subjective comments from clients and caregivers indicated that working with the university students one-on-one was one of the motivating aspects of the program for the participants. The clients felt respected, and they liked the individual attention and care they received from the student trainers. Caregivers reported that their family member with IDD looked forward to the sessions and to socializing with the other clients and the student staff. For many, it was the highlight of their week. Most clients were disappointed when the program ended and looked forward to the beginning of the next session.

We also received an overwhelmingly positive response from the student and volunteer staff, indicating that this was an enriching experience both professionally and personally. They reported that their confidence that they could work with clients with IDD increased, as did their openness to working with clients with IDD in their future careers. As one of the goals of Get FIT was to increase the capacity of the health promotion field to serve individuals with disabilities, this finding was encouraging.

Discussion

Despite the clear success of the Get FIT program, one of its challenges is in the area of helping clients to maintain proper nutrition outside the program. While we are able to reduce the risk of metabolic syndrome and increase fitness levels, the clinically non-significant weight loss is a concern because it is theoretically possible that, during a 10-week program, clients could lose up to 2 lbs per week, which would mean a clinically significant 5%–10% loss of body weight. This indicates that the clients are not incorporating the nutrition component of the program at home. They enjoyed the group education sessions and their individual sessions, but not many made changes to their diet. Post-intervention nutrition data showed that more clients were now in the preparation stage of change (thinking about changing in the next month) for eating more fruits and vegetables, but the food frequency data showed no change in their eating habits over the 10-week program (data not shown).

To assist the clients in this area, in 2012 we made significant changes to the nutrition education portion of the program. A pilot test of an instructor certification program for nutrition counseling using motivational interviewing was implemented, which includes 20 hours of training that incorporates hands-on practice using role playing and practice sessions with selected caregivers. Our goal with this new addition to the program is to affect positive dietary changes in the caregiver, which will then lead to positive dietary changes for the client with IDD. To date, nine health promotion students have been trained to serve as nutrition counselors, and the feedback thus far from both the students and caregivers has been positive.

To increase access to the Get FIT program, we have developed a portable version that can be implemented at a community site. We designed a fitness program that can be led by one instructor without the help of volunteers and can be implemented in an empty indoor space with the use of portable equipment such as dumbbells, stability balls, mats, and exercise bands. In this program, participants move from one station to another, performing different exercises at each station. The fitness program includes cardiovascular, strength-training, and flexibility components. We trained two health promotion student interns to lead the program and, currently, approximately 15 clients with IDD and their caregivers are participating at the community site. One staff member and three caregivers are being trained to lead the program at that site, which is important to ensure the continuity and sustainability of the program after the student interns complete their 10-week sessions. Each year we increase the number of community sites that have portable versions of Get FIT run by trained staff members, thus promoting sustainability of the program.

In summary, we believe that Get FIT is a much needed, effective physical activity and nutrition program that can be implemented at fitness centers and community sites with the right combination of volunteers and interested professional staff. The demand for the Get FIT program at Rowan University has grown steadily since its inception in 2008. Ongoing program evaluation of Get FIT has provided evidence that it is reaching all of its goals. Participants with IDD are showing improvements in their health, fitness, and social interaction; caregivers are showing improvements in health and fitness and appreciate being cared for (instead of always giving the care); and the health promotion students are increasing their confidence and interest in serving the IDD community in their future careers.

LESSONS LEARNED
- People with IDD can and do respond well to rigorous fitness programs typically offered only to the general population.
- People with IDD and their caregivers need a fitness and nutrition program separate from that for the general population and designed solely for their use.

- By working directly with people with IDD, student volunteers increase their confidence and willingness to work with this population in their future careers.
- A solid nutrition component focused on changing caretakers' behaviors is needed to affect the eating habits of their family member with IDD.

Acknowledgment

The Get FIT program is funded in part by the New Jersey Council on Developmental Disabilities.

References

1. Centers for Disease Control and Prevention. Racial/ethnic disparities in self-rated health status among adults with and without disabilities—United States, 2004–2006. MMWR Morb Mortal Wkly Rep. 2008 Oct 3;57(39):1069–73.
2. Krahn GL, Hammond L, Turner A. A cascade of disparities: health and health care access for people with intellectual disabilities. Ment Retard Dev Disabil Res Rev. 2006;12(1):70–82.
3. Rimmer JH, Yamaki K. Obesity and intellectual disability. Ment Retard Dev Disabil Res Rev. 2006;12(1):22–7.
4. U.S. Department of Health and Human Services, Office of the Surgeon General. The Surgeon General's call to action to improve the health and wellness of people with disabilities. Rockville, MD: Office of the Surgeon General, 2005. Available at: http://www.ncbi.nlm.nih.gov/books/NBK44667.
5. Grundy SM, Cleeman JI, Daniels SR, et al. Diagnosis and management of the metabolic syndrome: an American Heart Association / National Heart, Lung, and Blood Institute scientific statement. Curr Opin Cardiol. 2006 Jan;21(1):1–6.
6. Pinquart M, Sorensen S. Differences between caregivers and noncaregivers in psychological health and physical health: a meta-analysis. Psychol Aging. 2003 Jun;18(2):250–67.
7. Murphy NA, Christian B, Caplin DA, et al. The health of caregivers for children with disabilities: caregiver perspectives. Child Care Health Dev. 2007 Mar;33(2):180–7.
8. Temple VA, Frey GC, Stanish HI. Physical activity of adults with mental retardation: review and research needs. Am J Health Promot. 2006 Sep–Oct;21(1):2–12.
9. Cluphf D, O'Connor J, Vanin S. Effects of aerobic dance on the cardiovascular endurance of adults with intellectual disabilities. Adapt Phys Activ Q. 2001 Jan;18(1):60–71.
10. Rimmer JH. The conspicuous absence of people with disabilities in public fitness and recreation facilities: lack of interest or lack of access? Am J Health Promot. 2005 May–Jun;19(5):327–9, ii.
11. Wilhite B, Shank J. In praise of sport: promoting sport participation as a mechanism of health among people with a disability. Disabil Health J. 2009 Jul;2(3):116–27.
12. Baker A, Hanbridge J. Motivational interviewing: enhancing engagement in treatment for mental health problems. Behav Change. 2002;19(3):138–45.
13. Miller WR, Rollnick S. Motivational interviewing: preparing people for change. New York, NY: Guilford Press, 2002.

CHAPTER 24

The PILI 'Ohana Project
A Community-Academic Partnership to Eliminate
Obesity Disparities in Native Hawaiian and
Pacific Islander Communities

Joseph Keawe'aimoku Kaholokula, PhD, Claire Townsend, MPH,
Ka'imi Sinclair, PhD, Donna-Marie Palakiko, RN, MS, Emily Mahiki, MSW,
Sheryl R. Yoshimura, RD, MPH, JoHsi Wang, Puni Kekauoha,
Adrienne Dillard, MSW, Cappy Solatorio, Claire Hughes, DrPH,
Shari Gamiao, and Marjorie K. Leimomi Mala Mau, MD

Overweight and obesity affect 68% of the U.S. population.[1] The burden of over-weight and obesity is greater among some ethnic groups than others. Between 76% and 90% of Native Hawaiians / Pacific Islanders are overweight or obese,* compared with 57% of Whites and of the general population of Hawaii.[2,3] The consequences of obesity are also greater among Native Hawaiians / Pacific Islanders, with 19% having diabetes and over 30% having hypertension, compared with 4% and 14.6%, respectively, of Whites and 8.3% and 15.3% of the general population.[3-5] Complicating the prevention and treatment of overweight and obesity is that many individuals face social and economic challenges (e.g., discrimination, lack of livable wages) and live in obesogenic environments.[4]

To address overweight and obesity in Native Hawaiians / Pacific Islanders, in 2005 we formed a community-based participatory research (CBPR) project called the PILI

Joseph Keawe'aimoku Kaholokula, Claire Townsend, Ka'imi Sinclair, Puni Kekauoha, and Marjorie K. Mau are affiliated with the Center for Native and Pacific Health Disparities Research, Department of Native Hawaiian Health, John A. Burns School of Medicine, University of Hawaii at Mānoa; Emily Mahiki and Donna-Marie Palakiko, with the Ke Ola Mamo, Native Hawaiian Health Care System, in Honolulu; Sheryl R. Yoshimura and JoHsi Wang, with KōkuaKalihi Valley Comprehensive Family Services in Honolulu; Adrienne Dillard and Cappy Solatorio, with Kula no nā Po'e Hawai'i in Honolulu; and Claire Hughes and Shari Gamiao, with Hawai'i Maoli, Association of Hawaiian Civic Clubs, in Kapolei.

* Native Hawaiians / Pacific Islanders are people with ancestors among the original inhabitants of Polynesia (e.g., Native Hawaiians, Samoans), Micronesia (e.g., Chuukese), or Melanesia (e.g., Fijians). We included Filipinos, often arbitrarily classified as "Asian," given their similar risk for obesity and related diseases as well as their similar socioeconomic profile and disease outcomes in Hawaii.[4]

'Ohana Project,* comprising community and academic investigators from five organizations: (1) Department of Native Hawaiian Health in the John A. Burns School of Medicine, University of Hawaii at Mānoa, a clinical department focusing on health disparities disfavoring Native Hawaiians / Pacific Islanders; (2) Hawai'i Maoli of the Association of Hawaiian Civic Clubs, a nonprofit organization serving a confederation of 58 clubs across Hawaii and the continental United States; (3) Kula no nā Po'e Hawai'i, a nonprofit organization addressing the education and health needs of the Hawaiian Homestead communities of Papakōlea, Kewalo, and Kalāwahine; (4) Ke Ola Mamo, a nonprofit Native Hawaiian Health Care System for the island of 'Oahu providing health services primarily to low-income Native Hawaiians; and (5) Kōkua Kalihi Valley Comprehensive Family Services, a community-owned nonprofit providing health services to Pacific Islanders and immigrant Asians.[†] (See Nacapoy et al.[5] for more details.)

We received a grant from the National Institute on Minority Health and Health Disparities (NIMHD) for phases I and II of an 11-year CBPR initiative. This initiative is being implemented by NIMHD in three phases: phase I, a three-year planning phase (2005–8); phase II, a five-year intervention research phase (2008–13); and phase III, a three-year dissemination phase (2013–16). Currently in the final year of phase II, we describe here the activities, preliminary results, innovations, and lessons learned to date.

Phase I: Intervention Development

In phase I, we developed and pilot-tested a community-based overweight/obesity intervention for Native Hawaiians / Pacific Islanders. Community assessments were conducted to identify salient weight-related issues affecting Native Hawaiians / Pacific Islanders. Focus groups, informant interviews, surveys, and so-called windshield tours (i.e., walking/driving through a defined community to survey its infrastructure, condition, and available resources) were completed with 333 stakeholders. We used the information from the assessments and Social Action Theory[6] to translate the Diabetes Prevention Program's Lifestyle Intervention (DPP-LI)[7] for Native Hawaiian / Pacific Islander communities and to design a novel weight loss maintenance intervention to accompany the translated DPP-LI. With active involvement of our community partners, we adapted the DPP-LI into a three-month (eight lessons) intervention to initiate weight loss and designed a six-month (six lessons) family- and community-focused maintenance intervention.

Because we were more interested in weight loss maintenance than the initial weight loss itself, we wanted to compare the six-month family- and community-

---

* PILI is an acronym for Partnership for Improving Lifestyle Intervention; the Hawaiian word *pili* means "joining together." *'Ohana* is the Hawaiian word for "family." These words reflect values we uphold.

† Kalihi-Pālama Health Center, an outpatient health center offering primary care, behavioral health, and social services to primarily Pacific Islanders and immigrant Asians, was also a cofounding organization and participated in phase I.

focused intervention for weight loss maintenance with a six-month behavioral weight loss follow-up intervention having the same purpose. The former was specifically designed to engage participants in involving family and friends in their weight loss maintenance efforts and in identifying and taking advantage of community resources available to them. In doing so, participants learned how to apply and modify the strategies learned in the adapted three-month DPP-LI to their specific family and community context, in six lessons (one lesson per month) delivered in groups of 8–12 people. Each lesson was 1–1.5 hours in duration. In contrast, the standard weight loss follow-up intervention involved six phone calls (one call per month) made to individual participants to assist them with sustaining their weight loss efforts. Each call, lasting 15–20 minutes, involved a brief review of information and strategies learned from, as well as action plans developed, during their participation in the adapted three-month DPP-LI.

We conducted a pilot randomized controlled trial (RCT) with over 200 adult Native Hawaiians / Pacific Islanders to test our novel family- and community-focused weight loss maintenance intervention against the behavioral weight loss follow-up intervention, after all participants had completed the three-month adapted DPP-LI to initiate weight loss efforts. In the following discussion, we refer to the adapted three-month DPP-LI plus the six-month family and community intervention as the PILI Lifestyle Program (PLP) and to the three-month adapted DPP-LI plus six-month behavioral weight loss follow-up intervention as the Standard Behavioral Program (SBP). The interventions were delivered in the community setting of the participating community organizations: two community health centers, a Native Hawaiian Health Care System, a Hawaiian homestead community, and a civic club. (For more details, see Nacapoy et al.,[5] Mau et al.,[8] and Kaholokula et al.[9])

Our research was innovative in several ways. We incorporated strategies designed to influence participants' larger social systems to support their adoption and maintenance of healthy lifestyle behaviors. We capitalized on the importance of 'ohana (extended family/community) in daily living and decision making by involving family and friends and community resources in helping participants adopt sustainable healthy lifestyle behaviors.[10,11] We translated the DPP-LI to use in Native Hawaiian / Pacific Islander communities as a community-based and community-led intervention. Active participation by community stakeholders, as co-investigators, provided the contextual and cultural expertise to effectively translate the DPP-LI for use by Native Hawaiians / Pacific Islanders. Our community partners also expanded on the DPP-LI curriculum. They developed a lesson titled "Economics of Healthy Eating" to address the high cost of food in Hawaii. Another lesson incorporated by the community partners, "Talking with the Doctor," was intended to help participants effectively communicate with their health care providers. Mau et al.[8] provide more details about the DPP-LI adapted lessons and foci.

The RCT design and intervention delivery were also innovative. At the community investigators' insistence, all participants were offered the three-month DPP-LI adapted weight loss curriculum to ensure that all received an intervention. After completion of this curriculum, participants were randomized to receive either the PLP or the SBP. Both curricula were community-based and delivered by community health advocates

Blood pressure, body weight (kg), and height (cm) data were collected using standardized procedures. To assess physical functioning, participants completed a six-minute walk test, which measures the distance (in feet) a person is able to walk in six minutes.[12] Participants completed the brief Physical Activity Questionnaire to assess exercise frequency during the past month.[13] To estimate the amount of fat in participants' diets ($\leq 30\%$ vs. $> 30\%$ of daily fat in diet), a 39-item modified version of the Eating Habits Questionnaire was used to assess the frequency (1 = always to 4 = never) with which participants modified their meat consumption, avoided fat, replaced high-fat foods with low-fat alternatives, and consumed vegetables.[8,14]

Our initial findings are promising. The PLP was superior to the SBP: 51% of PLP participants met the $\geq 3\%$ weight loss goal of the study, compared with 31% of those in the SBP.[15] Among those who completed at least half of the prescribed lessons, PLP participants were five times more likely to maintain their weight loss than SBP participants.[9] Both PLP and SBP participants improved their physical functioning, blood pressure, and physical activity frequency, with PLP participants having greater improvements in these areas.

An unanticipated finding of our pilot study was the large ethnic differences in weight loss. Of the 100 participants who fully completed the pilot intervention study, 56% were Native Hawaiian, 22% were Chuukese, and 22% were a mix of other Pacific Islander ancestry, primarily Samoans and Filipinos. Sixty-four percent of Chuukese participants met the weight loss goal, compared with 35% of Native Hawaiians and 32% of Pacific Islanders.[15] Chuukese are mostly recent immigrants from Chuuk who face greater economic and acculturation challenges. The better outcome for the Chuukese participants may be related to (1) delivery of the lessons in their native language by bilingual Chuukese health workers, making the lessons more specific and relevant to their cultural context; (2) stronger community ties in this smaller immigrant community; (3) intervention strategies that may have been novel to them because they are recent immigrants and less embedded in lifestyle habits of their new country; and/or (4) differences in available resources across community types, as the Chuukese participants were recruited from community health centers where nutrition was heavily emphasized. It is important to note that only for the Chuukese participants was it necessary to deliver the intervention in a language other than English (as most were recent immigrants for whom English was a second language). The other ethnic groups had greater English fluency; for most, English was their primary and only language.

Based on the lessons we learned from phase I, it appears that one size does not fit all when it comes to a lifestyle intervention targeting overweight and obesity in Native Hawaiians / Pacific Islanders. Different intervention foci and strategies for weight loss might be needed to account for differences in acculturation-related factors, motivation to make dietary versus physical activity changes, and available community resources (e.g., trained health workers, exercise facilities).

Phase II: Intervention Research

Carrying forward the lessons learned and the innovations of phase I, we were successful in receiving continued support from NIMHD. We sought to refine and expand the PLP and definitively test its effectiveness. To gather information on how to improve the pilot-tested PLP, we convened seven focus groups with 63 former pilot intervention participants (6–14 per group) and 5 community health advocates (one group). The focus group was predominantly female (85.7%), with Native Hawaiians (64.7%), Samoans (10.3%), Chuukese (14.7%), and a mix of other Pacific Islanders (10.3%). The participants indicated that both the manner in which the intervention was delivered (face-to-face in a group setting) and the materials provided were culturally appropriate and relevant to the intent of the intervention. A majority specifically pointed to several strategies they found most useful, which included the 80/20 rule (defining success as meeting healthy lifestyle goals 80% of the time), the plate method (e.g., half of a nine-inch plate is vegetables, a quarter is protein, and a quarter is starch), cooking demonstrations, and integration of family and community supports into the program. The community health advocates stressed the importance of increasing interaction, simplifying handouts, and integrating family and community into the program. Overall, the feedback was positive and reinforced the intervention's acceptability and relevance. We found no differences in feedback among Pacific Islander groups.

Based on the focus group feedback and the lessons learned from phase I, we modified the intervention to include simplified handouts, additional space to take notes in the workbooks, a master action plan to organize/track participants' action plans across lessons, and addition of monthly community activities to increase contact time with participants and family and community involvement. We also expanded the PLP from a 9-month to an 18-month program to enhance the long-term maintenance of weight loss—consistent with what are currently understood to be best practices regarding weight loss maintenance.[16–18] As the number of sessions attended was associated with greater weight loss maintenance, it was also apparent from the pilot study in phase I that a deeper intervention was needed to improve the maintenance of weight loss. In expanding the PLP into an 18-month lifestyle program, we maintained the adapted DPP-LI 3-month component to initiate weight loss and expanded the 6-month family- and community-focused component to 15 months.

We also learned from the pilot study in phase I that many of the participants could not commit to or continue a formal lifestyle program with set schedules because of work-related challenges (e.g., shiftwork and working multiple jobs) and family obligations (e.g., childcare). To address this, the idea arose, from discussions with leading national scientists and our community partners, to test a DVD-delivered version of the family- and community-focused weight loss maintenance component of the PLP. We decided to test two versions of this component: (1) a face-to-face version delivered in a group setting with a community health advocate and (2) a DVD-delivered version in which the participant watches the lessons alone. In both versions, all participants receive the three-month adapted DPP-LI delivered face-to-face in a group setting by a community health advocate, then they are randomized either to continue with the face-to-face version or to receive the DVD-delivered version. The DVD lessons cover the same material and intervention strategies as the face-to-face version, using the same workbooks, handouts, and supplemental materials.

Both versions of the PLP are currently being tested in a three-arm RCT. All participants receive the three-month adapted DPP-LI (face-to-face) and, after completion, are randomized into one of three study arms for weight loss maintenance: the PLP delivered by community health advocates in group settings (arm 1); the PLP delivered via DVD technology, in which participants are given a DVD player to view the intervention on their own (arm 2); and a no-intervention control group (arm 3). We anticipated that the PLP, regardless of delivery mode, would be superior to the control (i.e., maintaining weight loss only through one's own effort). We further anticipated that the face-to-face mode would prove superior to the DVD-delivered mode, but with the former having less attrition.

We decided to include a no-intervention control group in phase II in order to definitively test the efficacy of the PLP. Although the community partners were opposed to having a no-intervention control in the pilot study of phase I, they recognized the importance of including one in phase II to ensure that efficacy can be established. Doing so would allow us to make the claim that our intervention, if found superior to control, is evidence-based, which would provide strong support for garnering additional resources and in influencing public health policy. The community partners are comfortable with randomizing some participants to a no–weight loss maintenance intervention because all participants at least receive the adapted DPP-LI component before being randomized. Thus, everyone receives a weight loss intervention.

The current RCT is being conducted with Native Hawaiians / Pacific Islanders who are clients of a large urban community health center (Kōkua Kalihi Valley), a Native Hawaiian Health Care System (Ke Ola Mamo), and a social service organization for Native Hawaiian children and families (Queen Liliʻuokalani Children's Center) who are members of the largest civic club in Hawaii (Association of Hawaiian Civic Clubs) and are residents of the oldest and only urban Native Hawaiian homestead communities (Kula no nā Poʻe Hawaiʻi). All of the lessons, with the exception of the DVD lessons, are delivered within these community settings by community health advocates from their organizations.

The 18-month PLP testing is in its final year of phase II, and over 330 adult Native Hawaiians / Pacific Islanders have been recruited. The final results are not yet in, but several successes are noteworthy. The leadership and wisdom of our community partners ensured successful recruitment and retention of participants in the study. The retention rates of participants in phases I and II, thus far, are comparable at around 70%, despite the lengthening of the PLP. The high rate of retention is due to the lessons learned from phase I and the capacity developed in the partnering community organizations.

We did several things that may have contributed to the relatively high retention rate in phase II. First, participants were asked to check in weekly (by phone, email, or text) with their community health advocate during the weight loss maintenance component, which involves reporting their weights for that week. If no check-in is completed by a participant for that week, the community health advocate follows up with that participant. This may have led to participants' greater commitment to the program, as well as helping to resolve problems early on so the participant does not drop out. Second, the level of group interaction among the participants was also enhanced, and games and activities were designed to keep them engaged; additionally, immediate positive reinforcements for their successes were incorporated into the intervention. Participant interaction is encouraged through ice-breaker activities to open each lesson. Some of these activities involve name games of fruits and vegetables and easy relay races involving passing/balancing of fruits and vegetables between participants. Another activity includes Menu-Makeover, in which groups of participants are assigned various local fast-food menus and asked to substitute healthier options, such as turkey dog for hotdog or tossed salad for macaroni salad. A popular group activity is Shopping on a Budget, where groups of participants plan a full day's meals on a predetermined amount, using sales ads from local grocery stores.

Overall, our community partners' ability to recruit Native Hawaiians / Pacific Islanders into an RCT and to retain a high number of them is remarkable. Like most ethnic minority communities, Native Hawaiians / Pacific Islanders often do not participate in RCTs, in part due to distrust of researchers' intentions.[19] Our community investigators have the credibility and cultural integrity needed to reach a population often thought of as unreachable or difficult to reach here in Hawaii.

Enhancing, Translating, and Disseminating the PILI Lifestyle Intervention

While testing of the 18-month version of the PLP is still underway, the community-academic partnership deemed the 9-month version that proved efficacious in phase I to be appropriate for enhancement and translation to other settings and for dissemination. To enhance the weight loss maintenance effects of the 9-month PLP, we are currently testing, in a two-arm RCT, the incremental effects of a home gardening component in which participants are given a home gardening kit and asked to grow fruits and vegetables of their choice at home for consumption by themselves and their family. Twenty-four participants have completed the three-month adapted DPP-LI and were randomized to receive either PLP alone (n = 12) or PLP plus home gardening (n = 12). This pilot study, called the PILI 'Āina Project ('āina means "land" in Hawaiian), is still underway and is also funded by NIMHD.

The PLP is being translated into a 12-month worksite-based lifestyle intervention, called PILI@Work, for employees of Native Hawaiian–serving organizations, in collaboration with 'Imi Hale: Native Hawaiian Cancer Network, which is funded by the National Cancer Institute. Using a CBPR approach, we worked with Native Hawaiian–serving organizations across several Hawaiian islands to test the effectiveness of PILI@Work over five years. Participants in this study, after receiving the three-month adapted DPP-LI, are randomized to receive either 9 months of the family- and community-focused component face-to-face or a DVD version of the same intervention. The intervention is delivered by a worksite wellness advocate (an employee of the organization), and randomization occurs by worksite to avoid cross-contamination. This project is currently in its third year (of a planned five years).

In preparation for phase III of NIMHD's 11-year CBPR initiative, we worked with the Office of Hawaiian Affairs on a two-year pilot dissemination project to build capacity in other Native Hawaiian communities and to test a community-to-community dissemination model. In testing this model, the original PILI 'Ohana Project community partners will mentor new community partners to develop capacity to address overweight and obesity in their communities through delivery of an effective lifestyle intervention. We are guided by the Social Action Model described by Minkler et al.,[20] a community-oriented model that focuses on increasing the problem-solving abilities of entire communities for the purpose of achieving social justice. The model promotes six key concepts: (1) empowerment (a social process that helps people gain mastery over their lives and communities), (2) critical consciousness (a mental state in which community members recognize the need for social change and are willing and ready to take action), (3) community capacity (a community's characteristics that affect its ability to mobilize and to identify and solve social problems), (4) social capital (community resources that exist through relationships between community members and between community organizations), (5) issues selection, and (6) participation and relevance (a community's ability to engage members and implement a plan of action).

Reflections from the Field

In our eight years of targeting obesity disparities in Hawaii, many valuable lessons have been learned about developing and sustaining a CBPR community-academic partnership; about building the capacity and social capital of Native Hawaiian / Pacific Islander communities for addressing their own health concerns; and about identifying and testing community-based and worksite lifestyle interventions for overweight and obese Native Hawaiians / Pacific Islanders. What we learned has implications for other Native (i.e., Native American and Alaska Native) and Pacific Islander populations elsewhere in the United States (summarized under "Lessons Learned," below).

We have learned much about engaging Native Hawaiians / Pacific Islanders in community-based and worksite lifestyle interventions to address overweight and obesity. Despite the poor socioeconomic circumstances and obesogenic environments of many Native Hawaiians / Pacific Islanders, they demonstrate the resiliency to overcome these barriers to healthy living. Our community-based 9-month PLP was effective in helping a majority of overweight or obese Native Hawaiians / Pacific Islanders to lose a significant amount of weight, and keep it off, and to improve their blood pressure and physical functioning. The 18-month version of the PLP that is currently being tested offers the promise of even greater weight loss maintenance.

We also learned the need for innovative ways of reaching Native Hawaiians / Pacific Islanders that take into consideration the competing demands on their time. Barriers to accessing traditional interventions for weight loss and its maintenance led us to an interest in using DVD technology as a mode of intervention delivery. Internet-based weight loss maintenance programs when compared with programs delivered face-to-face have resulted in similar weight loss maintenance outcomes.[21,22] By circumventing common obstacles such as time constraints, lack of transportation, and reduced financial resources, technology-based interventions offer the potential of targeting more people at a relatively low cost.[23] The use of DVD technology, a less costly everyday technology, could prove effective in delivering a lifestyle intervention, given the availability of DVD players in most homes, ease of use, and low cost, especially for people in socioeconomic circumstances where home computers are not as common as DVD players.[24]

Our CBPR approach and lessons learned in designing, testing, and disseminating community-based and community-led health promotion interventions have implications for other ethnic minority communities. We learned from our community-academic partnership that partners who share common goals and values and who are committed to the process of CBPR can be successful in implementing health-related interventions. Importantly, an enduring partnership requires a sustained effort by all partners to maintain a positive working relationship. It also requires a stable infrastructure within partner organizations, as well as stable leadership that encourages open and honest communication.

In sum, our partnership has come far in addressing the health concerns of Native Hawaiian / Pacific Islander communities because of our shared mission and vision, our adherence to traditional Native Hawaiian / Pacific Islander values that guide our relationship, and the CBPR principles that guide our work. ʻAʻohe hana nui ke alu ʻia (no task is too big when done together).

LESSONS LEARNED

On community-academic partnerships:
- A trusting community-academic partnership takes time to develop, requiring partners to work closely together all through the research.
- Including community leaders as co-investigators with coequal power and equitable resource sharing lessens the power hierarchy and social boundaries that often arise in scientific inquiry.

- Commitment to the project by all partners—for example, being flexible and adaptable to change; having a shared vision and mission and shared values—is vital.
- Active participation by community leaders can provide the contextual and cultural expertise needed to translate intervention research and incorporate community wisdom.
- Community partners can develop the expertise to combat health issues relevant to their communities and rally the human and material resources to do so.
- Working together and sharing resources enhances each community's reach and effectiveness.
- Successes early on provide data that support community partners in seeking additional resources.
- Academic partners' recognition of the value of working with communities can expedite the implementation of intervention research.
- Community-academic partnerships can contribute to social change within the communities and personal change for some community partners (e.g., seeking a college education and advanced degrees).

On intervention targeting overweight/obesity:

- Active involvement and strong leadership and commitment by community partners can ensure successful recruitment and retention of participants in RCTs.
- Different intervention foci and strategies may be needed to address differences in acculturation-related factors, motivation to make lifestyle changes, and available community resources.
- Group interaction, games, activities, and immediate positive reinforcements can increase participants' engagement and may contribute to enhanced weight loss maintenance.
- DVD technology and mobile computing technology offer an alternative and potentially effective means of delivering lifestyle interventions.

Acknowledgments

The authors thank the PILI 'Ohana Project participants, community researchers, and staff of the participating community organizations: Hawai'i Maoli—The Association of Hawaiian Civic Clubs, Ke Ola Mamo, Kula no nā Po'e Hawai'i, Kalihi-Pālama Health Center, Kōkua Kalihi Valley Comprehensive Family Services, Queen's Medical Center, Queen Liliu'okalani Children's Center, I Ola Lāhui: Rural Hawai'i Behavioral Health, Keiki o ka 'Āina, and Moloka'i Community Health Center. The CBPR projects mentioned in this chapter were supported by the National Institute on Minority Health and Health Disparities, for the PILI Lifestyle Program (grant number R24MD001660) and the PILI 'Āina Project (grant number U54RR026136); the National Cancer Institute, for the PILI@Work Project (grant number U54CA153459); and the Office of Hawaiian Affairs, for the pilot dissemination project. The content is solely the responsibility of the authors and does not necessarily represent the official views of the National Institute on Minority Health and Health Disparities, the National Institutes of Health, or the Office of Hawaiian Affairs.

References

1. Ogden CL, Carroll MD. Prevalence of overweight, obesity, and extreme obesity among adults: United States, trends 1960–1962 through 2007–2008. Atlanta, GA: Centers for Disease Control and Prevention, 2010. Available at: http://www.cdc.gov/nchs/data/hestat/obesity_adult_07_08/obesity_adult_07_08.pdf.

2. Mau MK, Sinclair K, Saito EP, et al. Cardiometabolic health disparities in native Hawaiians and other Pacific Islanders. Epidemiol Rev. 2009;31:113–29.

3. Salvail FR, Nguyen D, Liang S. 2010 State of Hawaii—by demographic characteristics. Behavioral Risk Factor Surveillance System. Honolulu, HI: Hawaii State Department of Health, 2010. Available at: http://hawaii.gov/health/statistics/brfss/brfss2010/demo10.html.

4. Mau MK, Wong KN, Efird J, et al. Environmental factors of obesity in communities with native Hawaiians. Hawaii Med J. 2008 Sep;67(9):233–6.

5. Nacapoy AH, Kaholokula JK, West MR, et al. Partnerships to address obesity disparities in Hawai'i: the PILI 'Ohana Project. Hawaii Med J. 2008 Sep;67(9):237–41.

6. Ewart CK. Social action theory for a public health psychology. Am Psychol. 1991 Sep;46(9):931–46.

7. Diabetes Prevention Program (DPP) Research Group. The Diabetes Prevention Program (DPP): description of lifestyle intervention. Diabetes Care. 2002 Dec;25(12):2165–71.

8. Mau MK, Keawe'aimoku Kaholokula J, West MR, et al. Translating diabetes prevention into native Hawaiian and Pacific Islander communities: the PILI 'Ohana Pilot project. Prog Community Health Partnersh. 2010 Spring;4(1):7–16.

9. Kaholokula JK, Mau MK, Efird JT, et al. A family and community focused lifestyle program prevents weight regain in Pacific Islanders: a pilot randomized controlled trial. Health Educ Behav. 2012 Aug;39(4):386–95.

10. Gibbons MC, Tyus NC. Systematic review of U.S.-based randomized controlled trials using community health workers. Prog Community Health Partnersh. 2007 Winter;1(4):371–81.

11. Norris SL, Chowdhury FM, Van Le K, et al. Effectiveness of community health workers in the care of persons with diabetes. Diabet Med. 2006 May;23(5):544–56.

12. ATS Committee on Proficiency Standards for Clinical Pulmonary Function Laboratories. ATS statement: guidelines for the six-minute walk test. Am J Respir Crit Care Med; 2002 Jul 1;166(1):111–7.

13. Marshall AL, Smith BJ, Bauman AE, et al. Reliability and validity of a brief physical activity assessment for use by family doctors. Br J Sports Med. 2005 May;39(5):294–7.

14. Kristal AR, Beresford SA, Lazovich D. Assessing change in diet-intervention research. Am J Clin Nutr.1994 Jan;59(1 Suppl):185–9S.

15. Kaholokula J, Townsend C, Ige A, et al. Sociodemographic, behavioral, and biological variables related to weight loss in Native Hawaiians and other Pacific Islanders. Obesity (Silver Spring). 2013 Mar;21(3):E196–203.

16. Perri MG, Corsica JA. Improving the maintenance of weight lost in behavioral treatment of obesity. In: Wadden TA, Stunkard AJ, eds. Handbook of obesity treatment. New York, NY: Guilford Press, 2002. Pp. 357–82.

17. Curioni CC, Lourenco PM. Long-term weight loss after diet and exercise: a systematic review. Int J Obes (Lond). 2005 Oct;29(10):1168–74.

18. Turk MW, Yang K, Hravnak M, et al. Randomized clinical trials of weight loss maintenance: a review. J Cardiovasc Nurs. 2009 Jan–Feb;24(1):58–80.

19. Kaholokula JK, Saito E, Mau MK, et al. Pacific Islanders' perspectives on heart failure management. Patient Educ Couns. 2008 Feb;70(2):281–91.

20. Minkler M, Wallerstein N, Wilson N. Improving health through community organization and community building. In: Glanz K, Rimer BK, Viswanath K, eds. Health behavior and health education: theory, research, and practice. San Francisco, CA: John Wiley & Sons, 2008. Pp. 287–312.

21. Wing RR, Tate DF, Gorin AA, et al. A self-regulation program for maintenance of weight loss. N Engl J Med. 2006 Oct 12;355(15):1563–71.

22. Harvey-Berino J, Pintauro S, Buzzell P, et al. Effect of internet support on the long-term maintenance of weight loss. Obes Res. 2004 Feb;12(2):320–9.

23. Berkel LA, Poston WS, Reeves RS, et al. Behavioral interventions for obesity. J Am Diet Assoc. 2005 May;105(5 Suppl 1):S35–43.

24. Day JC, Janus A, Davis J. Computer and internet use in the United States: 2003. Current Population Reports. Washington, DC: U.S. Department of Commerce, Economics and Statistics Administration, U.S. Census Bureau, 2005 Oct. Available at: http://www.census.gov/prod/2005pubs/p23-208.pdf.

CHAPTER 25

Nutrition Education at Mobile Markets

Community-Engaged, Evidence-Based Interventions
to Address Obesity in Low-Income Neighborhoods
in Milwaukee

Paul Hunter, MD, Courtenay Kessler, MS, David Frazer, MPH, Yvonne D.
Greer, MPH, RD, CD, David Nelson, PhD, Amy Harley, PhD, MPH, RD,
Rosamaria Martinez, MBA, RD, Michelle Thate, MPH, and Paulette Flynn

The starting point for this chapter, as for the rest of this volume, is fundamental facts such as these: Despite efforts to motivate individuals to eat healthy diets and exercise regularly, American obesity rates have risen since 1980[1] and racial and ethnic disparities persist.[2,3]* Efforts to increase access to affordable, healthy food have resulted in minimal increases in fruit and vegetable intake.[4] Stores in lower-income neighborhoods stock fewer healthy items, including fewer and lower-quality produce items, in comparison with stores in other neighborhoods.[5] Obesity levels are related, in part, to the community food environment and economic status of the household.[6] Combining nutrition education programming with increased access to affordable, healthy food in these neighborhoods is a promising strategy to change population behaviors.[7]

With adult obesity at 26.3% in 2010, Wisconsin ranks 30th most obese of the 50 states.[8] Almost 35% of adults in the Milwaukee neighborhoods with lowest socioeconomic status (SES) have a body mass index over $30 \, \text{kg/m}^2$, compared with 23% in

Paul Hunter, Courtenay Kessler, and David Frazer are affiliated with the Center for Urban and Population Health and the School of Medicine and Public Health, University of Wisconsin–Madison. Yvonne D. Greer is a Y-EAT Right Nutritional Consultant for Healthy Living. David Nelson is affiliated with the Center for Healthy Communities, Department of Family and Community Medicine, Medical College of Wisconsin; Amy Harley, with the Center for Urban and Population Health, University of Wisconsin–Madison, and the Zilber School of Public Health, University of Wisconsin–Milwaukee; Rosamaria Martinez, with the Department of Pediatric Gastroenterology and Nutrition, Medical College of Wisconsin; Michelle Thate, with Kansas City University of Medicine and Biosciences; and Paulette Flynn, with SHARE Wisconsin.

* See the introduction and the chapters in part I for more extensive presentations of recent trends in obesity and overweight in underserved populations in the United States.

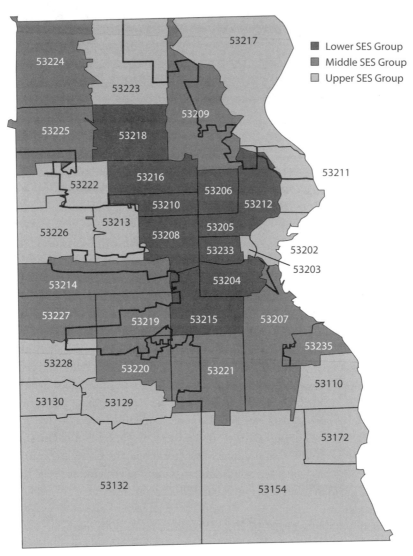

FIGURE 25.1. Socioeconomic status (SES) segregation in Milwaukee by zip codes. Source: Chen et al. (2011).[9]

higher-SES neighborhoods.[9] Milwaukee is highly segregated by SES (fig. 25.1),[9] and by some measures it is also the most racially segregated city in the United States.[10] The majority of African Americans in Milwaukee live in neighborhoods with the lowest SES in the city. Given Milwaukee's large disparity in rates of obesity coupled with its socioeconomically segregated,[11] racially and ethnically defined communities,[12] each neighborhood has its own particular needs, which means they require specific and targeted interventions.

Community-informed strategies are vital to the development and implementation of effective interventions. The objective of this project was to demonstrate that, with guidance from public health practitioners and academics, community organizations in low-income neighborhoods can use the evidence base and their community-specific knowledge to design and direct programming that combines distribution of healthy food with education about healthy eating. Both staff members and consumers at the community organizations can take part in such work.

Methods
Community-Academic Partners

To address both food security and nutrition education, a community-academic partnership was formed between SHARE (Self Help and Resource Exchange) Wisconsin, Center for Urban Population Health, and other community and academic organizations. SHARE Wisconsin brings healthy, affordable food to low-income neighborhoods in Milwaukee through mobile markets (MMs) hosted by community-based organizations.[13] SHARE is a nonprofit food-buying club that has helped families save 30%–50% on supermarket-quality food for over 25 years.[14] The Center for Urban Population Health worked with community and academic groups to implement community-informed, evidence-based nutrition programming at MMs.[15]

Program Planning

A Community Advisory Board (CAB) consisting of staff from community organizations hosting MMs and consumers at MMs guided the community perspective. Project staff met individually with potential CAB members to explain the project and invite them to join the board. The CAB represented the range of neighborhoods, organizations, and programs working with MMs, including members from social service agencies, health clinics, employment agencies, and public housing sites. Following initial community-building activities, the CAB reviewed recommended literature and commented on feasibility, relevance, and appropriateness for their neighborhoods. Members of the CAB also identified promising sites for nutrition education and developed proposals for programming. The board also provided expertise on the culture of the community served at each organization, considering race, ethnicity, language, gender, age group, income, and other relevant characteristics in program design and implementation.

A Technical Advisory Board (TAB) of public health researchers and practitioners identified promising evidence-based interventions for the CAB to consider for nutrition education programming at its sites. Research assistants used PubMed searches to identify programs combining healthy food access with education, focusing on urban, low-income, or racial/ethnic minority populations, that included weekly or monthly nutrition education sessions[16–18] and point-of-purchase interventions such as labels on store shelves to describe the nutritional content of food[19,20] or in-store education.[21] Interventions generally included incentives, sampling, and promotions.[21,22] The TAB also identified and reviewed two unpublished programs: (1) a regional social marketing campaign[23] and (2) a local intervention that we received permission to review prior to publication.[24]

To provide additional guidance to the CAB, the TAB and project staff developed a baseline survey to be administered at MMs to assess consumers' needs and interests related to food and nutrition. The University of Wisconsin–Madison Health Sciences Institutional Review Board exempted the survey (and project) from review. Project staff trained graduate and undergraduate students to administer the survey at MM sites. The survey included validated tools and the following topics: (1) consumption of fruits, vegetables, and fiber, using the Block Questionnaire;[25] (2) attitudes and beliefs about fruits and vegetables, using modifications of Sisters in Health[17] and Project FRESH[26] tools (J. V. Anderson, personal communication, 2010); (3) food security, based on the Survey on the Health of Wisconsin[27] and the Baltimore Healthy Stores[22] Consumer Impact Questionnaire (J. Gittelsohn, personal communication, 2010); (4) interests in nutrition education, including timing, location, topics, and teaching methods; and (5) self-reported health and zip code, using survey items from the Behavioral Risk Factor Surveillance System.[28] We calculated basic descriptive statistics (means, frequencies, and standard deviations) using the SAS 9.2 statistical package.[29]

We estimated fruit and vegetable consumption using an algorithm from Nutrition-Quest,[25] which requires participants' gender. Since gender data were not collected in

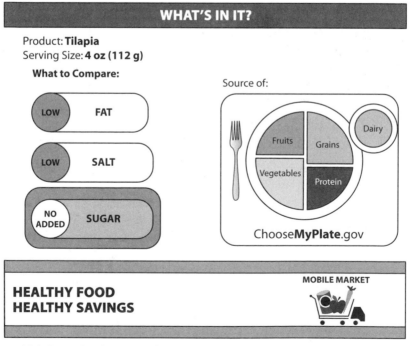

FIGURE 25.2. Example of a point-of-purchase food label used in mobile markets.

the baseline survey, we calculated estimates assuming first 100% male then 100% female populations. For all analyses, missing data were excluded. Two independent student reviewers analyzed open-ended questions using an inductive, data-driven approach.[30] The students then agreed upon a consistent codebook and recoded items using that codebook.

After six months of independent meetings, the CAB and TAB joined to review the survey results, prioritize information learned from the literature review, and establish a set of prioritized values and components for the proposed nutrition education. This integrated input from the TAB, CAB, and surveys guided the design of nutrition workshops and point-of-purchase labeling (fig. 25.2) at selected MM sites. Individual CAB agencies developed proposals for nutrition education, which were then reviewed by the TAB.

Outcomes

A total of 261 baseline surveys were collected. Table 25.1 shows characteristics of the survey respondents. Most were middle-aged. Based on zip codes, most (56%) lived in neighborhoods with low socioeconomic status.[9] Compared with other Milwaukee County residents, respondents reported poor to fair health twice as often.[31] While the surveys were offered in English and Spanish, only 2 of the 261 (< 1%) respondents selected the Spanish survey.

Table 25.1. Characteristics of mobile market customers responding to the project survey (n = 261)

Characteristic	Percent
Age distribution (years)	
Under 30	14
30–49	31
50–59	26
Over 60	29
Self-reported overall health status	
Excellent or very good	32
Good	38
Fair or poor	30
Zip code of residence	
City of Milwaukee = 97% of Wisconsin zip codes	
SES of residences in City of Milwaukee (tertiles)	
Lower	56
Middle	21
High	22

Source: For socioeconomic status (SES) of residences in City of Milwaukee: Chen et al. (2011).[9]

Fruits and Vegetables

Compared with a recommended 3.5–5 servings per day, survey respondents, on average, reported consuming 4.05 (SD = 2.00; assuming all participants were female) and 4.60 (SD = 2.00; assuming all male) servings. Ninety-seven percent of the respondents reported liking the taste of fruits and 93% liking the taste of vegetables. Eighty-nine percent reported ready access to fresh vegetables. Over half thought fruits and vegetables were expensive.

Food Security

Forty percent of respondents reported being concerned about having enough food for their families. Half reported having limited food choices because of their financial situation. A third reported having received emergency food in the past month.

Educational Interests

Seventy-four percent of survey respondents expressed interest in attending a nutrition education program. Topics of greatest interest included healthy cooking, stretching dollars for healthier food, cooking with healthier ingredients, and making healthy food taste better. Preferred methods of education included receiving recipes, participating in cooking demonstrations, attending group classes, and receiving pamphlets or other written materials.

Survey Summary

The baseline survey confirmed a need for food security in Milwaukee. However, reported fruit and vegetable consumption was unexpectedly high, suggesting that nutrition programming should incorporate topics beyond fruits and vegetables. The most commonly endorsed nutrition education techniques and topics were incorporated into the interventions.

Educational Interventions Designed

Five community organizations designed four pilot programs (table 25.2.) Sites included (1) a pair of WIC (Women, Infants, and Children Supplemental Food Program) clinics, (2) and (3) two public housing sites, and (4) an educational and social service center for families with young children (designated "early childhood"). These sites across Milwaukee County serve diverse populations, including Deaf or Hard-of-Hearing adults, middle-aged to elderly African American women, and Latino and African American families. Table 25.2 summarizes some of the key components at each site, including similarities and differences across nutrition education programs. Community organizations also recruited participants at their sites and provided meeting space.

Projects emphasized workshops involving food selection, label reading, and cooking demonstrations using foods from MMs. Staff of the Nutrition Education Program

Table 25.2. Characteristics of the mobile market intervention sites and program components

Characteristic	WIC clinics	Housing 1	Housing 2	Early childhood
Number of sessions	5	3	6	6
Length of session (minutes)	90	90	60	90
Focus population	Participants in Fit Families program at Health Dept.	All residents (elderly and disabled)	All residents (Deaf and Hard-of-Hearing)	Parents of children attending center
Primary ethnicities	Hispanic and African American	African American	Caucasian	African American
Primary language(s)	Spanish and English	English	English / American Sign Language	English
Partner resources	WIC nutritionists; reminder messages to parents; Spanish interpreter	Partnered with youth agency for physical activity; CAB member	Helped arrange for state waiver for interpreting services; MPH student intern	Site chef; program recruitment managers; health educator; reminder messages
Incentives	MM gift certificates	MM gift, certificates; kitchen utensils	MM gift certificates	MM gift certificates
Cooking demonstrations	Stir fry; smoothies; parfait	Stir fry	Casserole; smoothies; "cowboy caviar"	Stir fry; baked apple
Food tastings	Raw bok choy	"Cowboy caviar"	None	Banana pudding
Label reading	Yes	Yes	Yes	Yes
Food diaries	Yes—taught	Yes—resource	Yes—resource	Yes—taught
Health fair	No	Yes	No	No
Labeling MM food	Yes	Yes	Yes	Yes
Physical activity	Activities for children, using items around the house	Walking and other ways for adults to be active	Stretching; referrals to activities site exercise	Movement workshop (children and parents together)

Abbreviations: CAB, Community Advisory Board; MM, mobile market; MPH, master of public health; WIC, Women, Infants, and Children Supplemental Food Program.

of the University of Wisconsin Extension–Milwaukee County provided up to six hours of nutrition programming at each site. Additional components kept consistent across programs included (1) learner-centered didactic sessions, including food demonstrations; (2) curriculum related to food available at MMs and other easily accessible, healthy, affordable food; (3) use of Choose MyPlate in classes, food diary, and labeling; (4) physical activity demonstrations; and (5) labeling foods at MMs to highlight healthy choices (fig. 25.2). Staff of SHARE Wisconsin supported nutrition education programming by selecting food items to sell at MMs and assisting in implementing food labeling. Additionally, at some sites, participants in classes toured the MM and sampled food from the MM during class demonstrations.

Process Evaluation

Programs took place from November 2011 through April 2012. Hours of programming ranged from five to nine hours per site. Attendance ranged from 1 to 26 participants per session (excluding the health fair, attended by 48 participants). Based on 66 program pre-test surveys, most participants were female (table 25.3). Modifications to the original intervention plans included (1) adding an additional educational session in response to low attendance and (2) simplifying programming and evaluation tools to improve translation into American Sign Language for Deaf participants.

Participants completed satisfaction surveys at each session, including pre- and post-test surveys similar to the baseline survey. Program staff discussed challenges and successes at debriefings after the sessions. Challenges included logistics (childcare, transportation, timing) that limited attendance and retention. Anecdotal successes included (1) a child encouraging his reticent mother to try hummus, (2) an

Table 25.3. Mobile market participants' demographics and responses to satisfaction survey

	WIC clinics	Housing 1	Housing 2	Early childhood
From attendance records at educational sessions				
Total number of participants (total across sites = 143)	33	55	46	9
Average number of participants per session (overall 11.0; range = 1–48)	4.8 (range 2–11)	27.7 (range 9–48)	20.2 (range 16–26)	3.7 (range 1–6)
From pre-test survey of nutrition education participants (n = 66)				
Female (%)	93	79	80	100
Mean age (years)	30.4	53.7	69.6	33.4
From post-test survey of nutrition education participants (n = 46)				
Program worth participant's time (%)	100	95	85	100
Recommend program to a friend (%)	100	N.A.	85	100

Abbreviation: WIC, Women, Infants, and Children Supplemental Food Program.

increase in sales of brown rice, and (3) at the last session at each site, at least one participant asking when more sessions would be offered. Based on 46 post-test surveys, participants thought the programs were worth their time and worth recommending to a friend (table 25.3).

After attending classes, participants reported making changes that included (1) eating and physical activity behaviors, (2) learning about healthy food choices, and (3) reading food labels. Favorite program components included the teachers and learning about healthy choices. Only three changes were proposed, each named by only one participant: (1) more activities for children, (2) more participants, and (3) images of unfamiliar produce.

Discussion

The mobile markets project demonstrated the feasibility of combining education, product labeling, and bringing nutritious food into areas where healthy food options were lacking. A number of positive process results came out of the project (summarized under "Lessons Learned," below). First, due to the formation of the community-academic partnership, evidence-based strategies were vetted by community members to determine which strategies were feasible in and acceptable to the community. Community support was crucial and should be an integral component of future iterations. Second, regular and iterative coordination and evaluation allowed program adjustments and necessary corrections. Having project staff within the community helped to improve trust between community and academic partners. Finally, having even small incentives immediately reinforced nutrition programming.

Some limitations emerged. First, attaining regular and consistent attendance was challenging. With any voluntary, no-cost education, building capacity and attendance can be a challenge. The transience of MM customers at nonresidential sites and social stressors make obtaining regular attendance difficult. Second, we were concerned about the reliability of the survey results, based on unexpectedly high estimates for fruit and vegetable consumption and the apparently low literacy of respondents. Narrowing the focus, reducing the number of evaluation tools, and simplifying survey language may improve the quality of responses. Lastly, outcome evaluation will be critical in assessing the effectiveness of the program and making final recommendations for future directions.

More research is needed to understand successful methods to improve healthy eating behaviors in communities where healthy food options are limited. Increasing access alone is not enough; it needs to be combined with engaging, community-based, culturally appropriate education. To foster change, programs should combine access, education, and social support. Involving community members and identifying those who can influence their social contacts are keys to achieving future success. Engaging these opinion leaders and facilitating their participation may encourage consistent and increased attendance. Mobile markets and similar venues may also offer opportunities for informal nutrition education programming not involving enrollment in classes. This innovative project combined facets of access, engagement, and education in an attempt to improve nutritional status. We will continue to monitor access to the services provided and self-reported nutrition to further assess the needs and assets of the community.

LESSONS LEARNED

- Assemble a technical advisory board of professionals with diverse backgrounds and community experience.
- Work with food distributor(s) working in low-income neighborhoods.
- Plan sufficient time for recruiting community advisory board members.
- Meet early with potential CAB members to explain the role of the CAB in the project.
- Seek out community organizations with missions that align with the desired outcome of the project and that offer opportunities for genuine communication and relationships with their clients, rather than intermittent transactions of resources.
- Anticipate and address challenges to program success (e.g., staff turnover and lack of transportation for participants), both early in planning and throughout implementation.
- Limit process surveys to essential information; however, take care to ensure that outcome surveys are comprehensive.

Acknowledgments

A grant from the Ira and Ineva Reilly Baldwin Wisconsin Idea Endowment funded this project. The authors also acknowledge contributions from Stephanie Jones, Dwight Williamson, Sunny Peete, Nancy Castro, Diana Espino, Angela Check, Krystal Parsons, and Katie Voss (members of the Community Advisory Board); Kristen Malecki (Survey of Health of Wisconsin); Virginia Zerpa-Uriona (formerly of the Center for Urban Population Health); and Anthony Sturm, Allison Schaus, Esha Pillai, Kevin Smith, Madeline Lamb, Kelli Stader, Kathleen Ratteree, Iris Cruz, Kathryn Kelley, Holly Sage, Abigail Navarro, Lora Jorgenson-Tjornehoj, Abby Matthews, Dyango Zerpa, Kelsey Krentz, Jeanne Jean-Philippe, Tres Harris, Joshua Murphy, Katarina Grande, Ashley Snook, and Jessica Kowaleski (student interns and University of Wisconsin Population Health Fellows).

References

1. Ogden CL, Yanovski SZ, Carroll MD, et al. The epidemiology of obesity. Gastroenterology. 2007 May;132(6):2087–102.
2. Flegal KM, Carroll MD, Kit BK, et al. Prevalence of obesity and trends in the distribution of body mass index among US adults, 1999–2010. JAMA. 2012 Feb 1;307(5):491–7.

3. Ogden CL, Carroll MD, Kit BK, et al. Prevalence of obesity and trends in body mass index among US children and adolescents, 1999–2010. JAMA. 2012 Feb 1;307(5):483–90.

4. Casagrande SS, Wang Y, Anderson C, et al. Have Americans increased their fruit and vegetable intake? The trends between 1988 and 2002. Am J Prev Med. 2007 Apr;32(4):257–63.

5. Levi J, Vinter S, St. Laurent R, et al. F as in fat: how obesity threatens America's future. Washington, DC: Trust for America's Health. 2010. Available at: http://healthyamericans.org/reports/obesity2010/Obesity2010Report.pdf.

6. Whitacre PT, Tsai P, Mulligan J, et al. The public health effects of food deserts: workshop summary. Washington, DC: National Academies Press, 2009. Available at: http://www.nap.edu/catalog.php?record_id=12623.

7. Zoellner J, Connell C, Bounds W, et al. Nutrition literacy status and preferred nutrition communication channels among adults in the Lower Mississippi Delta. Prev Chronic Dis. 2009 Oct;6(4):A128.

8. Centers for Disease Control and Prevention. Adult obesity facts. Atlanta, GA: Centers for Disease Control and Prevention. Available at: www.cdc.gov/obesity/data/adult.html#States.

9. Chen HY, Baumgardner DJ, Galvao LW, et al. Milwaukee health report 2011: health disparities in Milwaukee by socioeconomic status. Milwaukee, WI: Center for Urban Population Health, 2011. Available at: http://www.cuph.org/mhr/2011-milwaukee-health-report.pdf.

10. Frey WH. Black-white segregation indices for metro areas. Ann Arbor, MI: University of Michigan Population Studies Center, 2011. Available at: http://www.psc.isr.umich.edu/dis/census/segregation2010.html.

11. Employment and Training Institute. Community indicators for Central City Milwaukee: 1993–present. Milwaukee, WI: University of Wisconsin–Milwaukee, 2012. Available at: http://www4.uwm.edu/eti/reports/indypage.htm.

12. Employment and Training Institute. Maps of the African American and white populations in the Milwaukee–Waukesha, WI PMSA. Milwaukee, WI: University of Wisconsin–Milwaukee, 2002. Available at: http://www4.uwm.edu/eti/integration/milwaukee.htm.

13. SHARE Wisconsin. Introducing SHARE. Butler, WI: SHARE Wisconsin, 2012.

14. SHARE Wisconsin. About SHARE's food. Butler, WI: SHARE Wisconsin, 2012.

15. Center for Urban Population Health. About us. Milwaukee, WI: Center for Urban Population Health, 2012. Available at: http://www.cuph.org/about.

16. Havas S, Anliker J, Greenberg D, et al. Final results of the Maryland WIC Food for Life program. Prev Med. 2003 Nov;37(5):406–16.

17. Devine C, Farrell T, Hartman R. Sisters in Health: experiential program emphasizing social interaction increases fruit and vegetable intake among low-income adults. J Nutr Educ Behav. 2005 Sep–Oct;37(5):265–70.

18. Kennedy BM, Champagne CM, Ryan DH, et al. The "Rolling Store:" an economical and environmental approach to the prevention of weight gain in African American women. Ethn Dis. 2009 Winter;19(1):7–12.

19. Lang JE, Mercer N, Tran D, et al. Use of a supermarket shelf-labeling program to educate a predominately minority community about foods that promote heart health. J Am Diet Assoc. 2003 Jul;100(7):804–9.

20. Sutherland LA, Kaley LA, Fischer L. Guiding Stars: the effect of a nutrition navigation program on consumer purchases at the supermarket. Am J Clin Nutr. 2010 Apr;91(4):1090–94S.

21. Paine-Andrews A, Francisco VT, Fawcett SB, et al. Health marketing in the supermarket: using prompting, product sampling, and price reduction to increase customer purchases of lower-fat items. Health Mark Q. 1996;14(2):85–9.

22. Gittelsohn J, Song HJ, Suratkar S, et al. An urban food store intervention positively affects food-related psychosocial variables and food behaviors. Health Educ Behav. 2010 Jun;37(3): 390–402.

23. Consortium to Lower Childhood Obesity in Chicago Children (CLOCC). 5-4-3-2-1 Let's Go. Chicago, IL: CLOCC, 2012. Available at: http://www.clocc.net/partners/54321Go/index.html.

24. Cronk CE, Hoffmann RG, Mueller MJ, et al. Effects of a culturally tailored intervention on changes in body mass index and health-related quality of life of Latino children and their parents. Am J Health Promot. 2011 Mar–Apr;25(4):e1–11.

25. Block G. Fruit/vegetable/fiber screener. Berkeley, CA: NutritionQuest, 2009. Available at: http://www.nutritionquest.com/wellness/free-assessment-tools-for-individuals/fruit-vege table-fiber-screener.

26. Michigan Department of Community Health. Project FRESH—farmer's market nutrition program. Lansing, MI: Michigan Department of Community Health, 2012. Available at: http://www.michigan.gov/mdch/1,1607,7-132-2942_4910_4921---,00.html.

27. Nieto FJ, Peppard PE, Engelman CD, et al. The Survey of the Health of Wisconsin (SHOW), a novel infrastructure for population health research: rationale and methods. BMC Public Health. 2010 Dec 23;10:785.

28. Office of Surveillance, Epidemiology, and Laboratory Services. Behavioral Risk Factor Surveillance System. Atlanta, GA: Centers for Disease Control and Prevention, 2012. Available at: http://www.cdc.gov/brfss.

29. SAS Institute. SAS 9.2 software key highlights. Cary, NC: SAS Institute Inc., 2010. Available at: http://www.sas.com/reg/wp/corp/12177.

30. Boyatzis RE. Transforming qualitative data: thematic analysis and code development. Thousand Oaks, CA: Sage Publications, 1998.

31. University of Wisconsin, Population Health Institute. County health rankings. Madison, WI: University of Wisconsin Population Health Institute, Robert Wood Johnson Foundation, 2011. Available at: http://www.countyhealthrankings.org/wisconsin/milwaukee.

CHAPTER 26

Report from a Pediatric Weight Management Program

Lessons Learned from Six Years of Experience with a Largely Medicaid-Based Population

Jessica M. Parrish, PhD, Elizabeth Getzoff, PhD, Kenneth Gelfand, PhD, Michelle Demeule, MS, RD/LDN, and Ann Scheimann, MD, MBA

A number of model treatment programs for pediatric obesity have been discussed in the literature.[1] Few of these programs, however, address the broad impact of community influences on program design or outcomes. The Weigh Smart (WS) program was developed in accordance with expert committee recommendations[2] and guidelines for model treatment programs[1] for pediatric obesity. In this chapter we report on lessons learned in a family-centered, hospital-based, interprofessional pediatric weight management program serving the Greater Baltimore area and surrounding communities in Maryland.* The Weigh Smart program serves a particularly diverse population. Given the limited physical activity opportunities in this environment, a physical therapist with the WS program works with the family and child to facilitate regular exercise.

Baltimore is a low-income, urban community with a large African American population and a growing Latino community, a population that is particularly at risk for obesity and related complications.[3,4] One study found higher rates of obesity among female schoolchildren in Baltimore than the national average.[5] Researchers have recognized the role of obesogenic environments in contributing to the rise of obesity among youths.[6] The obesogenic environments of urban, low-income communities such as Baltimore are often attributed, in part, to the limited availability of fresh food and limited opportunities for physical activity. Rural communities such as St. Mary's

---

Jessica M. Parrish, Elizabeth Getzoff, Kenneth Gelfand, and Michelle Demeule are affiliated with Mt. Washington Pediatric Hospital, Baltimore. Ann Scheimann is affiliated with the Division of Pediatric Gastroenterology and Nutrition, Johns Hopkins Hospital, Baltimore.

* This chapter might be read in conjunction with chapter 19, which begins with the same evidence-based recommendations and applies them in the very different setting of East Tennessee.

County and Western Maryland also face obstacles, with geographic barriers to specialized health care delivery for the treatment of pediatric obesity.

The Weigh Smart Program.

Weigh Smart staff at Mt. Washington Pediatric Hospital developed a pediatric obesity treatment program in the Baltimore community to address these disparities. Weigh Smart is a family-centered, interprofessional team approach to the treatment of pediatric obesity, employing a team composed of gastroenterology, psychology, nutrition, physical therapy, and nursing professionals. For those enrolled in the program, the entire family is required to make changes, rather than just the identified child. The program accepts children between the ages of 2 and 18 years who have a body mass index (BMI) above the 85th percentile. Weigh Smart sees approximately 200 new patients each year. Demographic data for WS participants are shown in table 26.1.

The initial intake visit is conducted jointly by a physician and a psychologist and includes medical, social, and psychiatric history, a physical exam, dietary recall, psychosocial questionnaires, and a review of physical activity. The families then receive individualized treatment recommendations and are referred to either the individual or the group program. The WS individual program allows children who are struggling with family conflict, mental health, or motivational issues to receive psychotherapy to address these issues, along with their family members, while they also receive assistance in implementing their weight management goals. The group program meets twice per week for 10 weeks, providing one hour of supervised exercise and one hour of class time per session. Seventy-nine percent of youths complete the 10-week WS program, which is defined as attending at least 16 of the 20 sessions. Sixty-three percent attend the one-month follow-up meeting. Preliminary examination of program outcomes suggests significant decreases in BMI, insulin, and triglycerides.

Nutrition education is tailored to the needs of the child and family based on individual medical issues. For the majority of families, the nutrition component of the WS program includes education on the Traffic Light Diet, an empirically validated

Table 26.1.   Demographics of Weight Smart
program participants (first six years)

Female (%)	67.0
Ethnicity (%)	
Caucasian	18.8
African American	68.0
Hispanic	5.1
Other or missing data	8.1
Living in a two-parent home (%)	34.0
Mean body mass index (kg/m^2)	36.8
Nonalcoholic fatty liver disease (%)	5.0

dietary intervention developed by Epstein and colleagues[7] that categorizes foods as red, yellow, or green. Given the limited health literacy of many families,[8] the Traffic Light Diet is particularly helpful as it includes specific categories of foods to consume and to avoid. Families learn about portion size, label reading, and making healthy choices when eating out at restaurants. Other nutrition education tools occasionally used include the plate method, which increases fruit and vegetable consumption by reserving half of one's plate for fruits and vegetables, and the low glycemic index diet.[9] Nutrition education alone, however, is rarely sufficient to produce long-term change. Behavioral support is often necessary to effectively change habits. As part of the team, psychology staff teach families behavioral techniques such as goal setting, modeling, problem solving, self-monitoring, and rewarding desired behaviors to facilitate behavioral change and improved parenting skills.

The flexibility of the WS program structure allows tailored treatment to serve families effectively. Caregivers are necessary targets of change in order to modify the child's food environment. Additional family members (e.g., grandparents) are invited to participate in treatment, based on their involvement in the child's care. Caregivers act as nutritional gatekeepers and model healthy habits for their children. Several studies have shown the superior effects on weight loss when parents are involved in the treatment.[10,11] In the WS group program, caregivers are required to attend all nutrition and psychology classes with their children and are invited to three exercise classes, so that they eventually can become their child's trainer through heart rate monitoring and motivational techniques. Caregivers have the opportunity to complete food and exercise logs and are expected to track their child's progress.

Barriers
We discuss here some challenges encountered by the WS program. Strategies developed to respond to these challenges, based on the program's six years of experience, are summarized under "Lessons Learned," below; these may be helpful to others engaged in similar efforts.

Sustainability
Financial viability is a problem in pediatric obesity programs, especially those serving underserved communities. As pediatric obesity programs often struggle to generate enough clinical revenue to be self-sufficient, they often rely on grant or institutional support for sustenance.[12] Each WS provider (medical, physical therapy, psychology, and nutrition) bills separately for his or her services, primarily based on comorbidities. Many of the participants in the WS program receive Maryland medical assistance (58.7%). Many others have few to no benefits for weight management services such as nutrition. In recognition that the cost of an interprofessional team can be onerous for many families, the hospital's foundation developed a grant to help families pay for treatment, in conjunction with a sliding scale fee. These measures help maximize the program's fiscal solvency.

Attrition

Effective treatment of pediatric obesity often requires long-term, intensive treatment. However, many of the families seen in the WS program face multiple stressors that make regular attendance at appointments difficult. The Weigh Smart staff has conducted surveys to determine how to meet participants' needs better and how to minimize attrition. Based on the feedback, group program hours were changed to the early evening and the number of sessions reduced from 13 to 10 weeks to be more convenient for families. Social work is critical in helping families get necessary resources, such as access to transportation to their appointments. Since distance is often a barrier for regular attendance at appointments, WS works with service providers (physicians and mental health professionals) who are located close to the family's home. To aid in reducing participants' time in the clinic and to decrease the no-show rate, families must complete an intake form and blood work prior to the initial appointment. Another factor leading to attrition is a family's level of motivation. The psychology professionals use motivational interviewing techniques to help improve the family's motivation and adherence.

Adherence

Another barrier often encountered in treating obesity is adherence to the treatment recommendations. One challenge is that many families have limited access to healthy foods. Many areas are characterized as "food deserts," or areas in which healthy food is difficult to find, according to the U.S. Department of Agriculture Economic Research Service's Food Locator.[13] An additional problem is that many healthier foods are more expensive. Because of these factors, some families purchase food for the entire month in a single supermarket visit and have limited access to fresh fruits and vegetables. Weigh Smart staff members have increasingly recognized the importance of asking families about their food shopping habits and tailoring recommendations accordingly. The program has also worked with Maryland Women, Infants, and Children Program (WIC) officials to alter the foods that WS participants are permitted to purchase with their WIC checks (e.g., nonfat instead of whole milk) to increase the healthfulness of foods made available to low-income families. A related problem is that many impoverished children rely on free or reduced-cost school lunches. Unfortunately, many schools offer predominantly high-fat, high-calorie options with few healthy choices. Attempts to communicate with schools about limiting lunch and snack time choices have had limited success, as federal school policy mandates that children must be allowed to select their own foods. One strategy developed to address this issue is to review school breakfast and lunch menus so that staff can help families make the healthiest choices.

Many families also struggle to get daily exercise.[2] Establishing regular exercise routines is often more difficult in urban communities due to safety concerns and limited resources. As part of the group program, children exercise twice weekly for an hour with a physical therapist. Many of these children are deconditioned, requiring attention from physical therapy prior to the group program. Children are exposed to a variety of exercises with the hope that they find some that they enjoy and can continue at home or by joining a center such as the YMCA. Each child receives three personalized at-home exercise routines that can be performed indoors with limited equipment. To help parents facilitate regular exercise in an environment with limited opportunities for physical activity, there are three family-based exercise sessions in which parents are trained to become their child's "trainer." They learn to monitor their child's heart rate and to motivate their children to exercise in the optimal fat-burning zone. The WS program has also worked with a local fitness facility to offer WS participants a reduced fee for gym membership. Weigh Smart is currently in the process of establishing a parent-led exercise group using social media to encourage physical activity.

Specialty Programs

In response to the increasing number of young children who are referred to the program, a Weigh Smart Jr. program has been developed to treat obesity in toddlers and children aged 2–7 years. These younger children tend to present as more overweight than older youths. Their treatment often requires a greater focus on providing their caregivers with behavior management strategies to improve their control of their child's daily routines, including sleep, eating, and exercise behaviors. A large part of treatment also focuses on increasing children's acceptance of healthy foods and teaching caregivers about the nutritional needs of younger children. In addition, work with younger children more frequently requires referrals to the social worker to help families with attending medical appointments and procuring necessary resources.

Following current population trends, the WS program has seen an increase in Latino patients. Latino youths, especially males, have been recognized in the literature as especially at risk for obesity and comorbidities.[14] The WS group curriculum has been adapted for use with Spanish-speaking groups. The dietary guidelines and food presentations are made more culturally relevant to Latino families. In addition, a greater number of family members are permitted to attend group sessions, given the important role of the extended family in Latino communities. One challenge that arose was that many of the Latino children eat a large meal after school. Thus, in delivering information about appropriate foods and servings for lunch and dinner, we were unknowingly encouraging four full meals a day. It was also interesting to observe that this population of caregivers was very satisfied with the camaraderie with other families and the health literacy education but appeared less invested in and attentive to their children's progress with weight loss. This has been addressed by holding family conferences midway through the program to problem-solve with families about potential barriers.

Future Directions

To increase the accessibility of Weigh Smart services, the program is striving to become more integrated into the community. Schools are particularly important targets for change and education, as many children consume a majority of their meals and snacks in the school environment. Weigh Smart works with local schools to deliver an after-school wellness program to decrease the risk of obesity and associated comorbidities.

Obesity is a chronic illness that affects more than a third of Maryland's youths. The WS program is designed to help children and families become healthier. In this chapter we have reviewed the distinctive characteristics of the population served and barriers such as financial sustainability, adherence, and attrition. The program's next steps include becoming more integrated into the community to provide care to an even greater number of children.

LESSONS LEARNED

- Identify strategies for helping children make healthy food choices at school.
- Help families with limited resources obtain healthy foods. Work with organizations that can be instrumental in providing increased access to healthy foods or exercise equipment.
- In addition to procuring healthy foods, families often benefit from instruction on how to plan and prepare healthy meals.
- Be flexible in structuring appointments and appointment times to meet parents' schedules and reduce attrition. Meeting with families in churches or schools can increase the number of families served.
- Be creative in finding exercise routines for families with limited access to safe, outdoor areas and physical activity opportunities.
- Understand cultural influences on meal planning, meal times, and meal time behaviors.
- Develop programming for younger children with an added focus on helping families access social services.
- Use multiple avenues to secure funding.

References

1. Davis AM, James RL. Model treatment programs. In: Jelalian E, Steele RG, eds. Handbook of childhood and adolescent obesity. New York, NY: Springer, 2008.
2. Barlow SE, Expert Committee. Expert Committee recommendations regarding the prevention, assessment, and treatment of child and adolescent overweight and obesity: summary report. Pediatrics. 2007 Dec;120 Suppl l4:S164–92.
3. Ogden CL, Carroll MD, Curtin LR, et al. Prevalence of high body mass index in US children and adolescents, 2007–2008. JAMA. 2010 Jan 20;303(3):242–9.
4. Moore DB, Howell PB, Treiber FA. Adiposity changes in youth with a family history of cardiovascular disease: impact of ethnicity, gender and socioeconomic status. J Assoc Acad Minor Phys. 2002 Jul;13(3):76–83.

5. Jehn ML, Gittelsohn J, Treuth MS, et al. Prevalence of overweight among Baltimore City schoolchildren and its associations with nutrition and physical activity. Obesity (Silver Spring). 2006 Jun;14(6):989–93.

6. Booth KM, Pinkston MM, Poston WS. Obesity and the built environment. J Am Diet Assoc. 2005 May;105(5 Suppl 1):S110–7.

7. Epstein LH, Wing RR, Koeske R, et al. Effects of diet plus exercise on weight change in parents and children. J Consult Clin Pyschol. 1984 Jun;52(3):429–37.

8. Kutner M, Greenberg E, Jin Y, et al. The health literacy of America's adults: results from the 2003 National Assessment of Adult Literacy. Washington, DC: National Center for Education Statistics, U.S. Department of Education, 2006. Available at: http://nces.ed.gov/pubs 2006/2006483.pdf.

9. Ludwig DS. Dietary glycemic index and obesity. J Nutr. 2000 Feb;130(2S Suppl):280–3S.

10. Golan M, Kaufman V, Shahar DR. Childhood obesity treatment: targeting parents exclusively v. parents and children. Br J Nutr. 2006 May;95(5):1008–15.

11. Epstein LH, Valoski A, Wing RR, et al. Ten-year outcomes of behavioral family-based treatment for childhood obesity. Health Psychol. 1990 Sep;13(5):373–83.

12. Slusser W, Staten K, Stephens K, et al. Payment for obesity services: examples and recommendations for stage 3 comprehensive multidisciplinary intervention programs for children and adolescents. Pediatrics. 2011 Sep;128 Suppl 2:S78–85.

13. Ver Ploeg M, Breneman V, Farrigan T, et al. Access to affordable and nutritious food—measuring and understanding food deserts and their consequences: report to Congress (Administrative Pub. No. AP-036). Washington, DC: U.S. Department of Agriculture, 2009.

14. Stovitz SD, Schwimmer JB Martinez H, et al. Pediatric obesity: the unique issues in Latino-American male youth. Am J Prev Med. 2008 Feb;34(2):153–60.

CHAPTER 27

Healthy Children, Strong Families

Obesity Prevention for Preschool American Indian Children and Their Families

Alexandra Adams, MD, PhD, Kate A. Cronin, MPH, and HCSF Community Research Group

National obesity rates among preschool American Indian (AI) children are among the highest of any racial or ethnic group (58.8%) and higher than for all racial/ethnic groups combined (30%).[1-4] Despite the decreases observed in other minority communities, the rates of obesity among AI preschoolers are not decreasing but rising.[5,6] Few obesity prevention trials have focused on preschool-age children, and effective programs targeting this neglected, critical developmental period—focusing on the family—are needed. The preschool years are crucial for long-term obesity prevention.[7]*

For the past 10 years, we have worked in community-based participatory research (CBPR) partnerships with four Wisconsin tribes on childhood obesity prevention.[8-12] Our early collaborative research with AI tribes in Wisconsin revealed a high prevalence of overweight (19%) and obesity (27%) among young children (ages 3–7) and their primary caregivers (> 75%).[8,13] In spite of the high prevalence of overweight and obesity, both concern about and recognition of the problem were low among caregivers, and few understood the connection between early obesity and later disease.[9] Our qualitative research revealed that AI communities take a much more holistic approach to health, which can render the disease model approach common to many public health interventions ineffective.[10,11]

Alexandra Adams is an associate professor in the Department of Family Medicine and director of the Collaborative Center for Health Equity, Institute for Clinical and Translational Research Health Sciences Learning Center, University of Wisconsin School of Medicine and Public Health (UW-SOMPH). Kate A. Cronin is affiliated with the Department of Family Medicine at UW-SOMPH. The Healthy Children, Strong Families (HCSF) Community Research Group includes multiple tribal mentors and staff who contributed to the work and gave feedback on the chapter.

* See chapter 1, in which Frisvold and Giri review the literature on early childhood education as a setting for obesity prevention. Here, we discuss an intervention designed for the home. See chapter 21 for additional work on obesity and overweight in American Indians.

Recent reviews of best practices in obesity prevention showed a limited number of interventions in the home[14,15] and a still rudimentary understanding of parental and family factors.[16] Of the available studies, only two of seven randomized trials for obesity prevention in preschool-age children were home-based, and only one, a 16-week trial, examined weight outcomes at ages younger than 5 years. This small trial (n = 40 mother-child pairs) was conducted with AI families and showed no significant change in weight-for-height z scores, but children in the intervention group did show a trend of decreased weight.[17]

To address the issue of childhood obesity while incorporating these factors, we collaboratively designed and tested a randomized trial of a home-visiting versus a mailed-only healthy lifestyle intervention for AI families with children ages 2–5: Healthy Children, Strong Families (HCSF).[18,19] In this chapter we discuss both the practical lessons learned from running a multitribal, multisite obesity prevention intervention with young AI families and the valuable feedback received from community mentors and HCSF participants that helped shape the direction of our future research interventions.

The HCSF Intervention

The original HCSF curriculum was developed in collaboration with partners at three Wisconsin tribes and the Great Lakes Inter-Tribal Council, Inc. (a consortium of 11 Wisconsin tribes), with substantive contributions from state and national early childhood experts and after extensive preliminary research with the tribal communities.[18] Healthy Children, Strong Families was a two-year, family-based, randomized controlled trial of the healthy lifestyle intervention with four Wisconsin tribes, enrolling 120 families. The intervention curriculum included 12 lessons targeting increased fruits and vegetables, increased physical activity, decreased screen time, and decreased added sugars. The 12 lessons included small incentive items intended to complement lesson themes, such as books, active games, and recipes. Lessons were supplemented with monthly newsletters. During year 1, trained community mentors worked with 2- to 5-year-old AI children and their primary caregivers to promote goal-based behavioral change through monthly home visits to deliver the HCSF nutrition and physical activity curriculum. Visits were scheduled at the participant's home at a time of the participant's choosing, and both the enrolled parent and the child were expected to be present. Other family members who were home were also invited to participate. Lesson delivery included at least one active learning component to engage the child, with the remaining portions of the visit dedicated to coaching the adult on newly adopted health behaviors and assistance with goal setting for newly introduced health topics. When the mentoring was consistent, it was well received, but issues such as participant no-shows and mentor turnover at some sites made home visiting challenging.

During year 2, families in the intervention group attended monthly group meetings. Families in the control group received monthly mailed materials only, with no home visits.[19] The intervention design is described elsewhere.[18,19]

Healthy Children, Strong Families is based on the AI model of elders teaching life skills to the next generation and reinforces cultural values of family interaction, healthy foods, and activity. The program aims to change behaviors not only through increased knowledge about healthy lifestyles but also through enhanced parenting skills and increased self-efficacy for behavioral change in diet, screen time, and physical activity.

Communities Involved in the Project

Four American Indian communities located in rural northern Wisconsin participated in this project. Intervention participants were primarily reservation based, and the four communities ranged in size from 2,000 to 8,000 tribal members. These communities have been collaborative partners with Alexandra Adams for 5–12 years. For all parts of the study, research approval was obtained from the University of Wisconsin Institutional Review Board and the relevant Tribal Councils.

Outcomes

The HCSF intervention was successful for several adult and child behavioral changes and showed other potential areas for modification.[20] An important finding was that delivering the intervention through mentors who visited families' homes appears to have little or no effect on the primary outcomes relative to sending the intervention through the mail. The effect of home visiting accounted for none of the variation in children's body mass index (BMI) z-scores and for less than 1% in adult caregivers' change in BMI. However, the curriculum itself seems to have brought about significant changes in several targeted behaviors and resulted in a mean decrease in adult BMI of $0.65 \, \text{kg/m}^2$, due to a significant decrease in measured weight of $1.53 \, \text{kg}$. Overweight/obese children (> 85th percentile, per Centers for Disease Control and Prevention [CDC] categories) showed a reduction in BMI z-score at 12 and 24 months compared with normal-weight children (< 85th percentile) at baseline. The CDC defines normal weight as 5th to < 85th percentile for BMI, overweight as 85th to < 95th percentile, and obese as ≥ 95th percentile, by age and sex growth charts.[21] In addition, both children and caregivers reported significant decreases in amount of time spent watching TV (by 27 minutes daily for adults, 15 minutes for children). Both children and adults also reported increased consumption of fruits and vegetables (in children, from 1.3 to 1.6 servings per day). Most other objective outcome measures were also in the direction of improved health. In the mentored group, a significant increase was observed in adults' self-reported self-efficacy for health behavior changes and health-related quality of life. Finally, CBPR principles were used throughout, and great success was achieved with engaging each community in lesson development, in developing local capacity for research delivery and evaluation, and in developing community advisory boards.

Discussion
Research Implementation

Honoring Community Preferences Can Affect Scientific Rigor Because none of the four tribal communities wanted to be a control community, participants were randomized by family within each community. With a small sample in our intervention group and multiple cases of extended family members in opposing study arms, this may have contributed to the lack of significant difference between the two arms. When implementing a randomized trial in small, close-knit communities, it is important to recognize this issue and take steps to minimize its effect on research results, if possible. Although randomization was effective, and both groups began with the same number of participants, we had a larger drop-out rate in the mentored intervention group, and we are hypothesizing that this was caused by mentor turnover at some sites and the difficulty of holding monthly meetings for a year in the intervention group.

Site Differences in Intervention Delivery Intervention delivery differed by site as a result of unforeseen and sometimes unavoidable impediments: mentor turnover due to personal problems, site preferences in types of mentors hired, and community problems interfering with hiring mentors and recruiting participants (e.g., a clinic fire). Overall, the most successful sites, defined as ones that recruited and retained the most participants, had committed mentors who were engaged over the entire study, or were already part of a wellness team at the clinic, or were specifically hired to coordinate the research at the local level. It is important to work closely with communities to develop realistic and sustainable staffing plans to accomplish research objectives, to develop local capacity for research, and to ensure fidelity to the research plan.

Multiple Communication Strategies to Successfully Track Participants Maintaining contact with participants in tribal communities proved to be challenging. Families frequently changed addresses and, even more frequently, phone numbers. Three strategies assisted with maintaining contact. First, we sent all participants (intervention and control groups) a monthly newsletter, which was part of the intervention curriculum, and returned newsletters triggered a phone call to obtain a new mailing address. This was especially important during year 2, when families in the control group had no contact other than the newsletters in the time between their post-study and their two-year follow-up measurement visits. Second, at the post-study visit, we asked participants to provide a *backup contact* whom we could call to obtain updated contact information for the participant if it became necessary. Finally, we set up a toll-free number that allowed participants to reach study staff without cost (although this became less important as more people began to use cell phones only).

Ultimately, we found that having multiple avenues to contact participants, coupled with the ability of local program staff to reach out to participants in everyday situations (e.g., running into a participant at the grocery store or at a community event), often made the difference in whether families stayed in the program throughout its duration. In a community-based research setting, this type of interaction is normative and, in our case, encouraged. No distinction was made between control and intervention status when these interactions occurred.

Incorporating Feedback

Community Mentor Feedback During the intervention period, study staff had formal and informal opportunities to solicit feedback from the home-visiting mentors. Study staff regularly checked in with mentors to support them and to monitor their progress with scheduling home visits. At six months and post-intervention, a formal structured interview was done with each home-visiting mentor, and at two of the participating sites, an end-of-program wrap-up session was held with the mentors.

Feedback from mentors revealed that, in some instances, active learning concepts in the curriculum could have reinforced negative rather than positive health messages. Based on this feedback, we immediately made changes to the lessons and implemented these with all families from then on. Other feedback from the mentors was used to modify the curriculum based on their overall experiences after the intervention period was complete. Important feedback from the mentors included requests for more interactive learning opportunities that engaged the entire family in each lesson, shorter lesson length, and more concrete tools, such as shopping lists and label-reading guides, to leave with families for their use between home visits.

HCSF Participant Feedback Feedback from HCSF participants was solicited formally through surveys at six months and at the one-year post-study visit. At two sites, focus groups were conducted at the end of the intervention. The results from five focus groups conducted with intervention and control group participants indicated good mastery and enjoyment of the lessons, and participants reported incorporating newly learned strategies for healthy behaviors into their daily lives. Favored family components included children's books on health topics, movement games, and easy recipes that allowed caregivers to cook together with their children. Many focus group participants reported enjoying the mentors' visits; however, participants' ability to make and keep monthly mentor appointments was inconsistent in many cases.

In addition to the planned benefits, a widely reported benefit of participation was an increase in family time—through walks, active play, reading with children, and preparing and eating meals as a family. Barriers to adopting healthy lifestyle behaviors included lack of social support for new behaviors and environmental barriers such as the perceived high cost of healthy foods and lack of time to practice healthy behaviors due to work and school commitments. Participants frequently mentioned that their child became a "change agent" by refocusing parents and extended family

Table 27.1. Healthy Children, Strong Families participant feedback

Increased family time:
- More active play and family walks
- Increased family meals and more child involvement in food preparation
- Increased reading, specifically at bedtime

Changes in health behaviors:
- More water, less sugar-sweetened beverages
- Increased attention to food purchases and food labels
- Less fast food / convenience food purchases

Health promotion:
- Child and adults shared newly learned nutrition information and physical activity opportunities within family and social networks
- Changes in types of foods shared at school functions and social gatherings
- Independently seeking out resources such as books with health topics as a fun way to learn new information together

Family bonding:
- Reports of feeling closer to child as program provided an opportunity to have "special time" with one child at a time
- Shift in activity choices for family time—less TV, increased preference for interactive pursuits (games, walks, crafts, etc.)

members on healthy behaviors and practices. A sample of positive changes reported by HCSF participants is given in table 27.1.

This family feedback was very useful in incorporating some of the unanticipated benefits into the revised curriculum, such as adding recipes and additional books. We have worked with people at one site to incorporate the modified curriculum into part of their Indian Health Service–funded diabetes prevention grant and have also incorporated it into their menu of wellness options for physician referral. Another site will be working with us in ongoing intervention research.

Conclusions

Healthy Children, Strong Families is a randomized healthy lifestyle intervention conducted in four America Indian communities. The intervention focuses on engaging the family and young child, focusing on family health and strength to reduce barriers to healthy lifestyles rather than on obesity prevention. This collaborative intervention has worked with community mentors and staff in a participatory process in intervention design, delivery, and evaluation. Healthy Children, Strong Families has had many successes and revealed many unexpected lessons. For example, the value of the monthly mailed lessons was unanticipated, as was the difficulty in showing a significant effect of the mentor's presence in the home. Despite the focus group feedback on the importance of the mentors, differences between the mentored and control groups were not significant in healthy lifestyle change. This may be due to both the unanticipated strength of the curriculum's impact and the difficulty with mentor turnover at several sites.

Targeting both the primary caregiver and the child was an important key to success, due to the intergenerational bonding and reinforcing of lessons learned. Unanticipated benefits of HCSF in the home included more family time, more reading, and more one-on-one time with preschool-age children. Having an attractive and flexible curriculum that was easily used by families in the home, accompanied by lesson supplies that were fun to use (such as children's books focused on health, games, and a versatile cookbook), was essential.

Using multiple methods of communication was critical to bridging communication gaps. Building local capacity for research delivery was also critical in retaining families and maintaining fidelity to the research objectives during the two-year intervention.

We believe that future obesity prevention and healthy lifestyle interventions should (1) focus on the family for intergenerational behavior modeling and change; (2) include fun, easy, interactive materials; (3) incorporate health-related children's books; and (4) focus on reducing both family and environmental barriers to change.

Families play a crucial role in obesity prevention, but the work on understanding family change is in its infancy. Healthy Children, Strong Families is the first multisite randomized trial of a healthy lifestyle intervention that targets both AI children and their caregivers. Our findings indicate that modifications of the well-received HCSF intervention may address early childhood obesity at a low cost to families among minority groups, and work on this is underway.

LESSONS LEARNED
- The use of good CBPR practices can affect scientific design and intervention implementation. Potential strategies such as using a delayed or active control and planning/budgeting for sustainable staffing at the local level can help address these issues.
- Multiple communication strategies and frequent contact with research participants can improve fidelity to the intervention and increase attendance at data-collection visits.
- Iteratively incorporating feedback from intervention staff and participants, during and after the intervention period, can both prevent potential negative issues and strengthen the intervention.
- Focusing on both adults and children in the family context is essential, due to mutual reinforcement of lifestyle changes.

Acknowledgments

The research reported in this chapter was supported by NHLBI/NIH U01HL087381. The authors thank the families and communities participating in the study.

References

1. Lindsay RS, Cook V, Hanson RL, et al. Early excess weight gain of children in the Pima Indian population. Pediatrics. 2002 Feb;109:E33.
2. Salbe AD, Weyer C, Lindsay RS, et al. Assessing risk factors for obesity between childhood and adolescence: birth weight, childhood adiposity, parental obesity, insulin, and leptin. Pediatrics. 2002 Aug;110(2 Pt 1):299–306.
3. Halpern P. Obesity and American Indians / Alska Natives. Washington, DC: U.S. Department of Health and Human Services, 2007.
4. Polhamus B, Thompson D, Dalenius K, et al. Pediatric nutrition surveillance 2004 report. Atlanta, GA: Centers for Disease Control and Prevention, 2006.
5. Centers for Disease Control and Prevention. Obesity prevalence among low-income, preschool-aged children—United States, 1998–2008. MMWR Morb Mortal Wkly Rep. 2009 Jul 24;58(28):769–73.
6. National Center for Health Statistics. Pediatric nutrition national surveillance summary of trends in growth and anemia indicators by race/ethnicity: children aged < 5 years. Atlanta, GA: Centers for Disease Control and Prevention, 2010.
7. Birch LL. Development of food preferences. Annu Rev Nutr. 1999;19:41–62.
8. Adams A, Miller-Korth N, Brown D. Learning to work together: developing academic and community research partnerships. WMJ. 2004;103(2):15–9.
9. Adams AK, Quinn RA, Prince RJ. Low recognition of childhood overweight and disease risk among Native-American caregivers. Obes Res. 2005 Jan;13(1):146–52.
10. Adams AK, Harvey H, Brown D. Constructs of health and environment inform child obesity prevention in American Indian communities. Obesity (Silver Spring). 2008 Feb;16(2):311–7.
11. Adams A, Prince R. Correlates of physical activity in young American Indian children: lessons learned from the Wisconsin Nutrition and Growth Study. J Public Health Manag Pract. 2010 Sep–Oct;16(5):394–400.
12. Adams A. Understanding community and family barriers and supports to physical activity in American Indian children. J Public Health Manag Pract. 2010 Sep–Oct;16(5):401–3.
13. Adams A, Prince R, Webert H. The Wisconsin Nutrition and Growth Study (WINGS), a participatory research project with three Wisconsin tribes. Great Lakes EpiCenter News. 2004;5(3):1–3.
14. Flynn MAT, McNeil DA, Maloff B, et al. Reducing obesity and related chronic disease risk in children and youth: a synthesis of evidence with "best practice" recommendations. Obes Rev. 2006 Feb;7 Suppl 1:7–66.
15. Monasta L, Batty GD, Macaluso A, et al. Interventions for the prevention of overweight and obesity in preschool children: a systematic review of randomized controlled trials. Obes Rev. 2011 May;12(5):e107–18.
16. Skouteris H, McCabe M, Swinburn B, et al. Parental influence and obesity prevention in pre-schoolers: a systematic review of interventions. Obes Rev. 2011 May;12(5):315–28.
17. Harvey-Berino J, Rourke J. Obesity prevention in preschool Native-American children: a pilot study using home visiting. Obes Res. 2003 May;11(5):606–11.
18. LaRowe TL, Wubben DP, Cronin KA, et al. Development of a culturally appropriate nutrition and physical activity curriculum for Wisconsin American Indian families. Prev Chronic Dis. 2007 Oct;4(4):A109. Epub 2007 Sep 15.

19. Adams A, LaRowe T, Cronin K, et al. Healthy Children, Strong Families: design of a family based healthy lifestyles intervention. J Prim Prev. 2012 Aug;33(4):175–85.
20. Adams A, LaRowe T, Cronin K, et al. Healthy Children, Strong Families: results of a randomized trial of obesity prevention for preschool American Indian children and their families. Presented at: Annual Meeting of the Obesity Society, Orlando, FL, 2011 Oct.
21. Centers for Disease Control and Prevention. About BMI for children and teens. Atlanta, GA: Centers for Disease Control and Prevention, 2011.

CHAPTER 28

A Structured Weight Management Program for Obese Patients in an Urban Safety-Net Hospital Center

Michelle McMacken, MD, Sarah Moore, MD, Diana Randlett, MD, and Lisa Parikh, MD

.

The U.S. Preventive Services Task Force[1] recommends that health care providers offer high-frequency weight loss counseling (two or more visits per month) to obese patients. Typically, however, primary care providers are consumed by managing the comorbid conditions that accompany obesity, leaving little time for detailed weight loss advice. Moreover, there are particular challenges to offering high-quality obesity counseling in culturally and linguistically diverse, underserved populations.

For these reasons, high-intensity weight loss counseling is impractical in many primary care settings. Our outpatient weight management program was designed to fill this resource gap by providing intensive multidisciplinary treatment for obese patients in our urban, safety-net hospital center.

Program Overview

The Bellevue Hospital Weight Management Clinic offers intensive nonsurgical weight management services for obese patients (body mass index [BMI] $\geq 30\,\text{kg/m}^2$). The focus is on individualized lifestyle education, behavioral counseling, and goal setting, with frequent follow-up visits to sustain motivation. We work closely with the hospital's bariatric surgery service to offer referrals for weight loss surgery when appropriate.

Setting

Bellevue Hospital Center, the nation's oldest public hospital, is a core New York University School of Medicine teaching facility serving a very diverse, medically

Michelle McMacken is an assistant professor of medicine in the Division of General Internal Medicine, New York University School of Medicine (NYU-SOM), and an attending physician at Bellevue Hospital Center, New York. Sarah Moore and Diana Randlett are clinical instructors in the Division of General Internal Medicine, NYU-SOM, and attending physicians at Bellevue. Lisa Parikh is an internal medicine resident in the Department of Medicine, NYU-SOM.

underserved population. Limited English proficiency is common (50%–60%). Approximately 46% of ambulatory care patients are Latino, 21% Black, 13% Asian, 12% White, and 8% other. Uninsured patients constituted 27% of outpatient visits to Bellevue in 2011. The remaining visits were for patients with Medicaid (44%), Medicare (15%), commercial health insurance (11%), or other (3%).

Referrals
Our referral criteria are (1) BMI $\geq 30\,kg/m^2$ and (2) interest in weight loss. Nearly 80% of our patients are referred to our program by their primary care providers. We also receive referrals from endocrinology, psychiatry, surgical specialties, and other ambulatory care clinics. Approximately 5%–10% of our referrals are from the bariatric surgery service, primarily for preoperative medically supervised weight management.

Staffing Model
Our program is staffed by three internal medicine attending physicians who have a strong interest in obesity medicine and years of experience in this field. These attendings also have a full-time primary care and inpatient practice, but 10% of their ambulatory care time is allotted to serve in the weight management clinic. Typically, only one attending physician is available to lead the clinic during its half-day-per-week session. One or two senior internal medicine residents rotate through the program each week. A part-time nutritionist, funded through a small grant, leads weekly group sessions for nutrition education in English and Spanish. Telephone interpretation services are provided by the hospital through the use of a dual-handset telephone in each examination room. A hospital-employed ancillary staff member is available to measure vital signs and make follow-up appointments. Program evaluation and other administrative tasks are performed by the attending physicians on nonclinic time.

Reimbursement
Our clinic visits are coded in the same manner as general medicine office visits. We document elements of the history of present illness, medical history, review of systems, physical exam, and assessment and plan as appropriate. We also document the amount of time spent face-to-face with the patient and in coordinating care.

The Initial Assessment
All patients receive an initial comprehensive medical evaluation. At this 45-minute visit, a thorough history is obtained using a standardized template as a guide (fig.28.1).

Medical History
In evaluating the medical history, we focus on obesity-related comorbidities and other medical conditions that may affect the patient's ability to make lifestyle changes. Most patients in our program have a primary care provider and have already been

Medical History
(diabetes/prediabetes, metabolic syndrome, obstructive sleep apnea, fatty liver disease, hypertension, osteoarthritis, hyperlipidemia?)

PCP _____   HbA1c or fasting glucose:_____

Referral source _____   Lipids:_____

Medications _____

     TSH:_____

Perceptions About Weight
What brings you to our clinic today? Would you like to change your weight?

Weight History/Social History
What is your lowest weight ever as an adult? What is your highest weight?
Were you overweight as a child or were there specific life events after which you gained weight (e.g., pregnancies, immigration to United States)?
Have you tried to lose weight before? If so, what did you do? Did it work? Did you gain weight back?
What things do you think cause you to be overweight?
What is your living situation (home, SRO, etc.)? How much support can your family and/or friends provide?

Motivation and Confidence
On a scale of 1 to 10 (where 1 is not at all important, and 10 is extremely important), how important is it to you to lose weight?
On a scale of 1 to 10, how confident are you that you can lose weight?
What are some things that will make it hard for you to lose weight?

Dietary Patterns (eating frequency, home vs. meals out, sweetened beverages, portion sizes, binge behavior, vegetables/high fiber foods)
Take me through what you ate yesterday (or on a typical day). (Include breakfast, lunch, dinner, snacks in between.)
Do you drink soda? Juice? Anything else from a bottle or can, or made from a powder?
What vegetables do you like?

Exercise Patterns
What do you do on a typical day?
How many hours of television do you watch each day?
How far can you walk without stopping?

Physical Exam (including weight and height; calculate BMI) – Cushingoid? Volume overload?

Setting Goals
How much weight would you like to lose?
Did you know that even if you lose only a small amount of weight, your health could improve a lot?
(A realistic goal should be to lose 5%–10% of body weight, over 6 months; 1 lb a week).
** Set a specific behavior goal for next time. Write it down on the 'My Behavior Change' sheet and give it to the patient. **

FIGURE 28.1. Template for patient's history at an initial visit to Bellevue Weight Management Clinic. BMI, body mass index; PCP, primary care provider; SRO, single room occupancy; TSH, thyroid-stimulating hormone.

evaluated for common obesity-related conditions, but when we identify gaps we refer the patient for screening as needed.

Medication Regimen

A careful review of the patient's medication regimen is a key element of the initial assessment. Numerous medications are associated with weight gain, including drugs commonly prescribed in the primary care setting, such as sulfonylureas, thiazolidine-diones, and certain antidepressants. Weight gain is also a major problem among patients being treated with atypical antipsychotics. In some instances, opportunities exist within U.S. Food and Drug Administration (FDA) guidelines to adjust the medication regimen to optimize weight loss or prevent further weight gain (e.g., using topiramate for migraine prophylaxis). In all cases of medication adjustments, we coordinate care with the patient's other providers. We have found almost no role for prescribing medications that are FDA-approved specifically for weight loss, as the benefits are transient, the side-effect profiles are poor, and the cost can be prohibitive.

Weight History

Many patients can name life events that resulted in weight gain and are aware of ongoing triggers such as anxiety or depression—insights that may guide the approach to behavior modification. It is also very illustrative to explore prior weight loss attempts, including what went well, what presented challenges, and potential reasons for weight regain. Some patients report previous use of extreme or fad diets; this revelation can provide an opportunity to highlight the benefits of gradual lifestyle change.

Motivation

Most of our patients are referred by their primary care providers because they expressed interest in losing weight; thus, many patients start our program with a high level of motivation to learn about lifestyle change. We use motivational interviewing techniques[2] to assess readiness to change and confidence; for example, providers can tease out possible barriers by asking questions such as, "You rated your confidence a 7 out of 10. What keeps you from calling it a 10?"

Social History

Social issues are explored at the initial visit as well. Although many of our patients have a spouse or partner who is also interested in losing weight, many others report that their families challenge their attempts to make behavioral changes such as serving healthier foods in the home. This barrier must be addressed, by involving the family in a future clinic visit, helping the patient brainstorm ways to negotiate, and/or supporting the patient in making behavioral changes independent of the family. Other common obstacles include financial constraints, poor access to healthful food, and housing problems.

Some patients are found to have significant barriers, such as untreated major depression or poorly controlled comorbid illness, that may prevent them from being able to commit to intensive lifestyle changes. In these cases, we refer the patient to mental health, social work, and other resources within the larger hospital network.

Diet and Exercise History

The dietary history is performed through a 24-hour recall or a review of the patient's typical day. Patients are specifically questioned about beverage choices, snacking habits, regularity of meals, portion sizes, consumption of fruits and vegetables, and restaurant/deli/takeout use. Beverages are particularly important, as many patients do not realize the contribution of sweetened or other caloric beverages to their energy intake.

Given the cultural diversity of our patient population, an individualized approach to dietary assessment and counseling is critical. Most patients do not follow a typical American diet. Sometimes the cuisine involves foods unfamiliar to the weight management provider. This challenge is typically addressed by devoting much of the initial dietary history to exploring the components of the patient's usual diet—through direct interviewing or a review of food diaries, or both. It is helpful for the provider to assess which traditional foods are high in simple or refined carbohydrates, which vegetables and fruits are typically eaten, how foods are prepared (e.g., fried, cooked with oils), and what beverages are consumed (such as homemade juices or sugar-sweetened drinks). This understanding allows the provider to offer dietary counseling within the framework of the typical cuisine—in particular, increasing the proportion of any low-calorie, nutrient-dense vegetables typically found in the patient's diet while reducing simple carbohydrates and/or liquid calories. During a recent visit, for example, a provider unfamiliar with a patient's traditional West African diet spent time using Internet resources to explore how fufu, a staple dish, is made. Discovering it is high in starch, the provider counseled the patient not to consume other high-starch foods in the same meal and to decrease the portion size in order to lose weight.

The exercise history involves an assessment of the patient's exercise tolerance, specific barriers to physical activity, and current level of physical activity.

Approach to Treatment
Weight Loss Goal

We work with patients to set a realistic weight loss goal, usually 5%–10% of initial body weight over 6–12 months. We acknowledge that this modest degree of weight loss may not meet personal goals for some patients, but it does confer significant health benefits.[3] Our emphasis is on practical, sustainable lifestyle changes.

Behavior Change Goals

Based on what we have learned about the patient in the initial assessment, we define several broad categories in which the patient has room for positive lifestyle change (e.g., eating regular meals, reducing portion sizes, adding more vegetables to the diet, eliminating liquid calories, limiting takeout or restaurant meals, or increasing physical activity). We then ask the patient to select one category from this list. The remainder of the visit is spent creating specific, measurable, concrete goals. This motivational interviewing approach, emphasizing the spirit of evocation and autonomy, anchors the goals in areas in which the patient is ready to make changes. For example, if the patient chooses the category of reducing portion sizes, a specific goal could be to use a half-cup measuring cup to serve rice and other carbohydrates. For liquid calories, a specific goal could be to switch from regular sodas to unsweetened seltzer water or from juice to whole fruit.

In the absence of dietary changes, the amount of physical activity required to promote weight loss usually exceeds the 150 minutes of weekly exercise recommended in current national guidelines.[4] This level of physical activity is not feasible for many of our patients due to orthopedic, cardiopulmonary, or other comorbid conditions. However, exercise does enhance dietary interventions for weight loss, has important cardiovascular and other health benefits, and is critical for preventing weight regain.[5] We individualize our recommendations on intensity and duration of exercise to each patient's exercise tolerance and capability. Because of its safety and accessibility, we recommend walking as the preferred form of exercise for most patients. Pedometer-based step tracking and exercise diaries can enhance motivation. For those patients able to join a fitness facility, we suggest strength training and aerobic activity, including stationary bikes and other low-impact equipment.

Our counseling techniques are tailored to each patient's educational and health literacy status. For example, the portion-control plate is more instructive for low-literacy patients than teaching about food labels or calorie counting.

Self-management Strategies

At the end of the visit, patients are given a "prescription" that lists the behavior change goals agreed on during the visit (fig. 28.2). The patient's weight is also recorded on this sheet. We promote self-management skills including food diaries, exercise calendars, and, if possible, regular home weighing.

Follow-up Visits

High-frequency follow-up visits are offered (weekly, biweekly, or monthly), in a combination of group and individual visits. During the individual follow-up visit, we check the patient's weight and review the specific behavior change goals set during the previous visit. A patient-centered, collaborative approach is used to identify significant barriers and to set new, small behavior change goals. A new prescription is created to reflect the updated goals.

All patients are encouraged to attend our weekly Healthy Lifestyle groups, which provide support, motivation, and detailed nutrition education. Weight is also checked at this weekly visit, which helps promote accountability.

```
┌─────────────────────────────────────────┐
│ Name_____       │
│ Date _____      │
│ Today's Weight _____       │
│ Next Appointment_____        │
└─────────────────────────────────────────┘
```

My Behavior Change Plan

Exercise Goals

____I will (check one)

    ___Walk ___Swim ___Bike

    ___Dance ___Other_____

        I will do this _____minutes/day

        I will do this _____days/week

        Which days (circle all that apply): Sun M T W Th F Sat

____I will buy a pedometer and record the number of steps I take each day

Diet Goals (check one or two)

____I will use a smaller plate (9 inches or a salad plate). I will wait 20 minutes to make sure I'm really hungry before serving myself seconds.

____I will eat more vegetables: half of my lunch or dinner plate

____I will drink WATER instead of fruit juices, sweetened tea, bottled drinks, and/or soda

____I will bake, broil or steam my foods instead of frying when possible

____I will eat smaller portions of the following foods:

_____

____I will switch from simple starches to complex starches like:

    a. lots of vegetables

    b. brown rice instead of white rice

    c. whole wheat bread instead of white bread

    d. whole wheat pasta instead of regular white pasta

    e. other_____

____I will eat regular meals including breakfast

____I will keep a food diary to record what I eat

____I will cook more at home instead of eating out

____Other_____

____Other_____

____Other_____

Bellevue Weight Management Clinic

FIGURE 28.2. Patient's behavior change plan used at Bellevue Weight Management Clinic.

Physician Education and Training

A significant proportion of primary care physicians do not feel competent in obesity counseling and treatment.[6] This lack of confidence and training may be magnified in the setting of cross-cultural communication.

Resident physicians who rotate in our program learn valuable skills in obesity medicine, lifestyle counseling, and motivational interviewing. Each clinic session begins with a 45-minute orientation led by the attending physician, including a discussion of key points in obesity management, pharmacology, and bariatric surgery. Subsequently, the resident physicians see patients directly and present cases to the attending preceptor, giving them an opportunity to apply their skills.

These skills translate into residents' primary care practice, not only in obesity management but in other areas as well. Furthermore, exposure to our program helps correct misconceptions about obesity and weight loss. Resident feedback has been very positive; most are happy to have the time outside their usual continuity clinic to sharpen their counseling skills and gain a better understanding of treatment options for obese patients.

Outcomes

Between January 2006 and July 2010, 323 patients attended our program for an initial visit. More than one-third carried an axis I psychiatric diagnosis. The racial/ethnic breakdown mirrored that of the general Bellevue population: 58% Latino, 23% Black, 11% White, 3% Asian, and 5% other.

Approximately half of these patients kept a follow-up appointment after the initial visit. In general, younger patients and patients using medications associated with weight gain were more likely to return for additional visits. Among patients with at least two visits to our program, one-third achieved clinically significant weight loss (5% or more of initial body weight). Weight loss paralleled the number of visits.

Future Directions

As in most weight management programs, preventing attrition and weight regain is a major challenge. Nearly half of our patients do not return for a second visit. For patients who do continue in our program and lose weight, maintaining that weight loss often proves difficult—a finding consistent with previous studies on nonsurgical weight loss.[7,8] We are exploring various methods of keeping patients engaged in the weight loss process and preventing weight regain. Potentially viable options are technology-based supports such as text messaging or telephone reminders, brief check-in visits with ancillary staff, incentives such as free pedometers, and peer support systems.

Cross-cultural dietary counseling presents another challenge; when the provider is unfamiliar with the patient's typical cuisine, it is very difficult to make culturally relevant recommendations on dietary change. Moreover, data are limited on effective weight loss counseling strategies for many of the cultural/ethnic groups we serve. More information is needed on what treatment and counseling approaches work best for different cultural/ethnic groups.

Our model demonstrates that successful weight loss counseling is possible in a culturally diverse, underinsured population that lacks access to commercial weight loss programs. We do not have specific funding beyond the modest (less than 10%) time commitment of our attending physician providers. It is our hope that our program can be reproduced in other urban, diverse, socioeconomically challenged areas.

LESSONS LEARNED

- Successful weight loss counseling, with a focus on setting small behavior change goals, is possible in a culturally diverse, underinsured population.
- Approximately half of the patients in this program returned for a second visit. Potential causes of attrition (personal, scheduling conflicts, lack of interest/motivation, program dissatisfaction, or others) must be identified and addressed.
- Weight loss parallels the number of visits to the program.
- The program filled a gap in the internal medicine curriculum around treatment of obesity. It is consistently a favorite rotation for the house staff.

References

1. U.S. Preventive Services Task Force. Screening for obesity in adults: recommendations and rationale. Ann Intern Med. 2003 Dec 2;139(11):930–2.
2. Rollnick S. Behaviour change in practice: targeting individuals. Int J Obes Relat Metab Disord. 1996 Feb;20 Suppl 1:S22–6.
3. McTigue KM, Harris R, Hemphill B, et al. Screening and interventions for obesity in adults: summary of the evidence for the U.S. Preventive Services Task Force. Ann Intern Med. 2003 Dec 2;139(11):933–49.
4. Donnelly JE, Blair SN, Jakicic JM, et al. American College of Sports Medicine Position Stand: appropriate intervention strategies for weight loss and prevention of weight regain for adults. Med Sci Sports Exerc. 2009 Feb;41(2):459–71.
5. Jakicic JM, Davis KK. Obesity and physical activity. Psychiatr Clin North Am. 2011 Dec;34(4):829–40.
6. Jay M, Kalet A, Ark T, et al. Physicians' attitudes about obesity and their associations with competency and specialty: a cross-sectional survey. BMC Health Serv Res. 2009 Jun;9:106.
7. Dansinger ML, Tatsioni A, Wong JB, et al. Meta-analysis: the effect of dietary counseling for weight loss. Ann Intern Med. 2007 Jul 3;147(1):41–50.
8. Wing RR, Tate DF, Gorin AA, et al. A self-regulation program for maintenance of weight loss. N Engl J Med. 2006 Oct 12;355(15):1563–71.

CHAPTER 29

Creating Safe Neighborhoods for Obesity Prevention
Perceptions of Urban Youth

Semra Aytur, PhD, MPH, Rebecca Butcher, MS, PT, MPH,
Cynthia Carlson, PE, PhD, and Karen Schifferdecker, PhD, MPH

Obesity is a complex systems problem, requiring comprehensive efforts to support healthy social and physical environments.[1] Recent recommendations include broadening the concept of evidence to consider new forms of information, especially when existing evidence is limited.[2] Little is known about lower-income/refugee adolescents' perceptions of relationships between safety, active living, and healthy eating in the context of their daily lives. Our study solicited these underrepresented voices, using Photovoice, to inform the evidence concerning obesity prevention.

The Photovoice Project

The city of Manchester, New Hampshire, has combined chronic disease prevention with evidence-based criminal justice initiatives to bring citizens, law enforcement, and other partners together to create safer, activity-friendly neighborhoods. The city developed institutional policies, originating from a Weed and Seed (W&S) grant from the Department of Justice in 2001,[3] that simultaneously support violence prevention and obesity prevention. This chapter focuses on a Photovoice project that was conducted within a community-based participatory research study of institutional policy change. Photovoice, a participatory action research method, enables people with little power to assess community strengths and concerns and communicate their views to decision makers.[4-7] The project was conducted in two neighborhoods: (1) an officially designated W&S target neighborhood ("designated"); and (2) a neighborhood

Semra Aytur is affiliated with the Department of Health Management and Policy, University of New Hampshire (UNH), in Durham; Rebecca Butcher, with the Center for Program Design and Evaluation at Dartmouth Medical School, in Hanover, and the Graduate School for Public Health at UNH–Manchester; Cynthia Carlson, with the Department of Environmental Science at New England College in Henniker, NH; and Karen Schifferdecker, with the Department of Community and Family Medicine, Dartmouth Medical School.

that was not a W&S target area but was undergoing neighborhood revitalization and had adopted several W&S strategies ("undesignated").[8,9] Based on 2010 Census data, 517 adolescents resided in the designated neighborhood; 518 in the undesignated neighborhood. The study protocol was approved by the institutional review boards of two universities.

Both neighborhoods experience higher percentages of first-graders with elevated body mass index than the city average (designated, 26%; undesignated, 20%). Approximately 23%–36% of the population is below the federal poverty level, in the undesignated and designated neighborhoods, respectively.[9,10] A growing population of refugees and immigrants resides in these neighborhoods; Manchester has six times more refugees than Boston in proportion to the cities' overall sizes. It is estimated that one-third of all refugees in New Hampshire come from Africa (13% from Sudan, 7% from Somalia, and 13% from other African countries). Initially, most immigrants and refugees receive assistance from federal and state agencies to help with housing, job training, and other services; however, this assistance greatly diminishes after the first year. There is no long-term follow-up with needs such as housing. With Manchester's resources stretched thin during the economic recession, refugee issues have become contentious politically. In 2012, policymakers unsuccessfully tried to request from the State Department a reduction in the number of refugees.

Seventeen English-speaking youths (ages 13–18) were initially recruited to the Photovoice project (designated: seven boys and three girls; undesignated: five girls and two boys). However, one girl in the undesignated neighborhood withdrew, and we were unable to publish data from two boys in the undesignated neighborhood because we could not confirm written parental permission to share the photos. Thus, we used data from 14 adolescents for the analysis: 12 were from African refugee families (from various countries, including Sudan, Somalia, Tanzania, and Rwanda), 1 was White, and 1 was African American.

Participants attended Photovoice sessions once a week for six weeks during the summer or fall of 2011. In the first five sessions, they were provided with cameras and asked to take photos of their neighborhoods, focusing on health and safety issues. Participants also received safety training and were instructed not to place themselves at risk while taking photographs.

In sessions 1–6, participants discussed four to eight photos per session, using the *SHOWeD* method (What do you *See* here? What's really *Happening*? How does this relate to *Our* lives? *Why* does this problem/strength exist? What can we *Do* about this?),[5,7] and they wrote captions to share with community stakeholders. Field notes and audio recordings were collected to capture their dialogue.

Outcomes

Overall, each participant took approximately 24 pictures. Of these, 54 pictures were selected for discussion and analysis. Due to the unbalanced sample sizes, gender-specific findings from the two neighborhoods should not be interpreted as directly comparable.

Adolescents' images and narratives revealed a holistic view of health, including mental, physical, social, and environmental phenomena. Positive neighborhood assets were identified, but participants also revealed gendered behavioral adaptations to signs of social disorder and violence.

Physical Activity and Environment

Boys described playing basketball as the most common physical activity, and their photos revealed diverse recreational locations, including parks, indoor courts, and schools. However, boys noted that facilities were often in disrepair and indoor facilities were sometimes unaffordable.

Boys' narratives and photos demonstrated fairly unrestricted mobility across the city. Older boys (older than 15 years) reported generally feeling safe in their neighborhoods. They took photos of police and used these to illustrate that the city was "doing a good job." However, younger boys identified neighborhood parks and locations that they avoided because of drug dealings, people smoking or drinking outside, or older boys dominating the basketball courts. Younger boys adapted by walking long distances and crossing major roadways to use courts in a low-income housing project that they described as "not cared for" and "dangerous."

Girls' photos and stories revealed a more complex dynamic influencing physical activity and feelings about health, safety, and quality of life. While girls communicated the importance of free access to school sports facilities, they described few other recreational options. They connected increased crime, drug use, racism, religious intolerance, smoking, and graffiti with the lack of safe spaces for teens. Girls also reported more household and childcare responsibilities than boys, which limited their free time and often put them in roles frequently thought of as being for adults (e.g., translating for parents, negotiating with landlords, or keeping siblings safe from criminal activity).

Girls demonstrated their own behavioral adaptations to perceived neighborhood power differentials. They reported keeping together on the streets and limiting activities to places and situations where safety levels were predictable, thereby constraining their geographies. Photographs of vacant lots, suspected drug houses, and street corners where people congregated to smoke illustrated places that the girls avoided. Unlike the boys, the girls did not share confidence in the effectiveness of police. They viewed law enforcement as fairly ineffective, both at enforcing rules on drug use and smoking on school grounds and as "never being around when they should be" in places perceived as well-known drug hangouts or locales for crime.

Although both boys and girls included images and descriptions of how aesthetic features influenced their feelings about the environment, boys focused mostly on outdoor, public areas, whereas girls included images and narratives of their homes and schools. Participants frequently voiced frustrations with landlords and housing issues (e.g., broken doors and windows) and disappointment with signs of disorder in schools (e.g., trash, cigarette butts, broken lockers).

Food Environment

Participants described many fast-food restaurants and convenience stores in their neighborhoods, but no supermarkets within walking distance. Both boys and girls expressed concern that teens are targets for prominently displayed beer and cigarette advertisements at neighborhood corner stores. They noted that teens were easily influenced by words such as *pleasure* and *rich*.

Both girls and boys described sources of healthy (e.g., farmer's market) versus nonhealthy foods, but girls spoke more of the importance of local food pantries, food stamp programs, community gardens, and the neighborhood food truck, which provides fresh ingredients that they used to prepare meals. Boys spoke less about food sources, food preparation, and family food occasions and reported frequently buying fast food when they wanted a snack.

Community Engagement

Participants generally felt disempowered to change their neighborhoods and were often unaware of the mechanisms to effect change. They were particularly disturbed by signs of vandalism to homes, schools, and businesses, which suggested that people "didn't care," that gangs were active, and that adults had not created enough activities or recreational opportunities for youths. Two boys knew that the city had something called a Graffiti Van for graffiti removal, but none of the boys expressed personal responsibility in initiating or participating in neighborhood clean-ups. Girls voiced reluctance to share concerns or recommendations with adults, stating, "They never listen to us." Fears of retribution and being shunned by peers were cited as reasons that they "could not do anything" about crime and disorder in schools and neighborhoods.

As sessions progressed, the participants began to discuss the possibility of initiating change. Boys voiced higher comfort levels in reporting crime and disorder to police. Girls began speaking about reaching out to resettlement mentors, guidance counselors, teachers, and even the school newspaper and student council to offer recommendations for their schools. However, the girls remained reluctant to share concerns about crime and disorder with police.

Challenges and Suggestions for Improvement

What we learned from this study ranged from practical adaptations of the Photovoice process to considerations of how future interventions could be tailored for this population. First, as observed by other researchers,[11] Photovoice protocols for immigrant and refugee youths may need to be modified. We learned that having separate discussions for girls and boys can help participants feel more comfortable, especially if culturally sensitive gender issues arise; similarly, sensitivity to power differentials between older and younger participants is needed. Second, we advise planning ahead for additional time for recruiting, obtaining consent/assent, following up with participants, and retrieving cameras. We found that it was necessary to hold meetings in a variety of locations that were accessible to participants with different transportation needs; walking was the only form of transportation for many participants, while others depended on bus schedules. None received rides from parents, who often worked multiple jobs. Third, Photovoice can be conducted more efficiently if meetings are embedded in existing curricular settings (e.g., classroom or after-school activities) or if "gatekeeper" community-based organizations help with the process, but we found no centrally coordinated organizations connected to this population that were able to take on this role during the study timeframe. Overall, these constraints created limitations for our research; for example, we were unable to obtain written parental consent to use two boys' photos because we did not have translators/research assistants available to meet with parents around their work shifts.

Despite these challenges, we learned important lessons to help inform future obesity prevention efforts. First, we confirmed the importance of working with immigrant and refugee youths to understand their concerns about physical activity and healthy eating. Second, Photovoice provided an effective way to discuss complex issues related to these behaviors, contributing to a multisectoral dialogue about relationships between social determinants of health and obesity in this community. Results of our work informed the following obesity prevention initiatives in Manchester:

1. Establishing a Community School model,[12] which uses schools as safe havens, bringing multisectoral partners together to offer a range of educational, health, and social services to youths, families, and communities. This model creates a supportive, stable environment for students to live, learn, and play.
2. Adopting organizational policies that allow schools to remain open for community use after normal school hours (e.g., joint-use agreements allowing the use of school facilities for physical activity).
3. Developing innovative strategies to support physical activity as part of everyday life, including a new Local Park Improvement concept, a "Livable Alleyways" initiative, Health Impact Assessment to promote health and equity in neighborhood revitalization projects, and drafting an ordinance to address absentee landlord issues.
4. Improving access to healthy, affordable foods through community gardens and a Healthy Corner Store Initiative.

Discussion and Conclusions

Prior research suggests that perceptions of neighborhood environments are associated with obesogenic behaviors,[13] even after controlling for objectively measured environmental characteristics and other confounders. The literature has demonstrated that youths from certain racial/ethnic groups, especially African American girls, are at greater risk of becoming physically inactive[14] during adolescence. However, with few exceptions,[11,15] there is a paucity of research on the perceptions of immigrant/

refugee youths as they relate to obesity prevention. Understanding how low-income immigrant and refugee adolescents perceive access to food and physical activity in the context of their daily lives can help us understand predisposing factors for obesity and how these factors may increase obesity risk during the acculturation process.

Our findings provide insights regarding potential associations that require further study to determine links between obesity risk and perceptions of safety, power differentials, physical activity, and food access in this population. In our study, boys and girls adapted their behavior in different ways to navigate their social and physical environments. Boys' unrestricted mobility across the city and their positive feelings toward law enforcement contributed to their more active lifestyle compared with girls. Fewer recreational options, compounded by perceptions of greater vulnerability and time constraints imposed by household/childcare responsibilities, placed girls at increased risk of obesity. Earlier research suggests that girls are less likely than boys to use parks for physical activity,[16] as observed in our study. However, the girls in our study showed resilience and positive adaptations to neighborhood environments, using photographs to highlight places they considered "beautiful" and to showcase colorful ethnic meals they had prepared. Compared with boys, girls participated in more sedentary after-school activities (e.g., homework club). While this may increase obesity risk in the short term, there may be a net benefit in the long term by improving upstream social determinants of health (e.g., education).

Earlier research suggests that youths are less likely than others to feel empowered to mobilize resources and reduce barriers to healthy eating and active living.[17] Although participants in our project initially felt disempowered to communicate their views or effect change, the Photovoice process enabled them to begin discussing ideas for policy/environmental change. For example, participants recommended greater attention to improving neighborhood safety, converting vacant lots into community gardens and recreational spaces, repairing sidewalks, cleaning up graffiti and litter, fixing storefronts, transforming unused buildings into affordable housing, and locating healthier food stores within walking distance of neighborhoods. Participants identified a need for more teen-centered recreational opportunities, especially for girls, and for eliminating cigarette advertisements from areas where kids play. Photovoice conducted with Latina girls has identified similar themes regarding concerns about safety and security, the central role of family relationships, and sensitivity to advertising/messaging.[18] However, in contrast to the findings for Latina youths, in our study, the importance of education and preparing for college emerged as a central theme, particularly for girls. Thus, tailored interventions that build upon correlations between better school performance and physical activity[19] may hold promise for this population.

Youth perspectives are currently being shared with Manchester decision makers and residents. City health and youth leaders also participated in Photovoice training. Other cities are now developing youth-led obesity prevention initiatives.[20–22]

Because residents' participation and cross-sector collaboration are central to the city's initiative, the importance of empowering youths to voice their perspectives is recognized. By highlighting the perceptions of underrepresented groups, Photovoice can provide contextually sensitive forms of evidence to inform obesity prevention interventions at the local level.

LESSONS LEARNED

- Include immigrant and refugee youths in planning, implementing, and evaluating obesity prevention strategies.
- Modify Photovoice protocols according to cultural context.
- Use participatory action research methods such as Photovoice to promote discussions linking the social determinants of health to obesogenic behavior.

Acknowledgments

This work was supported by the Robert Wood Johnson Foundation through an Active Living Research grant (68495) and by the Centers for Disease Control and Prevention through Prevention Research Center grant 1U48DP001935-01. The authors are grateful to the City of Manchester, representatives from city departments, and residents and youths who generously worked with them on this project with the hope of making Manchester a safe and healthy place to live. The authors also thank Rob Wilson, Richard Madol, Elizabeth Madol, and Suen Odueyungbo for their assistance with Photovoice.

References

1. Kumanyika SK, Parker L, Sim LJ, eds. Bridging the evidence gap in obesity prevention: a framework to inform decision making. Washington, DC: National Academies Press, 2010.
2. Huang TT, Drewnosksi A, Kumanyika SK, et al. A systems-oriented multilevel framework for addressing obesity in the 21st century. Prev Chronic Dis. 2009 Jul;6(3):A82. Epub 2009 Jun 15.
3. Franzini L, Elliott MN, Cuccaro P, et al. Influences of physical and social neighborhood environments on children's physical activity and obesity. Am J Public Health. 2009 Feb; 99(2):271–8. Epub 2008 Dec 4.
4. Catalani C, Minkler M. Photovoice: a review of the literature in health and public health. Health Educ Behav. 2010 Jun;37(3):424–51. Epub 2009 Oct 1.
5. Strack RW, Magill C, McDonagh K. Engaging youth through photovoice. Health Promot Pract. 2004 Jan;5(1):49–58.
6. Nykiforuk C, Vallianatos H, Nieuwendyk LM. Photovoice as a method for revealing community perceptions of the built and social environment. Int J Qual Methods. 2011;10(2): 103–24.
7. Wang C, Burris MA. Photovoice: concept, methodology, and use for participatory needs assessment. Health Educ Behav. 1997 Jun;24(3):369–87.
8. Ewing R. Can the physical environment determine physical activity levels. Exerc Sport Sci Rev. 2005 Apr;33(2):69–75.

9. New Hampshire Health Department. Health and socioeconomic indicators. Manchester, NH: New Hampshire Health Department, 2010.

10. U.S. Census Bureau. Population finder. Washington, DC: U.S. Census Bureau, 2000.

11. Vaughn LM, Rojas-Guyler L, Howell B. "Picturing" health: a Photovoice pilot of Latina girls' perceptions of health. Fam Community Health. 2008 Oct–Dec;31(4):305–16.

12. Coalition for Community Schools. Community schools in the Race to the Top. Washington, DC: Coalition for Community Schools, 2009 Nov. Available at: http://www.communi tyschools.org/assets/1/AssetManager/RTT_Making_the_Case_11_30_09.pdf.

13. Hoehner CM, Brennan-Ramirez LK, Elliott MB, et al. Perceived and objective environmental measures and physical activity among urban adults. Am J Prev Med. 2005 Feb;28 (2 Suppl 2):105–16

14. Gordon-Larsen P, McMurray RG, Popkin BM. Adolescent physical activity and inactivity vary by ethnicity: the National Longitudinal Study of Adolescent Health. J Pediatr. 1999 Sep;135(3):301–6.

15. Renzaho AM. Fat, rich and beautiful: changing socio-cultural paradigms associated with obesity risk, nutritional status and refugee children from Sub-Saharan Africa. Health Place. 2004 Mar;10(1):105–13.

16. Roemmich JN, Epstein LH, Raja S, Yin L. The neighborhood and home environments: disparate relationships with physical activity and sedentary behaviors in youth. Ann Behav Med. 2007 Feb;33(1):29–38.

17. Adkins S, Sherwood N, Story M, et al. Physical activity among African-American girls: the role of parents and the home environment. Obesity Res. 2004 Sep;12 Suppl:38–45S.

18. Walia S, Leipert B. Perceived facilitators and barriers to physical activity for rural youth: an exploratory study using Photovoice. Rural Remote Health. 2012;12:1842. Epub 2012 Jan 23.

19. Singh A, Uijtdewilligen L, Twisk JW. Physical activity and performance at school: a systematic review of the literature including a methodological quality assessment. Arch Pediatr Adolesc Med. 2012 Jan;166(1):49–55.

20. Kramer L, Schwartz P, Cheadle A, et al. Promoting policy and environmental change using photovoice in the Kaiser Permanente Community Health Initiative. Health Promot Pract. 2010 May;11(3):332–9. Epub 2009 Oct 20.

21. Dorfman L, Wallack L. Moving from them to us: challenges in reframing violence in youth. Enola, PA: National Sexual Violence Resource Center, 2009.

22. Healthy Eating, Active Communities. Photovoice as a tool for youth policy advocacy. Oakland, CA: Healthy Eating, Active Communities, 2009.

CHAPTER 30

Peer Influence on Obesity-Related Behaviors

Design and Rationale of the Waipahu HART Project

Camonia R. Long, PhD, CHES, Heather Glow, MPH, CHES, and Claudio Nigg, PhD

In the State of Hawaii in the first decade of the twenty-first century, 25.5% of Filipino students in grades 9–12 were ranked as obese.[1] The Waipahu Health Action Research Training (HART) project addresses the issue of adolescent obesity among high school students in the community of Waipahu, Hawaii, a predominantly Filipino population.*

Waipahu is a former sugar plantation town where various cultures and races have taken root in the course of history. It is a semi-urban low-income community located on the leeward side of O'ahu and has an estimated population of 38,216, predominantly Asian nationals, who make up 66% of the population.[2] U.S. Census results show that the Waipahu population is primarily composed of young people aged 18 and under and adults aged 25–44 years. Females make up about 50% of the population, with a female-to-male ratio of 100:97.6.[2] The community of Waipahu was chosen for this program due to an already established working relationship and the community's need and support. The Waipahu Community Coalition and Waipahu High School have played large roles in supporting the HART project and in supporting community health. Focusing on this community for obesity prevention for Pacific Islanders, as well as for similar communities in the mainland United States, highlights the idea that culturally sensitive and sustainable programs are needed to promote positive behavioral change among often-forgotten communities.

This project uses existing classroom activities and assignments to address the feasibility of delivering a curriculum on obesity prevention behaviors (namely, physical

---

Camonia R. Long is a postdoctoral fellow with the University of Hawaii Cancer Center and principal investigator of the Waipahu HART project. Heather Glow is the program manager of the Waipahu HART project at the University of Hawaii Cancer Center. Claudio Nigg is an associate professor in the Department of Public Health Sciences at the University of Hawaii Manoa.

* This report is a companion to chapter 24, which also concerns Native Hawaiians/Pacific Islanders, and to other chapters that focus, as a whole or in part, on adolescents: chapters 2, 3, 11, 13, 14, 17, 19, 26, 27, and 29.

activity and nutrition) to high school students. The obesity curriculum was specifically designed to address community need and based on previous data collected by the students. The intervention is tailored to the individual suggestions, needs, and culture of the students in this community.

The project uses a modified version of the FLASH (Fun Learning for Student Health) peer influence approach.[3] This approach involves peers to influence obesity prevention behaviors among high school students. Students from the Waipahu High School Senior Health Careers course are trained and participate in the project as health educators and assessors (in this way learning about the research process). Juniors from four of the Waipahu High School Health Classes receive the curriculum. The main activities in the project include baseline measurements and discussion, a four-week peer-led obesity prevention curriculum (focusing on topics of general health, nutrition, and physical activity), further discussion, and post-intervention assessment. The design and rationale of this project may be used to propose larger community interventions in Waipahu with similar peer-led designs.

According to the Centers for Disease Control's data from the National Health and Nutrition Examination Survey (NHANES), 16.9% of children and adolescents (12.5 million) aged 2–19 years are obese.[4] The obesity rate has tripled among children and adolescents since 1980.[5] These facts demonstrate the need for more focused public health research that identifies effective overweight and obesity prevention efforts.

The Healthy People 2010 initiative identified the status of overweight and obesity as 1 of 10 leading health indicators on which action should be taken.[6] Calling for a reduction in the proportion of children and adolescents who are overweight or obese, Healthy People 2010 also reports that the United States has made little progress toward the target goal.[6] Healthy People 2020 lists healthy nutrition and weight status as main objectives of concern; the report emphasizes the importance of prevention for obesity and obesity-associated health consequences.[7] Data from the NHANES report on overweight and obesity rates show significant racial and ethnic disparities in obesity prevalence among U.S. children and adolescents.[4] The data categorize race/ethnicity in three ways: non-Hispanic White, non-Hispanic Black, and Mexican American.[4] Due to these grouping categories, national data remain limited for overweight and obese children and adolescents of Filipino and Native Hawaiian descent.

The Filipino and Native Hawaiian cultures and people are special. The first Filipino immigrants to Hawaii arrived on the islands around 1906 to work on the sugar plantations.[8] Census data for Hawaii show an estimated population of 328,880 individuals of Filipino or mixed Filipino descent.[9] Today, Filipinos constitute the fourth largest ethnic group in Hawaii, approximately 13% of the 1.2 million total population.[8] Many Filipinos in Hawaii still follow their traditional culture, religion, and holidays and eat traditional Filipino foods. Filipino culture is often displayed through traditional dances as well as stories passed down through the generations. Native Hawaiians also share their traditional culture through storytelling and dance. Native Hawaiians share strong cultural beliefs, values, and pride in their culture.

Traditional mainland approaches may not reach this population's needs. This underscores the importance of identifying specific health intervention efforts that address preventable health risk behaviors among Filipino and Hawaiian-born children and adolescents.

Obesity Interventions

Many intersecting phenomena contribute to childhood obesity. Theory-based interventions combating childhood obesity have proven successful in addressing many of these factors.[10] Theory-based research is very important in that it categorizes data in terms of psychological, behavioral, and contextual variables.[10] Thus, such research can target the most salient characteristics of behavioral change systematically. The most widely used theories for physical activity have been the Theory of Reasoned Action / Planned Behavior, the Transtheoretical Model of Behavior Change, Social Cognitive Theory, and Self-Determination Theory.[10]

The Theory of Planned Behavior (TPB) developed by Ajzen[11] focuses on the constructs of attitude, subjective norms, perceived behavioral control, and intention. *Intention* is the precursor of behavior, and intention, in turn, is predicted by attitude, subjective norms, and perceived behavioral control. *Attitude* is determined by an individual's beliefs about the outcomes or characteristics of engaging in the behavior.[12] It is important to address the particular attitude of the individual and to weigh the positive and negative beliefs about the behavior. This allows a better understanding of the individual and how to help that individual make positive behavioral change. *Subjective norms* are determined by the individual's normative beliefs and whether or not influential individuals approve or disapprove of performing the behavior.[12] By building on an individual's subjective norms, an intervention may draw attention to highly regarded individuals who engage in the positive behavior and thus induce the individual to engage in it as well. This is especially important when dealing with children and adolescents. They often look to their peers for social modeling. For exercise interventions, peer modeling of positive exercise and healthy nutrition behavior can help frame exercise and healthy nutrition as fun and "cool."[11]

Perceived behavioral control is determined by the individual's control beliefs, the control of an individual's beliefs about the presence of factors that may impede or facilitate performance of the behavior.[12] For an intervention focusing on exercise and nutrition, it is essential to acknowledge these barriers and facilitators.[11] Working with the individual to overcome the perceived barriers and acknowledge the facilitators is essential for achieving immediate as well as lifelong behavioral change.

Research based on TPB has shown promise in applying this theory as a means of combating childhood obesity.[13] Promising research conducted in a school-based setting used a school-based nutrition and physical activity intervention focusing on the use of the constructs of TPB.[13] The core of the study consisted of a survey of TPB and the use of this survey to design focus areas of the intervention. The study showed decreases in sweets and fat intake as well as increased long-term physical activity.

The researchers attribute their success to focusing on the individual barriers and attitudes associated with nutrition and exercise. Further research focused on the impact of TPB and parental involvement in childhood obesity.[14] Results showed that parent's body mass index (BMI) predicted the BMI of the child and that the parent's attitudes and own health behaviors served as predictors of the child's attitude and health behaviors. The Theory of Planned Behavior has also been used to evaluate barriers and attitudes to fruit and vegetable consumption among college students.[15] Results showed that attitude and perceived behavioral control were the most important factors in the students' fruit and vegetable consumption.

Project Design and Rationale

The Waipahu HART project was designed as an evaluative pilot study with the purpose of assessing a physical activity and nutrition curriculum in order to garner feasibility data on interventions targeting physical activity and nutrition behaviors among high school students. This project, as described above, was based on the Theory of Planned Behavior and the FLASH peer modeling approach. The design and rationale came from a modified version of the FLASH peer influence approach.[3] The FLASH approach provides peer engagement and influence during curriculum-guided health activities. The main goal in using this approach was to examine the feasibility of using Waipahu High School senior-year health careers students to influence preventive behaviors in physical activity and nutrition health among their high school peers.

For the initial project design, researchers found it important to understand the attitudes, beliefs, and barriers concerning physical activity and nutrition among the high school students in Waipahu. The foundation for the design was built by engaging the students about their personal needs and the health status of their community. Researchers on the Waipahu HART team have been working with Waipahu High School students for the past two years to develop a sound understanding of the individual health needs of the students and the community. For the students and community to feel ownership in the project, the students themselves collected and disseminated the data. The researchers served as facilitators and as a knowledge base for the students. An additional goal was to train and engage students in the research process. We have found that a community-based project delivers the most honest and useful data from which to build this school intervention.

As noted, the majority of the background research was conducted by the students. At the beginning of the project, students were asked to conduct so-called *windshield assessments*, in which students drove through their community to quickly view health opportunities and barriers. This information gave us a snapshot of the overall community from students' point of view. Students also participated in community mapping, during which they walked around their neighborhood and school and used the Internet and other mapping resources to draw a map of their community. The results provided a more detailed, personal view of the community. Finally, students participated in classroom focus groups.

The primary rationale for the project came from individuals in the Waipahu community itself. Throughout the research process, the team developed a collaborative working relationship with Waipahu High School. The data collected from the students and the community provided the rationale for developing a school-based obesity intervention curriculum focusing on physical activity and nutrition. The topics chosen for the curriculum emerged from the data obtained from the windshield assessments, community mapping, and focus groups conducted by the students on their individual and community needs. Specific topics to be included in the intervention curriculum were (1) nutrition and physical activity (energy balance); (2) general health and nutrition (using FITT: *frequency, intensity, time, and type* of physical activity principle); (3) "eating the rainbow" and variety and intensity of physical activity; and (4) eating out and working out. The intervention curriculum was designed to foster peer-based learning and included many group activities as well as visual aids. The Filipino community of Waipahu encourages a positive attitude toward family and culture, which made it natural for this intervention to choose students from the senior-year Waipahu High School Health Careers Class to be intervention leaders, delivering the curriculum to the junior-level health classes.

At the beginning of the project, the senior-student health educators receive orientation to the research process: conducting quantitative and qualitative research, delivering a health curriculum, and analyzing data (phase 1). This initial training lasts for five class periods. These trainings are held to ensure that student health educators are both familiar and comfortable with the teaching material. Student health educators are also assured that they will be accompanied into the classrooms by one member of the research staff during their teaching periods; the research staff member serves as a source of support during the teaching sessions.

Developing the Physical Activity and Nutrition Curriculum

After being introduced to the entire curriculum during the training, seniors are divided into four groups, with one group representing each intervention week, and are asked, as individual groups, to select a curriculum topic. Once each senior has been assigned to a group and each group has selected a topic, a group of six to seven seniors facilitates discussion of the selected topic each week, for four weeks.

Each group is trained in proper survey administration techniques and in confidentiality and research ethics through CITI (Collaborative Institutional Training Initiative) training. Groups practice their scripts and develop visual aids for their presentation. The seniors practice delivering their topics several times in front of the whole senior class and the researchers to develop confidence and to improve their delivery. Once all the groups feel comfortable delivering their material, they are scheduled to deliver it to the juniors. This preparation typically entails three to four practice sessions.

Each group is provided with a folder for its week. Each curriculum folder (labeled week 1, 2, 3, or 4) contains three main items: (1) an outline of the group's session,

(2) a script of the entire session, and (3) specific worksheets and/or handouts for the session. Because the intervention is intended to assess the feasibility of a peer-led intervention, the folders also include questionnaires for the student participants to complete.

The outline of each session includes a warm-up, an activity, and a cool-down. The warm-up is delivered through an icebreaker (week 1) or discussion of the previous week's activities (weeks 2–4). The session outline also provides specific timeframes that students are to follow during the session; each session is designed to be delivered in less than one hour of class time. The activities for each week vary, depending on the topic to be covered, but range from lessons about the Food Guide Pyramid to types of physical activity, making healthy food choices, and eating healthy food when eating out. The cool-down for each week includes explanations of the homework for the next week and dissemination of the questionnaire, if necessary.

The script for each week's curriculum follows the session outline for that particular week. Included in the script for each week is a section for each group of seniors to introduce themselves and introduce their lesson. During training, seniors are encouraged to memorize their scripts and to adjust them as they see fit when they are talking to the juniors. Seniors are also encouraged to ask questions and to discuss any concerns about their scripts when they practice with the Waipahu HART team. The worksheets and/or surveys that accompany each session depend on that particular session's topic.

Delivering the Curriculum to the Junior Health Class

After orientation, the senior-class students deliver the curriculum to the student participants. The junior-class student participants complete a baseline demographic survey and a physical activity and nutrition questionnaire. Implementation of the four-week peer-led curriculum follows, with the senior students acting as health educators and the junior students as participants (phase 2). After implementation of the curriculum, a group meeting is scheduled to discuss experiences with the peer-led curriculum and to complete the post-intervention questionnaire on physical activity and nutrition (phase 3). During the group meeting, students are guided through systematic research procedures to identify relevant consistencies within the curriculum, leading to a group discussion summarizing the curriculum sessions overall. Participation in the curriculum is a mandatory component of the health teacher's classroom curriculum, and the teacher grades participation. Participation in the pre-post surveys and discussions is voluntary. Alternative assignments are established for the students who opt not to participate in the survey and discussions, at the discretion of the health teacher. The three phases of the program are summarized in figure 30.1.

Successes and Challenges

Through ongoing development of the Waipahu HART project, students and members of the Waipahu community reported that the students learned new ideas that might

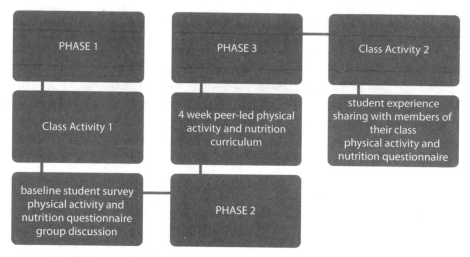

FIGURE 30.1. Waipahu Health Action Research Training (HART) project design.

help improve their physical activity and nutrition. In the researchers' view, students demonstrated their increased comfort with sharing information about what their community needs and how these needs can be addressed. Students were excited about participating in the project and developed their own ideas about what the project should look like. Staff from the Waipahu High School, including the Health Careers Class teacher and the school principal, expressed their excitement about the potential impact of the project on both the students and the larger community.

We believe that the key factors contributing to the successful design of the Waipahu HART project include (1) beginning the project by engaging the students about their personal needs and the health status of the community, (2) developing a sound understanding of the individual health needs of the students and the community, and (3) developing a collaborative working relationship with Waipahu High School.

Continuing challenges include developing new ways to approach students and families. Most parents in the community of Waipahu have little unscheduled time to devote to physical activity and nutrition education. However, it is essential that both students and parents are made aware of physical activity and nutrition options and knowledge in order to promote the health of this community. Lastly, working within both university and public school system timeframes can be challenging when attempting to complete community-based intervention work. Despite these challenges, the design and rationale of this project may offer promise for interventions on similar health topics and in communities similar to Waipahu.

LESSONS LEARNED
- A well-received educational intervention is possible by following these guidelines:

- —Begin the project by engaging the students about their personal needs and the health status of the community.
- —Develop a sound understanding of the individual health needs of the students and the community.
- —Develop a collaborative working relationship with students in the community.
- The Filipino-Hawaiian community of Waipahu responded enthusiastically to a peer-led educational intervention on nutrition and physical activity in the high school.

Acknowledgments

The authors thank the students, parents, and faculty of the Waipahu High School for their assistance with the project. This research was supported by National Institutes of Health / National Cancer Institute grant no. R25 CA90956.

References

1. Hawaii Health Data Warehouse. Overweight or obese, for state and selected ethnicities, by county, gender, BRFSS age group, education level, employment status, marital status, poverty level, healthcare coverage, for the years 2000–2010. Mililani, HI: Hawaii Health Data Warehouse, State of Hawaii Department of Health, 2012. Available at: http://www.hhdw.org/cms/uploads/Ethnicity_Reports/LHI_Overweight_Obese_1.pdf.
2. U.S. Census Bureau. Profile of general population and from housing characteristics: 2010 demographic profile data DP-1. Washington, DC: U.S. Census Bureau, 2010. Available at: http://factfinder2.census.gov/faces/tableservices/jsf/pages/productview.xhtml?pid=DEC_10_DP_DPDP1&prodType=table.
3. Venditti EM, Elliot DL, Faith MS, et al. Rationale, design and methods of the HEALTHY study behavior intervention component. Int J Obes (Lond). 2009 Aug;33 Suppl 4:S44–51.
4. Ogden C, Carroll M. Prevalence of obesity among children and adolescents: United States, trends 1963–1965 through 2007–2008. National Health and Nutrition Examination Survey data. Hyattsville, MD: U.S. Department of Health and Human Services, Centers for Disease Control and Prevention, National Center for Health Statistics, 2010. Available at: http://www.cdc.gov/nchs/data/hestat/obesity_child_07_08/obesity_child_07_08.pdf.
5. Centers for Disease Control and Prevention. Data and statistics: obesity rates among all children in the United States. Atlanta, GA: Centers for Disease Control and Prevention, 2012. Available at: http://www.cdc.gov/obesity/childhood/data.html.
6. National Center for Health Statistics, Centers for Disease Control and Prevention. Healthy People 2010: leading health indicators at a glance. Atlanta, GA: Centers for Disease Control and Prevention, 2011. Available at: http://www.cdc.gov/nchs/healthy_people/hp2010/hp2010_indicators.htm.
7. U.S. Department of Health and Human Services, Office of Disease Prevention and Health Promotion. Healthy People 2020. Washington, DC: U.S. Department of Health and Human Services. Available at http://www.healthypeople.gov/2020/default.aspx.

8. Labrador RN. Performing identity: the public presentation of culture and ethnicity among Filipinos in Hawai'i. Cultural Values. 2002;6(3):287–307.

9. U.S. Census Bureau. Selected population profile in the United States: 2008–2010 American Community Survey 3-year estimates (S0201). Washington, DC: U.S. Census Bureau, 2010. Available at: http://factfinder2.census.gov/faces/tableservices/jsf/pages/productview.xhtml ?pid=ACS_10_3YR_S0201&prodType=table.

10. Nigg CR, Paxton RJ. Conceptual perspectives. In: Smith AL, Biddle SJH, eds. Youth physical activity and sedentary behavior. Champaign, IL: Human Kinetics, 2008.

11. Ajzen I. The theory of planned behavior. Organ Behav Hum Decis Process. 1991;50: 179–211.

12. Ajzen I. From intentions to actions: a theory of planned behavior. In: Kuhi J, Beckmann J, eds. Action-control: from cognition to behavior. Heidelberg, Germany: Springer-Verlag, 1985. Pp. 1–39.

13. Angelopoulos PD, Milionis HJ, Grammatikaki E, et al. Changes in BMI and blood pressure in after school based interventions: the CHILDREN study. Eur J Public Health. 2009 Jun;19(3):319–25.

14. Andrews KR, Silk KS, Eneli IU. Parents as health promoters: a theory of planned behavior perspective on the prevention of childhood obesity. J Health Commun. 2010 Jan;15(1): 95–107.

15. Blanchard CM, Fisher J, Sparling PB, et al. Understanding adherence to 5 servings of fruits and vegetables per day: a theory of planned behavior perspective. J Nutr Educ Behav. 2009 Jan–Feb;41(1):3–10.

CHAPTER 31

Walking Groups
A Simple, Affordable Intervention Program for Public Housing Developments

Deborah J. Bowen, PhD, Aurelia Rus, MPH, Clelia Beltrame, MPH,
Mathilda Drayton, Mary Jane Williams, MS, and Rachel Goodman, MA

An adult body mass index (BMI) of 25.0 -29.9 kg/m² is classified as overweight, and a BMI of 30 kg/m² or greater is classified as obese.[1-4] Data from NHANES (National Health and Nutrition Examination Survey) II, NHANES III, and NHANES 1999–2000 show consistent increases in obesity among adults aged 20–74, standardized to the 2000 Census age distribution.[4] Data from the Behavioral Risk Factor Surveillance System suggest that, in Boston, public housing residents have a much higher prevalence of chronic disease risk factors than the city's general population. Women living in public housing reported twice the prevalence of obesity and more than three times the prevalence of diabetes compared with women living in the city overall.[1] Regular physical activity brings many health benefits, including reduced risk of illness from such chronic diseases as coronary heart disease, stroke, and type 2 diabetes, as well as reduced risk of fall-related injuries and reduced occurrence of premature death.[5-10] Massachusetts residents (adults and children) fall far short of the recommended physical activity standards.

Environmental Influences on Obesity-Related Health Behaviors and Choices

The adjective *obesogenic* was coined to describe environments that promote unhealthy eating and discourage physical activity.[11]* Obesogenic neighborhood characteristics

Deborah J. Bowen, Aurelia Rus, Clelia Beltrame, and Mathilda Drayton are affiliated with Boston University School of Public Health; Mary Jane Williams, with the Boston Public Health Commission; and Rachel Goodman, with the Boston Housing Authority.

* The perspective taken here, in which the environment of people's daily lives looms large in the account of trends in obesity and overweight, conforms well with the perspective of this volume as a whole. See the introduction and chapter 7 for further elucidation. Also see chapter 8, on the role of safety in obesity prevention, for a general discussion of the observations that underlie the intervention described in this chapter (and other interventions like it).

produce increasing opportunities for energy intake and decreasing opportunities for physical activity. Factors that affect energy intake include (1) increased portion sizes in restaurants; (2) decreased consumption of fruits and vegetables; (3) increased consumption of take-out prepared food; (4) less choice of groceries; and (5) increased consumption of alcoholic and soft drinks.[12,13] The built environment has also been associated with eating choices and activity in several studies,[14-16] especially in low-income neighborhoods where the availability of healthy choices may be limited compared with suburban areas. Among low-income minority women, significant environmental barriers to exercise include lack of a sense of safety and lack of places to exercise.[17-19] Little research exists on the effect of public housing's built environment and building design on the healthy choices of the residents, yet research in other settings suggests that the built environment is a powerful influence on behaviors.[11] Previous work indicates that population density, median household income, employment density, and establishment density may be associated with obesity risk.[20]

A program to foster increased exercise in an environment that may be hostile to physical activity is the walking for fitness program. Walking regularly (5–7 times per week) has been shown to change obesity levels, reduce chronic disease risk factors, and reduce the likelihood of diabetes and heart disease.[2-4] Walking is a simple activity, requiring no specialized equipment, memberships, or training. Models of encouraging walking exist in the literature, although none has been tested in public housing settings. The lack of strong public health intervention outcome data, together with the dearth of information on how to enhance walking among residents of public housing family developments (PHFDs), led us to propose feasibility studies for different types of walking programs to engage public housing residents in regular walking.

Prevention Research Center: Training and Procedures

Our understanding of public housing residents has developed from our engagement over a number of years in working with this population in research and programmatic efforts. The Partners in Health and Housing–Prevention Research Center, funded since 2001 by the Centers for Disease Control and Prevention, focuses exclusively on prevention research among PHFD residents. It is a partnership between the Boston University School of Public Health, the Boston Housing Authority, Boston Public Health Commission (Boston's city health department), and the Community Committee for Health Promotion (comprising PHFD residents and representatives of agencies and organizations that work in PHFDs). The Boston Housing Authority oversees 24 PHFDs with almost 30,000 residents (over 18,000 adults) in 13,937 units or apartments; 68% of adult residents are female. On average, Boston Housing Authority PHFDs have more than 300 units. Hispanics (35%) are the most common ethnic group in the PHFDs, followed by Blacks (32%) and Whites (21%). English (52%) and Spanish (33%) are the primary languages spoken in PHFDs. Average annual household income is $13,700, which is below the poverty line for a household with one adult and one child.

Each of the PHFDs is unique in its physical structure and function. Only low-rise to medium-rise buildings are allowed as PHFDs in Boston. Some consist of multiple buildings with a central courtyard, while others are decentralized and sprawling. Some have a single entrance and exit, while others have multiple entrances that are locked to all but residents. The dramatic differences in the built environment in PHFDs mean that we have the opportunity to measure and understand the role of differing living structures in residents' choices.

Staff from the Prevention Research Center (PRC) recruited and trained Healthy Living Associates (HLAs) to deliver the intervention. The primary source of HLA recruitment was graduates of the existing Resident Health Advocate (RHA) Program of the PRC. The RHAs receive 14 weeks of training that includes modules on leadership skills development, health promotion, determinants of health, priority health topics such as asthma and depression, cultural competence, outreach education, and navigating the health system. The RHA trainees serve a six-month internship of six hours per week providing health information at a PHFD, working directly with individual residents, and interacting with neighborhood health centers. There is a strong interest in full-time employment among RHAs who finish their internship. Minimum hiring criteria included (1) demonstration of successful health advocacy in the community, (2) being a nonsmoker, (3) ability to understand and speak English well (some speak Spanish as well, if the PHFD houses many Spanish-speakers), and (4) demonstration of basic writing skills. We hired one to four RHAs per development as HLAs, and they conducted the intervention activities. The Training and Education Core of our Prevention Research Center supported the training of all HLAs.

HLA Training

The trainees attended one session that included (1) basic principles and processes of research, including data collection; (2) principles of confidentiality and informed consent, including National Institutes of Health certification in human subject protections and Health Insurance Portability and Accountability Act regulation training; and (3) overview and description of study goals and activities. The trainees completed the two-day course on basic skills for working on healthy behaviors as well as coursework in specific skills related to intervention implementation. This course was given in conjunction with the Prevention Research Center's ongoing RHA training. The course covers (1) public health implications of obesity; (2) health consequences of obesity and benefits of weight reduction; (3) treatment of obesity and success or failure; (4) PHFD-wide activities and how to conduct them; (5) how to support women in reducing weight; (6) how to prevent relapse by relying on environmental support; and (7) how to remotivate continued attempts after relapse. The trainees took a post-test immediately after training to ensure competency in knowledge, correctly answering all questions prior to participating in additional training.

Public housing family developments were eligible for selection as one of our study sites if they had at least 100 women residents living with children; 25 PHFDs (representing 80% of all adult PHFD residents in Boston) met these criteria. We selected four of these PHFDs, of comparable overall size, minority resident status, and building structure. We adhered to the principles of community-based participatory research in our activities to develop this project.[21,22]

Walking Group Leaders

Walking group facilitators were project coordinators hired by the PRC to serve as HLAs from each development. Study staff met weekly with the HLAs to collect forms, discuss participant recruitment strategies, discuss comments and feedback about the walking groups, and provide support to the HLAs. Leaders recruited participants from within their development and scheduled and led the walking groups.

Forms collected by the facilitators included weekly sign-in sheets, walk leaders' time sheets, start-up forms from each resident at his or her first walk, a log of walk leaders' weekly activities, and ending forms at the end of the 12-week walking period.

The main recruitment strategies employed were referrals from PRC health screenings, word of mouth, and flyers. Flyers were distributed in a variety of ways, including door-to-door, posting on community flyer boards, posting in the mailroom, placing in mailboxes, and distributing at community events. At the end of each week, HLAs submitted a form detailing their recruitment activities for that week.

Walking Group Procedures

Walking group participants gathered at a meeting place, such as a community room, within their development that was determined by the group leaders. When participants arrived, they signed in. The first time each participant attended the walking group, he or she completed a screening form that asked for information about current health status and readiness for walking. In addition, 25 participants were selected from each development to serve as an evaluation cohort by completing a longer baseline survey asking about physical activity and related variables. Each participant was given a pedometer and shown how to operate it. After participants arrived at a walk, the group leaders initiated and guided a light stretching session. The groups then proceeded with their walks. Walk length varied by development and by the weather. After each walk, leaders and participants returned to the meeting place for a post-walk stretching session.

Each of the four developments was assigned one of four different conditions: trail markers, map, buddy system, or pedometer only (control). In the trail marker condition, trail markers were placed around the development and the surrounding neighborhood to mark different paths that the walking group could take. In the map condition, walk routes in the community were mapped out and followed during the walk. In the buddy system, participants were encouraged to find a buddy and walk with him or her during every walk. In the pedometer condition, participants received no special instructions.

At the end of the walking group trial period, each cohort participant was asked to fill out an ending survey. Surveys were distributed by facilitators and walking group leaders, and participants received a gift certificate after returning each of the baseline and ending surveys.

Survey Contents

Both the startup and the ending forms measured walking behavior using an adapted and simplified form of the International Physical Activity Questionnaire[23] to measure frequency of walking. We also measured days of the week for walking and self-reported time spent walking. We adapted other measures from the Twin Cities walking program.[24] We measured self-confidence for walking at both time points, specifically, walking self-efficacy; residents' judgments about the quality of the neighborhood surrounding the development for walking, to assess how easy or hard the residents might see walking in groups near the development to be; and development-level social cohesion, to look at the effects of a walking group on larger social interactions in the development. Finally, we asked walkers for their opinions on how the groups were conducted.

Outcomes

Table 31.1 provides descriptive information for the four PHFDs recruited for the walking program. The developments were ethnically diverse and of moderate size, with, in two of the developments, a tenant task force that supported residents and helped them obtain needed services from the Boston Housing Authority when needed.

Figure 31.1 shows participation in the walking groups over the 12-week program for each of the developments. Participation was relatively high for the first scheduled walk, then smaller for the next few, then steadily climbed across the remaining weeks of scheduled walks. We calculated the percentage of new walkers at each walking time point, and the average across the 12 weeks was 42% new walkers (people who had never been to a walking group) per week.

Table 31.2 provides some background data on the walkers selected for the evaluation cohort that represents the walking program. The walkers reflected the diversity of the residents. Predominantly, walkers were female, were Black or Hispanic, and reported relatively low education levels. Self-rated health was rated across the spectrum, with many residents rating their health in the fair or poor categories. Table 31.3 presents data showing the differences in responses of the evaluation cohort before and after the walking program. Many of the measured variables were differently reported before and after the program. For 65% of the walkers, this was at least a six-week period. Generally, walkers differed in the proportion who defined themselves as regular walkers and in the number of days per week they walked. Two other variables that differed between baseline and follow-up were walking self-efficacy and development of social cohesion, both of which increased in cohort members between

Table 31.1. Characteristics of four participating public housing family developments in walking groups, Boston

Development	No. of units and households	Structure of building	Tenant task force?	% Hispanic residents	No. of resident health advocates previously trained
A	366 units	Townhouse, mid-rise, and low-rise	No	58.46	3
	345 households				
B	421 units	Townhouse and mid-rise	Yes	47.59	6
	349 households				
C	386 units	Townhouse and low-rise	Yes	49.57	8
	329 households				
D	354 units	Townhouse and low-rise	No	56.3	2
	289 households				
Total	1,527 units 1,312 households	—	—	—	19

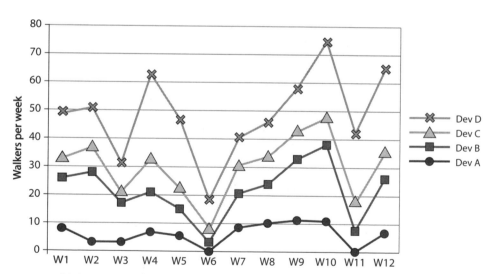

FIGURE 31.1. Walking group participation over time (12 weeks) in four public housing family developments in Boston.

Table 31.2. Characteristics of participants joining
walking groups in public housing family
developments, evaluation cohort (n = 102)

Characteristic	Percent (n)
Gender	
Female	84 (86)
Male	16 (15)
Age	
<25 years	24 (23)
25–40 years	28 (26)
41–76 years	48 (53)
Highest grade completed	
Up to some high school	27 (27)
High school diploma	35 (35)
Some college or technical	22 (22)
College degree or other education	16 (16)
Race/ethnicity	
White	9 (8)
Black / African American	52 (51)
Hispanic	41 (40)
Other	2 (1)
Employed	
Yes	36 (36)
Self-reported health	
Excellent	11 (10)
Very good	7 (6)
Good	56 (50)
Fair	15 (14)
Poor	11 (10)

before and after the walking program. No other variables were reported as changed
from before to after the walking group.

Discussion

We began this program to see whether holding walking sessions for public health
family development residents would result in residents walking more and participating in walking programs. The residents did participate. Ultimately, approximately
20% of Boston's PHFD residents participated in walking programs. This is a large
proportion, comparing favorably with participation rates in other health promotion
programs.

Most residents who reported being walkers walked in the neighborhood or around
the development. Few reported using nearby parks. The reasons for this are not known
but could include accessibility of parks and fears about lack of safety in parks. Future

Table 31.3. Differences in physical activity and related variables for participants in walking groups in public housing family developments, evaluation cohort (n = 102)

Characteristic	Percent at baseline (n)	Percent at follow-up (n)
Self-rated regular walker	25 (100)	67 (101)
Days per week you walk?		
None	75 (20)	33 (35)
1–2	4 (1)	49 (42)
3	12 (3)	16 (12)
4 or more	8 (2)	9 (6)
Method of activity (for "active rated people" only)		
Walking	88 (89)	95 (96)
Running	14 (13)	14 (14)
Exercise	30 (30)	32 (37)
Biking	10 (10)	10 (10)
Swimming	7 (7)	6 (6)
Other	11 (11)	10 (9)
Where people walk		
Around development	70 (70)	80 (80)
In neighborhood	51 (50)	85 (86)
To school	13 (13)	13 (13)
To church	4 (4)	3 (3)
Local park	31 (31)	40 (40)
	Baseline mean (SD)	**Follow-up mean (SD)**
Walking self-efficacy	3.5 (0.4)	4.2 (0.5)
Social cohesion	2.7 (0.7)	4.2 (0.6)
Neighborhood walking quality	2.3 (0.8)	2.4 (0.8)
Program evaluation (follow-up only)		
Difficulty of walks	—	3.2 (0.5)
Usefulness of walk leaders	—	4.2 (0.5)
Physical benefit of walking	—	4.5 (0.6)
Social benefit of walking	—	4.0 (0.7)

research must attend to these and other issues that prevent residents from moving around their neighborhoods and walking for health.

This was an uncontrolled feasibility study, and therefore we cannot assess from these data how much residents changed due to attention, interaction with each other and the walk leaders, or other changes that occurred during the time of the walking group. The data do support expanding the scale of this project and setting up walking programs throughout the city in developments for groups such as families, seniors, and children. This will be possible, given our collaboration with the Boston Housing Authority, Boston Public Health Commission, and the community of public housing residents. With these partnerships we were able to implement this small feasibility study to learn what works in housing developments. Expanding the scope necessitates more resources, more time, and more staff to work with HLAs to encourage walking in developments.

Residents reported that they liked the walking groups, the walk leaders, and the idea of walking in the neighborhood. This is a positive step toward enabling residents to leave their homes and engage in neighborhood interactions. Unpublished data collected from residents indicate that their number one concern was the safety of their developments. Many residents told us that they are afraid to go out in their hallways for fear of attack by neighbors. This fear may have diminished with walking, in that people's sense of neighborhood cohesion appeared to increase overall after participation in the walking groups.

LESSONS LEARNED

- Public housing residents can be supported to participate in active walking sessions.
- Participation in walking sessions seems to improve overall physical activity, as well as social interactions.
- The sustainability of these programs still must be evaluated.

References

1. Brooks DR, LA Mucci. Support for smoke-free restaurants among Massachusetts adults, 1992–1999. Am J Public Health. 2001 Feb;91(2):300–3.
2. National Institute of Diabetes and Digestive and Kidney Diseases (NIDDK). Understanding adult obesity. Bethesda, MD: NIDDK Weight-Control Information Network, National Institutes of Health, 2008. Available at: http://win.niddk.nih.gov/publications/PDFs/understandingobesityrev.pdf.
3. World Health Organization. Obesity: preventing and managing the global epidemic. Report of a WHO consultation. Geneva, Switzerland: World Health Organization, 2000.
4. National Center for Health Statistics. Prevalence of overweight and obesity among adults: United States, 1999–2000. Hyattsville, MD: National Center for Health Statistics, 2002.
5. Ball K, Crawford D. Socioeconomic status and weight change in adults: a review. Soc Sci Med. 2005 May;60(9):1987–2010.
6. Morland K, Wing S, Diez Roux A. Neighborhood characteristics associated with the location of food stores and food service places. Am J Prev Med. 2002 Jan;22(1):23–9.
7. Yen IH, Kaplan GA. Poverty area residence and changes in physical activity level: evidence from the Alameda County study. Am J Public Health. 1998 Nov;88(11):1709–12.
8. Humpel N, Owen N, Leslie E. Environmental factors associated with adults' participation in physical activity: a review. Am J Prev Med. 2002 Apr;22(3):188–99.
9. Reidpath DD, Burns C, Garrad J. An ecological study of the relationship between social and environmental determinants of obesity. Health Place. 2002 Jun;8(2):141–5.
10. Klesges RC, Obarzanek E, Klesges LM, et al. Memphis Girls Health Enrichment Multisite Studies (GEMS): phase 2: design and baseline. Contemp Clin Trials. 2008 Jan;29(1):42–55.

11. Hill JO, Peters JC. Environmental contributions to the obesity epidemic. Science. 1998 May 29;280(5368):1371–4.

12. McTigue KM, Garrett JM, Popkin BM. The natural history of the development of obesity in a cohort of young U.S. adults between 1981 and 1998. Ann Intern Med. 2002 Jun;136(12): 857–64.

13. French SA, Jeffery RW, Story M. Pricing and promotion effects on low-fat vending snack purchases: the CHIPS Study. Am J Public Health. 2001 Jan;91(1):112–7.

14. Ellaway A, Macintyre S. Does where you live predict health related behaviours? A case study in Glasgow. Health Bull (Edinb). 1996 Nov;54(6):443–6.

15. James WP, Nelson M, Ralph A. Socioeconomic determinants of health: the contribution of nutrition to inequalities in health. BMJ. 1997 May 24;314(7093):1545–9.

16. Mooney C. Cost and availability of healthy food choices in a London health district. J Hum Nutr Diet. 1990;3(2):111–20.

17. Brownson RC, Baker EA, Houseman RA, et al. Environmental and policy determinants of physical activity in the United States. Am J Public Health, 2001 Dec;91(12):1995–2003.

18. Eyler AA, Baker E, Cromer L, et al. Physical activity and minority women: a qualitative study. Health Educ Behav. 1998 Oct;25(5):640–52.

19. Nies MA, Vollman M, Cook T. African American women's experiences with physical activity in their daily lives. Public Health Nurs. 1999 Feb;16(1):23–31.

20. Lopez RP. Neighborhood risk factors for obesity. Obesity (Silver Spring). 2007 Aug;15(8): 2111–9.

21. Minkler M, Wallerstein N, eds. Community based participatory research for health. San Francisco, CA: Jossey-Bass, 2002.

22. Israel BA, Schulz AJ, Parker EA, et al. Review of community-based research: assessing partnership approaches to improve public health. Annu Rev Public Health. 1998;19:173–202.

23. Craig CL, Marshall AL, Sjostrom M, et al. International physical activity questionnaire: 12 country reliability and validity. Med Sci Sports Exerc. 2003 Aug;35(8):1381–95.

24. Transit for Livable Communities. Bike walk Twin Cities. St. Paul, MN: Transit for Livable Communities, 2012. Available at: www.bikewalktwincities.org.

INDEX

access to healthy foods, 51, 81, 82, 99, 100, 170, 194, 243, 325, 327, 330, 340, 342, 356, 366–67
acculturation: definition of, 81; dietary, of Hispanics, 80–102; Latino childhood obesity and, 48
Acculturation Rating Scale for Mexican Americans, 84, 87, 99
Achterberg, C., 222
adolescent obesity, 7; interventions for Mexican American youth, 128, 134–40; Migrant Middle School Media Nutrition Project, 221–26; Photovoice project for refugee/immigrant youth, 362–68; prevalence of, 4–6, 25, 43; Waipahu HART Project for, 370–77. *See also* childhood obesity
advertising/marketing: of beer and cigarettes, 365, 367; of foods to African Americans, 154; Latino childhood obesity and, 47, 51–53, 57
African American Collaborative Obesity Research Network (AACORN), 151–55, 158–59
African American girls, 63–76; culturally tailored interventions for, 64, 73, 74; double jeopardy phenomenon affecting, 74; future directions for studies of, 74; health/social consequences of obesity in, 75; lessons learned from studies of, 76; methodology for inclusion of studies of, 64–65, 73; need for race- and gender-based interventions for, 74–76; parental involvement in interventions for, 72; racial disparity between obesity in White girls and, 63–64; results of treatment/prevention studies in, 65–72; social cognitive theory in interventions for, 72, 73–74; strengths/limitations of studies in, 75
African Americans / Blacks, 1, 8, 80, 194; BMI compared with Whites, 164; childhood obesity in, 44, 45, 63; contextual factors affecting obesity interventions for, 151–59; Fine, Fit, and Fabulous for, 263–72; high calorie consumption by, 154; impact of early education programs on obesity in, 29, 31, 32–33, 39; incarcerated, 108–9; in military, 181; physical activity and obesity in, 164; safe

neighborhoods for physical activity by, 154, 157, 158, 162–71; SOPHE diabetes intervention for, 290–97; Weight Smart program for children, 337–42; W.O.W. Wellness program for women, 214–20
Ajzen, I., 372
Akresh, I. R., 84
Alaska Natives, 29, 44; SOPHE diabetes intervention for, 290–97
alcohol consumption, 88, 95, 109, 114, 195, 380
Alliance for a Better Community (ABC), 229–33
Alliance for a Healthy Border (AHB), 243–52; characteristics of border communities in, 245–46; community health centers participating in, 245, 247–48, 249, 252; development and implementation of, 244–49; evaluation of, 246, 249; lessons learned from, 252; location and context of, 244; outcomes of, 249; strengths, challenges, and possibilities for replication of, 249–51
American Academy of Pediatrics, 222
American Collaborative Obesity Research Network, 151
American Correctional Association (ACA), 113
American Diabetes Association, 293, 294; Risk Test, 268
American Dietetic Association, 29
American Heart Association, 113, 139, 293, 309
American Indians, 1, 8, 194; childhood obesity in, 44, 344; Head Start children, 29; Healthy Children, Strong Families for, 344–50; SOPHE diabetes intervention for, 290–97
American Medical Association (AMA), 3, 117
Anderson, S. E., 44
antipsychotics and weight gain, 277, 356
anxiety, 46, 111, 216, 241, 356
Appalachian communities: Cherokee Health Systems and Changes for Life in, 205n, 275–79; Community Appalachian Investigation and Research Network Learning Paradigm in, 205–12; obesity epidemic in, 205–6, 282; West Virginia PEIA Weight Management Program in, 282–88

Army Nurse Corps, 179
Army Physical Fitness and Weight Control
    Program (AR 600-9), 178, 179–81
arthritis, 3, 111
Ashida, S., 127, 133–34
Asian Americans, 1, 29, 45
asthma, 3, 46, 111, 263, 381
Avila, P., 127, 130
Ayala, G. X., 84, 96

Bachman, K. H., 111
Bandura, A., 73
Baranowski, T., 69, 71
Barkin, S., 128, 138–39, 181
Barrera, M., Jr., 98, 99
Batis, C., 83, 85, 95
Beech, B. M., 70
Behavioral Risk Factor Surveillance System
    (BRFSS), 5n, 183, 205, 216, 328, 379
Bellevue Hospital Weight Management Clinic
    (New York), 353–61; future directions for,
    360–61; initial patient assessment in,
    354–57; lessons learned from, 361; outcomes
    of, 360; physician education/training in,
    359–60; referrals to, 354; reimbursement for
    care in, 354; setting of, 353–54; staffing of,
    354; treatment approach of, 357–59
BeLue, R., 46
Bem, S. L., 74
Binswanger, I. A., 109–10
Blacks. See African Americans / Blacks
body mass index (BMI), 3, 25, 379; of Changes
    for Life participants, 277–78; changes in
    Migrant Middle School Media Nutrition
    Project, 223–25; of children/adolescents, 43,
    44–45; of Compañeros en Salud participants,
    237; diabetes and, 291; effect of exercise in
    African American vs. White girls on, 63–64;
    effect of interventions for Mexican Ameri-
    cans on, 127–37, 139; of Fine, Fit, and
    Fabulous participants, 268; health care costs
    and, 111; in Health of Houston Survey 2010,
    198; of Healthy Children, Strong Families
    participants, 346; Hispanic dietary
    acculturation and, 82, 84–89, 95, 96–98, 99;
    impact of early education programs on,
    29–32, 33, 35–36, 37; of incarcerated
    persons, 109; of military personnel, 179;
    and socioeconomic status in Milwaukee,
    325–26; of Weight Smart participants, 338;
    of West Virginia PEIA Weight Management
    Program participants, 283, 284; of Whites vs.
    Blacks, 164; of W.O.W. Wellness participants,
    217–18
Bopp, M., 127, 132

breastfeeding, 94, 97, 255–56, 257, 258, 259,
    260
Bronx Health REACH Coalition, 263–70
Bucholz, E. M., 29, 30, 32, 33
bullying, 46, 300
Bussey, K., 73

California Healthy Kids Survey, 140
cancer, 3, 46, 111, 123, 164; Health Disparity
    Index for, 195, 199
cardiovascular disease, 3, 46, 75, 99, 123, 300;
    Health Disparity Index for, 195, 199; income
    inequality and, 195; inmate deaths from, 111,
    112; physical activity and, 164, 176; Project
    Joy and, 157; in Southwest Bronx, 263;
    WISEWOMAN project for, 112, 156
Carneiro, P., 28
Casazza, K., 67
Cason, K., 91, 97
Centers for Disease Control and Prevention
    (CDC), 4, 5n, 43, 44, 194, 196; Behavioral
    Risk Factor Surveillance System, 5n, 183,
    205, 216, 328, 379; BMI growth charts, 6,
    277, 278, 346; cooperative agreement with
    SOPHE project, 292, 293, 296; definition of
    healthy weight, 196, 217, 346; definition of
    obesity/overweight, 194, 346; Division of
    Nutrition, Physical Activity, and Obesity,
    283; Family Healthware tool, 133; National
    Health and Nutrition Examination Survey, 4,
    5, 6, 30, 32, 44, 63, 83, 85, 106, 123, 183,
    194, 371, 379; on obesity in military, 180,
    183; obesity prevalence data, 5, 6, 43, 177,
    183; on physical activity for persons with
    disabilities, 306, 307; REACH program, 263;
    Task Force on Community Preventive
    Services, 168; WISEWOMAN project, 112,
    156
Centers of Excellence in the Elimination of
    Disparities (CEEDs), 263, 292
Changes for Life (Tennessee), 275–80; design
    and implementation of, 276–77; lessons
    learned from, 280; limitations of, 279;
    methods for evaluation of, 277–78; modifica-
    tions of, 278–79; outcomes of, 277–78
Cherokee Health Systems (CHS), 205n, 275–79
childhood obesity, 7; in American Indians, 344;
    Changes for Life for, 275–80; Comienzo
    Sano: Familia Saludable for, 255–60; among
    girls in Baltimore, 337; Healthy Children,
    Strong Families for, 344–50; in homeless
    shelter settings, 300; impact of early
    education programs on, 25–40; in Latinos,
    43–57; Let's Move campaign for, 53–54;
    physical activity and, 177; prevalence of, 4–6,

7, 25, 28, 43, 44–45, 255, 275, 299–300, 371;
race/ethnicity and, 8, 44–45, 164, 371;
socioeconomic status and, 275; Weight Smart
for, 337–42. *See also* adolescent obesity
Children's Hospital of Philadelphia, 299, 302, 303
cholesterol level: of African American girls, 69;
of Alliance for a Healthy Border participants,
245, 248, 250; of Compañeros participants,
239; effect of weight loss interventions on,
127, 130; of Fine, Fit, and Fabulous participants, 266, 271; of incarcerated women, 112,
113; metabolic syndrome and, 237, 310; of
Mexican American children, 55; of persons
with intellectual and developmental
disabilities, 306, 310; of W.O.W. Wellness
participants, 216, 218
Clark, L., 54
Clarke, K. K., 127, 130–31
Comienzo Sano: Familia Saludable (California),
255–60; development of, 256–59; educational topics for, 258; evaluation of, 259;
health implications of, 259–60; lessons
learned from, 260; participants in, 258
Community Appalachian Investigation and
Research Network (CAIRN) Learning
Paradigm (West Virginia), 205–12; lessons
learned from, 212; pragmatic objectives of,
206; progress report of, 210–11; role of
community research associates in, 207–10;
tiered diffusion model of learning in, 206–10
community health centers (CHCs), 244; in
Alliance for a Healthy Border, 245, 247–48,
249, 252; Cherokee Health Systems, 274–75;
in PILI'Ohana Project, 315, 316, 318
community partnerships / community-based
participatory research (CBPR) projects, 186;
African American Collaborative Obesity
Research Network, 151–55, 158–59; Alliance
for a Healthy Border, 243–52; in Boston
public housing developments, 380, 386;
Changes for Life, 276; Community Appalachian Investigation and Research Network,
205–12; Fine, Fit, and Fabulous, 263–72;
Healthy Children, Strong Families, 344–50;
Idaho Partnership for Hispanic Health,
236–41; joint use of school facilities (Los
Angeles), 230–34; nutrition education at
mobile markets (Milwaukee), 325–34; for
obesity interventions in Latino youths, 56,
57; Photovoice project (New Hampshire),
362–68; PILI'Ohana Project, 313–22; for
promotion of safe neighborhoods, 170, 171;
SOPHE diabetes interventions, 290–97; West
Virginia PEIA Weight Management Program,
284; W.O.W. Wellness, 214–20

Compañeros en Salud (Idaho), 236–41;
community change and dynamics affected
by, 240–41; history of, 237–38; lessons
learned by, 241; outcomes and evolution of,
239–40; oversight of, 237; participants in,
237; replication and resource sharing by, 241;
structure of, 238–39
computer-based interventions, 134, 135, 142,
143, 144
contextual factors in African American
communities, 151–59; challenges
presented by, 155–57; community-based
participatory research on, 155; implications
of, 158–59; opportunities presented by,
157–58; safe neighborhoods for physical
activity, 154, 157, 158, 162–71; shifting
thinking toward people and communities,
152–54
Convergence Partnership, 170
correctional facilities, obesity in, 8, 106–20;
consequences of, 111–12; current nutritional
practices and, 113–14; disparities within
incarcerated population, 107–9; health
care costs in, 106, 112; lessons learned
from studies of, 120; methodology for
literature review of, 107; nutrition and
lifestyle interventions for, 112–13; nutrition improvement efforts and, 116–17;
prevalence of, 109–10; sample menus and,
114–16; vocational programs and, 117–19;
WISEWOMAN project for, 112; in women,
110–11
counseling: for African American girls, 65, 66;
in Bellevue Hospital Weight Management
Clinic, 353, 357, 358, 359–61; in Get FIT
program, 308, 311; for Latinos, 50, 53, 128,
131, 257; in West Virginia PEIA Weight
Management Program, 284, 285
Cousins, J. H., 126–27, 129, 143
Crespo, C. J., 54
crime: in African American communities, 154,
155; cortisol level and, 167; diet and fear of,
167–68; in Mexican American communities,
140; physical activity and fear of, 162,
164–66, 168–69; in schools and neighborhoods, 168–69, 170, 364, 365. *See also*
violence
Cuidando el Corazon, 126
culturally tailored interventions: for African
American girls, 64, 73, 74; for Hispanics,
123–24, 144
curanderos, 54, 57

Dance for Health, 134–35
Davis, J. N., 128, 137–38

Dean Ornish Program for Reversing Heart
Disease, 282
deaths: among American Indians/Alaska
Natives, 291; from cancer, 111; in correctional facilities, 111–12; diabetes-related, 244,
291; from heart disease, 111; obesity paradox
and, 184; obesity-related, 3; physical activity
for prevention of, 379
Dennison, B. A., 36, 37
depression, 216, 356, 357, 381; in African
American girls, 63; of incarcerated persons,
110; income inequality and, 195; Latino youth
obesity and, 46; among persons in shelters,
300, 303
diabetes, 300; in African Americans, 4,
290–97; in Alliance for a Healthy Border
participants, 244, 247–48; in American
Indians / Alaska Natives, 4, 290–97, 349; in
Appalachia, 205, 207, 210, 211, 282; benefits
of physical activity, 164; in Cherokee Health
Systems participants, 276, 277, 279;
childhood obesity and, 43; in Compañeros en
Salud participants, 236, 237, 238; Fine, Fit,
and Fabulous prevention program for, 264,
265, 268, 271; gestational, 7, 258; Health
Disparity Index for, 195, 199; in Hispanics, 4,
46, 57, 123, 124, 133, 236, 237, 238, 244, 255;
in incarcerated persons, 106, 111, 114, 119;
metabolic syndrome and, 306; in Native
Hawaiians / Pacific Islanders, 313, 314;
prevalence of, 106; race/ethnicity and, 46,
290–91; in Southwest Bronx, 263; testing for,
186; trends in prevalence of, 106; type 2,
obesity and, 3, 4, 46, 75, 123, 124, 205, 207;
walking for reduction of, 380; in West
Virginia PEIA Weight Management Program
participants, 282, 283; among women living
in public housing, 379; in W.O.W. Wellness
participants, 216, 218
Diabetes Prevention Program, 4, 265, 314
Diaz, V. A., 123, 141–42
dietary acculturation of Hispanics, 80–102,
124, 144; acculturation measures and proxies
in studies of, 81, 83, 84–94, 98; associations
between acculturation, diet, and obesity,
83–96; barriers to healthy eating, 97–99;
BMI and, 82, 84–89, 95, 96–98, 99; dietary
measures in studies of, 83, 84–94, 98; health
effects of, 99; healthy immigrant selectivity,
80; Hispanic paradox, 80; among Hispanic
subgroups, 82, 83, 101; length of residence in
U.S. and, 99–100; lessons learned from
studies of, 102; limitations of research on,
100–102; methodology for literature review
of, 82; obesity interventions for, 99; physical

activity and, 101; qualitative studies of,
91–94, 96–99, 101; selective, 100; socioeconomic status and, 100
Dietary Guidelines for Americans, 113, 117, 265,
266
dietary intake, 7; access to healthy foods, 51, 81,
82, 99, 100, 170, 194, 243, 325, 327, 330, 340,
342, 356, 366–67; of fiber, 55, 81, 85, 117,
138, 225, 328; of Head Start children, 32, 33;
of inmates, 113–17; Latino childhood obesity
and, 47–48, 50–51
Dietary Reference Intakes (DRI), 113, 116,
117
disabilities, 1, 3, 8
disparities: definition of, 193; elimination of,
193; Healthy Weight Disparity Index, 193,
196–200; indices of, 195–96; in obesity, 1–3,
193–95; race/ethnicity and, 290
Domel, S. B., 127, 129
double jeopardy phenomenon, 74

early childhood education (ECE) programs,
25–40; Head Start and supplemental
interventions, 29–34; impact on obesity, 26,
28, 29–39; lessons learned from, 40;
methodology for literature review of, 27–28;
other childcare programs, 34–38; research
agenda for, 39–40
Early Childhood Longitudinal Study: Birth
Cohort, 28, 44; Kindergarten Class of
1998–1999 (ECLS-K), 34, 35–36, 37, 47
Eating in Emotional Situations
Questionnaire, 51
Eck, J. E., 164, 165
Eisenhower, Dwight D., 176, 177, 185
environmental factors, 7–8, 229, 379–80; in
African American communities, 151–59,
162–71; as barriers to physical activity,
162–63, 379–80; Hispanic dietary acculturation and, 81; in public housing family
developments, 379–87; safety concerns (see
crime; safe neighborhoods for physical
activity; violence)
epidemic of obesity, 1, 4, 9, 63, 64, 177, 243.
See also prevalence of obesity/overweight
Epstein, L. H., 339

faith-based interventions: factors affecting
success of, 269–71; Fine, Fit, and Fabulous,
263–72; for Hispanic adults, 127, 132; Project
Joy, 157; W.O.W. Wellness, 214–20
Faith-Based Outreach Initiative (FBOI), 264,
265, 267, 269, 270
Faithful Footsteps, 132
Family Resource Network, 307, 308

hypertension, 106, 123, 301; chronic stress and, 167; in Fine, Fit, and Fabulous participants, 268, 271; in Hispanics, 124, 239, 247–48; in incarcerated persons, 111, 112, 114, 119; Latino childhood obesity and, 43, 55; metabolic syndrome and, 237, 306, 309; in military personnel, 179; in Native Hawaiians / Pacific Islanders, 313, 316, 321; in persons with intellectual and developmental disabilities, 306; physical activity for, 164; in West Virginia PEIA Weight Management Program participants, 283; in W.O.W. Wellness participants, 216, 218

Idaho Partnership for Hispanic Health (IPHH), 236–41
immigrant Hispanics, 47, 226; breastfeeding by, 255; Compañeros en Salud for, 237; dietary acculturation of, 80–102; healthy immigrant selectivity, 80; from Mexico, 124, 141–42
Improving Head Start for School Readiness Act, 26–27
income inequality indices, 195
Institute for Family Health, 263
Institute of Medicine, 113, 117, 167
insulin, 67, 69, 128, 136, 143, 338
intellectual and developmental disabilities (IDD), persons with, 306–12; caregivers for, 307; Get FIT program for, 307–12; health of, 306–7
Interactive Multimedia for Promoting Physical Activity (IMPACT), 135
International Physical Activity Questionnaire, 383
Intertribal Friendship House, 292

Jackson, Thomas "Stonewall," 178
Jacobson, N. S., 142
joint use of school facilities (Los Angeles), 230–35; lessons learned from, 234–35; Mendez Learning Center pilot project, 231–33; policy and systems change for, 230–31; schools as health hubs, 230; sustainability and scalability of, 233–34
J.U.G.A.R. initiative (Los Angeles), 230–34
junk foods, 84, 91, 95, 97. See also fast foods

Kaiser Family Foundation, 52
Kaplan, M. S., 100
Kimbro, R. T., 46
King, R. S., 108
Klesges, R. C., 68

Latino childhood obesity, 43–57, 221; acculturation and, 48; barriers to effective interven-

tions for, 53, 57; biological factors and, 53; Comienzo Sano: Familia Saludable for, 255–60; epidemiology of, 44–46; food habits and, 47, 50–51; media/marketing influences on, 47, 51–53; Migrant Middle School Media Nutrition Project for, 221–26; parental/familial factors and, 47, 48–50, 57; prevalence of, 44–46, 57; promising interventions for, 53–55; research agenda for, 55–57; risk factors for, 46–47; social/economic factors and, 47–48; Weight Smart for, 337–42
Latino Health Project, 45
Latinos/Hispanics, 1, 8; Alliance for a Healthy Border for, 243–52; children, 8; children of migrant farmworkers, 221–26; culturally sensitive interventions for, 123–24, 144; dietary acculturation of, 80–102, 124, 144; Fine, Fit, and Fabulous for, 263–72; health effects of obesity in, 43, 46, 99, 123; healthy immigrant selectivity in, 80; Hispanic paradox in, 80; Idaho Partnership for Hispanic Health for, 236–41; impact of early education programs on obesity in, 29, 31, 32–33, 34, 35, 37, 39; incarcerated, 108–9; interventions for Mexican Americans, 55, 99, 123–45; in military, 181; obesity and socioeconomic status of, 47, 100, 124; obesity prevalence in, 123, 194, 243; population growth of, 43, 46, 124, 221; safe neighborhoods for physical activity by, 53, 56, 143, 144, 163, 256; subgroups of, 124, 143–44. See also immigrant Hispanics; Mexican Americans
Let's Move campaign, 53–54
life-course perspective, 7
Lin, H., 89, 96
Littman, A. J., 179, 183–84
liver disease, 3, 46, 111, 112, 338
LiveWell Northeast Denver, 170
Loukaitou-Sideris, A., 164, 165
Lumeng, J. C., 29, 30, 32, 33, 34, 35
Lutfiyya, M. N., 45

Maher, E. J., 34, 35
Mauer, M., 108
Maurino, L., 118
McArthur, L. H., 47
McAtee, M. J., 180
McAuley, P. A., 184
media influences: Hispanic acculturation and, 81, 87, 94; Latino childhood obesity and, 47, 51, 52–53, 57; Migrant Middle School Media Nutrition Project, 221–26; military obesity and, 182; Photovoice project for refugee/immigrant youth, 362–68; physical activity program, 137. See also television viewing

race/ethnicity, 1–2, 6, 7; BMI and, 164; childhood obesity and, 8, 44–45, 164; diabetes and, 46, 290–91; of Head Start children, 29; of incarcerated persons, 107–9; of military personnel, 181; obesity prevalence and, 1–2, 6, 7, 80, 194, 243, 325

Ramirez, A., 221

refugee/immigrant youth, Photovoice project for, 362–68

Relative Index of Inequality, 195

resistance training, 128, 136–37, 142, 143, 145

Resnicow, K., 66, 125

Reynolds, K., 128, 135–36

Robert Wood Johnson Foundation, 57, 186

Robin Hood index, 195

Robinson, T. N., 69, 70

Romero, A. J., 128, 139–40

Romero-Gwynn, E., 82

Rowan University, 307, 308, 311

Rush, Benjamin, 178

safe neighborhoods for physical activity, 8, 163n, 229n, 379n; in African American communities, 154, 157, 158, 162–71; correlation with obesity, 164–68; in early childhood education programs, 26; future directions related to, 169–71; in homeless shelter settings, 301, 302; joint use of school facilities in Los Angeles, 229–35; in Latino communities, 53, 56, 143, 144, 163, 256; for Maryland Weigh Smart Jr. program, 340–42; for military personnel, 182, 186; partnerships for promotion of, 170, 171; perceived and objective measures of, 166; in Photovoice project, 364; poverty and, 229; syndemics approach to, 169–70; traffic safety and, 162, 165–66, 168, 171; in urban settings, 163, 169; walking groups and, 380, 385, 387

Salud America!, 57

Sarnecky, M. T., 179

Satcher, D., 4

Schlundt, D., 181

school-based interventions: breakfast and lunch program, 28, 113, 340; joint use of school facilities, 230–35; for Latino children, 55, 56; physical education classes, 25; for refugee/immigrant youth, 366; Waipahu HART Project, 370–77

school safety, 168

Seaton, Fred, 176

sedentary behavior, 4, 177, 199, 243; among African Americans, 63, 154; of girls vs. boys, 8, 367; among Hispanics, 93, 101, 125, 128, 129, 136, 137; of inmates, 114; among persons with intellectual and developmental

disabilities, 306. *See also* physical activity/fitness

Selective Service Act, 178

Shaibi, G. Q., 128, 136–37, 143

SHARE Wisconsin, 327, 332

Short Acculturation Scale for Hispanics, 86, 87

Silver Sneakers, 286

sleep apnea, 46, 283, 300

smoking, 364; by Hispanics, 82; by inmates, 110, 111, 112, 113; in West Virginia, 282

Social Action Model, 320

Social Cognitive Theory of Gender-Role Development and Functioning, 73

Society for Public Health Education (SOPHE) diabetes interventions, 290–97; aims of, 292; collaborative partnerships for, 292–94, 296; for Jenkins County, Georgia, African Americans, 291, 294; lessons learned from, 296–97; for San Francisco Bay Area American Indians / Alaska Natives, 291–92, 294–95

socioeconomic status (SES): childhood obesity and, 275; correlation with obesity, 1, 4, 6, 7, 194, 243, 325–26; of Head Start children, 29; healthy immigrant selectivity and, 80; of Hispanics, 47, 100, 124, 129, 142, 144; indices of income inequality, 195; of inmates, 110, 119; and obesity in Milwaukee, 325–26; poor health and, 2. *See also* poverty

Spruijt-Metz, D., 128, 137

stigmatization, 3

Stolley, M. R., 68

Story, M., 71

stress eating, 167

stroke, 123, 124, 237, 271, 379

structural factors, 7–8, 9

Sturgeon, J., 176

sugar-sweetened beverages, 26, 50, 63, 68, 81, 97, 222, 269, 276, 279, 349, 357, 358

Summer Food Service Program, 222

Supplemental Nutrition Assistance Program (SNAP), 194

Survey of Inmates in Local Jails, 109

Survey of Inmates in State and Federal Correctional Facilities, 109

Sussner, K. M., 94

Swidler, A., 185

syndemics, 169–70

Syndemics Prevention Network, 169

Tekin, E., 34–37

television viewing, 56, 159; among African Americans, 70, 154; Changes for Life and, 278; childhood obesity and, 26, 31, 34, 36, 37,